Practical Endocrinology and Diabetes in Children

To our wives and children

Practical Endocrinology and Diabetes in Children

SECOND EDITION

JOSEPH E. RAINE

MD, FRCPCH, DCH
Consultant Paediatrician
Whittington Hospital
Highgate Hill
London, UK

MALCOLM D.C. DONALDSON

MD, FRCP, DCH
Senior Lecturer in Child Health and Consultant Paediatric Endocrinologist
Royal Hospital for Sick Children
Yorkhill
Glasgow, UK

JOHN W. GREGORY

MBChB, MD, FRCP, DCH, FRCPCH
Professor of Paediatric Endocrinology
Department of Child Health
Wales College of Medicine
Cardiff University
Heath Park
Cardiff, UK

MARTIN O. SAVAGE

MA, MD, FRCP, FRCPCH
Professor of Paediatric Endocrinology
Department of Endocrinology
St Bartholomew's and the Royal London School of Medicine and Dentistry
West Smithfield
London, UK

RAYMOND L. HINTZ

MD
Professor of Pediatrics
Stanford University Medical Center
Stanford, CA, USA

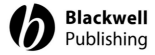

Blackwell
Publishing

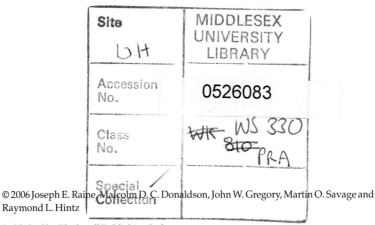

© 2006 Joseph E. Raine, Malcolm D. C. Donaldson, John W. Gregory, Martin O. Savage and Raymond L. Hintz

Published by Blackwell Publishing Ltd
Blackwell Publishing, Inc., 350 Main Street, Malden, Massachusetts 02148-5020, USA
Blackwell Publishing Ltd, 9600 Garsington Road, Oxford OX4 2DQ, UK
Blackwell Publishing Asia Pty Ltd, 550 Swanston Street, Carlton, Victoria 3053, Australia

First published 2001

Library of Congress Cataloging-in-Publication Data

Practical endocrinology and diabetes in children / Joseph E. Raine . . .
  [et al.].—2nd ed.
    p. ; cm.
  Includes bibliographical references and index.
  ISBN-13: 978-1-4051-2233-7
  ISBN-10: 1-4051-2233-1
  1. Diabetes in children 2. Pediatric endocrinology. I. Raine, Joseph E.
  [DNLM: 1. Endocrine System Diseases—Child. 2. Diabetes Mellitus—Child. WS 330 P8955 2005]
  RJ420.D5D52 2005
  618.92'462—dc22   2005014108

ISBN-13: 978-1-4051-2233-7
ISBN-10: 1-4051-2233-1

A catalogue record for this title is available from the British Library

Set in 8.5/11.5 Palatino by SNP Best-set Typesetter Ltd., Hong Kong
Printed and bound in Singapore by Fabulous Printers Pte Ltd

Commissioning Editor: Alison Brown
Editorial Assistant: Saskia van der Linden
Development Editor: Vicki Donald
Marketing Manager: Phil Wright
Production Controller: Kate Charman

For further information on Blackwell Publishing, visit our website:
www.blackwellendocrinology.com

The publisher's policy is to use permanent paper from mills that operate a sustainable forestry policy, and which has been manufactured from pulp processed using acid-free and elementary chlorine-free practices. Furthermore, the publisher ensures that the text paper and cover board used have met acceptable environmental accreditation standards.

Contents

Colour plate sections appear between pages 20 and 21

Preface to the Second Edition

The new edition has been completely updated and some chapters, for example the diabetes chapter, have been extensively revised. Additional growth charts for specific syndromes have also been added to the appendix. We have also added a new section to each chapter entitled 'Potential pitfalls'. This edition also incorporates a new editor, Professor Raymond Hintz, from Stanford University, California. Professor Hintz has helped to provide a North American perspective for the book which we hope will increase its relevance and international appeal.

JER, MDCD, JWG, MOS, RLH

Preface to the First Edition

There are very few books that bridge the gap between the large detailed endocrine reference book and the short review of aspects of endocrinology. The aim of this book is to provide a practical, concise and up-to-date account of paediatric endocrinology and diabetes in a readable and user-friendly format.

Given the importance of diabetes in clinical practice, particular emphasis has been placed on its practical management. At the end of each chapter there are guidelines for which conditions should be discussed with a specialist centre and an outline of controversial areas. We have also included interesting cases at the end of each chapter to illustrate diagnostic difficulties and also to help those studying for postgraduate examinations, such as the MRCPCH, which include such 'grey cases'.

The book is aimed primarily at paediatricians in general hospitals and at junior paediatric staff with an interest in paediatric endocrinology and/or diabetes. However, we also hope that the book will be useful to medical students, nurses working on paediatric endocrinology wards and to diabetes nurse specialists.

JER, MDCD, JWG, MOS

Acknowledgements

The authors would like to thank Dr David Levy, Consultant Diabetologist, Whipps Cross Hospital, London; Dr Jill Challener, Consultant Paediatrician Hinchingbrooke Hospital, Cambridgeshire; Dr Joanna Walker, Consultant Paediatrician, St Mary's Hospital, Portsmouth; Dr Faisal Ahmed, Consultant Paediatric Endocrinologist, Mr Stuart O'Toole, Consultant Paediatric Surgeon, and Ms Wendy Paterson, Auxologist, Royal Hospital For Sick Children, Glasgow; Professor Robert Fraser, MRC Blood Pressure Unit, Western Infirmary, Glasgow; Dr Helen Lyall, Consultant Gynaecologist and Dr Mike Wallace, Consultant Clinical Scientist, Biochemistry Department, Glasgow Royal Infirmary, for their help and advice with different sections of the book.

Foreword to the First Edition

Endocrinology is the science of communication. Between distant glands and organs in the body, between neighbouring cells or tissues, and between the cell surface and the intracellular target molecules. With the advance of the knowledge of such chemical signal transduction outside and inside cells, endocrinology may seem like a field inaccessible to the junior staff member, the general practitioner or anyone that has not achieved experience in the clinical management of endocrine disorders. Modern molecular biology has widened the knowledge in endocrine details in an exponential manner, and comprehensive textbooks are growing in size to such an extent that they are inaccessible to most practising doctors.

Putting endocrinology in the context of the growing child and the maturation of the adolescent girl or boy adds another dimension to the subject. Correct diagnosis, treatment and family interaction may be decisive for the future development of the child. Although many endocrine disorders in childhood are of a chronic nature, in most cases a knowledgeable management can support the development of the child into a normally functioning adult, not compromised by any physical or mental restraints. Therefore, it is mandatory that endocrine disorders in childhood are detected, treated and followed up in a professional way. In rare diseases, this can only be achieved with the help of clinically experienced physicians, specialist nurses and other members of the paediatric endocrine team. However, due to the rarity of many of the paediatric endocrine disorders, such expertise cannot be present everywhere. Therefore the practising paediatrician and the junior hospital staff needs a guide to the basics in the field, a guide that gives a practical help in management and advise on who should be referred to a tertiary unit.

The four authors of the present volume have set out to produce such a practical guide into paediatric endocrinology. Instead of collecting a large group of world experts, each covering a narrow field, they have compiled the es-

sentials into a textbook written in a structured way. The chapters are problem- rather than disease-based; topics like short and tall stature, disorders of pubertal development or sexual differentiation and obesity are each given their own treatise. The recommendations given reflect those of the four authors—others might have a slightly different view on each topic. The authors have tried to indicate this by ending each chapter with one subheading on 'Future developments' and also 'Controversial issues'. This invites further reading, which can be started with the 'Recommended reading' at the end of each section. This generally refers to recent reviews. This book does not contain extensive lists of references to original work. Therefore the reader should consider this as the basics of the field. It can preferably be complemented by literature search on a computerized database like Medline or Pubmed, that are now so easily accessible to most readers.

In line with the practical approach, this volume gives indications on when it is appropriate to refer the patient to a specialist centre for paediatric endocrinology. This certainly varies with the structure and organisation of medical care—in some countries this threshold is lower, in others it is higher. Thus, the opinions expressed reflect the status in the UK. So do some of the treatments (or non-treatments) suggested. In spite of a growing internationalization of medical care, treatment approaches are still anchored in national traditions. In paediatric endocrinology this is obvious in areas that deal with variants of normal development, like short or tall stature, early or late puberty. This book takes a rather conservative attitude in most issues like this.

Although the authors in their preface state that this book is aimed primarily at paediatricians in the UK that are not specializing in paediatric endocrinology, it contains numerous detailed practical instructions on how to work up patients with more or less rare disorders or symptoms. In close collaboration with a paediatric endocrinologist, I think that it will be of great help in improving the early detection and correct management of endocrine disorders in childhood and adolescence. Although the authors repeatedly refer to the situation in UK, I am convinced that many readers in other parts of the world will find this book to be of great help in their daily work with endocrine problems.

Martin Ritzén
Stockholm, April 2001

1 Diabetes mellitus

Definition

Diabetes is diagnosed in the presence of either a blood glucose concentration of >11.1 mmol/L [200 mg/dL] or a fasting glucose concentration of >7 mmol/L [126 mg/dL]. The diagnosis of diabetes when symptoms are present is usually straightforward and a glucose tolerance test is rarely needed. Glucose tolerance testing may be indicated following the identification of a borderline blood glucose concentration (e.g. in the sibling of a child with diabetes, or in children with disorders such as cystic fibrosis predisposing to diabetes which, in the early stages, may be asymptomatic). The protocol for and interpretation of results from an oral glucose tolerance test are shown in Table 1.1.

Diabetes is a heterogeneous condition which may be classified on the basis of pathogenesis (Table 1.2). Most of this chapter will focus on type 1 diabetes which is by far the most common form of diabetes in children. Other types of diabetes are discussed on pages 25 and 29.

Incidence

The incidence of type 1 diabetes in children (0–14 years) is approximately 13.5/100 000 in the UK (prevalence 1 in 1200) but varies from 0.6/100 000 in China to 42.9/100 000 in Finland. The reasons for these large variations are unclear but may include genetic factors given the evidence of variations in the incidence of diabetes in different ethnic groups (e.g. in the USA, white people have a higher incidence than non-whites). There is a family history of type 1 diabetes in 10% of cases. The risk of developing type 1 diabetes for an individual with an affected relative is outlined in Table 1.3. If a twin develops type 1 diabetes the lifetime risk to a non-affected monozygotic twin is approximately 60%, whereas that for a dizygotic twin is 8%. Environmental effects are probably important as the incidence rises in the winter months. A number of countries have documented an increase in the incidence of diabetes particularly in children under 5 years of age although the peak incidence occurs in those aged 11–14 years.

Table 1.1 Protocol for the oral glucose tolerance test.

Indications
Confirmation of the diagnosis of diabetes mellitus in
  uncertain cases and diagnosis of impaired glucose tolerance

Preparation
Perform in the morning after an overnight fast

Procedure
1 Pre-test — plasma glucose sample
2 0 min — administer oral glucose 1.75 g/kg (up to a maximum
  of 75 g) diluted with water (consume over 5–10 minutes)
3 +2 hours — plasma glucose sample

Interpretation
1 Fasting plasma glucose >7.0 mmol/L [>126 mg/dL] or 2 hours
  concentration >11.1 mmol/L [>200 mg/dL] are diagnostic of
  diabetes
2 2-hour plasma glucose concentration >7.8 mmol/L [>140 mg/
  dL] and <11.0 mmol/L [<198 mg/dL] suggests impaired
  glucose tolerance
3 Fasting plasma glucose >6 mmol/L (>108 mg/dL) and
  <7 mmol/L (<126 mg/dL) suggests impaired fasting
  glycaemia

Table 1.2 The American Diabetes Association Classification
of Diabetes.

Type 1	Immune-mediated and idiopathic forms of β-cell dysfunction which lead to absolute insulin deficiency
Type 2	A disease of adult or occasionally adolescent onset which may originate from insulin resistance and relative insulin deficiency or from an insulin secretory defect
Type 3	Includes a wide range of specific types of diabetes including the various genetic defects of β-cell function, genetic defects in insulin action and diseases of the exocrine pancreas (e.g. cystic fibrosis)
Type 4	Gestational diabetes

Aetiology and pathogenesis

The precise cause of type 1 diabetes is unknown but there
are a number of possible contributory factors.

Autoimmune
Several autoantibodies have been identified in newly
diagnosed cases of type 1 diabetes. These include islet cell
antibodies (60–90% of new patients), glutamic acid decar-

Table 1.3 The risk of developing type 1 diabetes for an
individual with an affected relative.

Relative with type 1 diabetes	Risk to individual (%)
Sibling	8
Mother	2–3
Father	5–6
Both parents	30

boxylase antibodies (65–80%) and insulin autoantibodies
(30–40%). Type 1 diabetes is also associated with other
autoimmune disorders such as Hashimoto's and Graves'
disease (3–5%), coeliac disease (2–5%) and Addison's
disease (<1%).

Genetic
Numerous susceptibility loci — genes that predispose to
type 1 diabetes — have been found. Several of these loci
are located in the major histocompatibility complex
(MHC) region on the short arm of chromosome 6 which
contains genes that regulate the immune response.
For example, the presence of DR3 and DR4 are associated
with a high risk of developing diabetes. The homozygous
absence of an aspartate residue at position 57 on the DQB
chain leads to an approximate 100-fold increase in the risk
of developing type 1 diabetes. Conversely, there are also
protective alleles such as DRB1*1501 and DQB1*0602.
Genetic factors play a greater part in the aetiology of type
1 diabetes in children diagnosed under the age of 5 years.
The risk of a sibling developing diabetes is therefore
higher in this group, being 12% by the age of 20 years.
Genetic and autoimmune markers have been used in
research studies to try to predict the risk of siblings of
patients with type 1 diabetes developing the disease.

Viral
Epidemics of viral infections in the autumn and winter
months are associated with an increase in the incidence of
diabetes. Several viruses (e.g. coxsackie B, enteroviruses,
rubella, mumps and cytomegalovirus) have been implicated in the aetiology of type 1 diabetes. Possible mechanisms for their effect include molecular mimicry in which
the immune response to the infection cross-reacts with
islet antigens. Alternatively, viral infections, including
those occurring antenatally, may have more direct effects
on β-cells.

Nutritional

Breast-feeding seems to provide protection against the risk of developing type 1 diabetes. Whether this is a direct effect of breast milk or is related to the delayed introduction of cow's milk is unclear. Many new patients with type 1 diabetes have IgG antibodies to bovine serum albumin, a protein in cow's milk with similarities to the islet cell antigen. This protein may stimulate autoantibody production leading to islet cell destruction as a result of molecular mimicry.

Chemical toxins

Ingestion of the rodenticide Vacor is associated with development of type 1 diabetes.

Stress

Prior to the onset of type 1 diabetes, adults have been shown to experience more 'severe life events' than a control group. The cause for this effect is unclear but may relate to stress-induced impairment of resistance to infection in genetically susceptible individuals.

Biochemistry

Insulin is an anabolic hormone with a key role in glucose metabolism (Fig. 1.1) and important effects on fat and protein metabolism. Following a meal, circulating concentrations of insulin rise, facilitating the entry of glucose into cells via glucose-specific transporters, particularly in the muscles and adipose tissue. Insulin stimulates glycogen synthesis in the liver and muscle, inhibits gluconeogenesis in the liver and stimulates fat and protein synthesis. Conversely, during fasting, glucose concentrations and insulin secretion fall leading to absence of glucose uptake in muscle and adipose tissue, with stimulation of glycogenolysis in the liver and muscles and hepatic gluconeogenesis (from amino acids and ketones).

In subjects with type 1 diabetes, insulin deficiency results in hyperglycaemia which, when the renal threshold for glucose is exceeded, leads to an osmotic diuresis causing polyuria and secondary polydipsia. When fluid losses exceed intake, particularly when vomiting occurs, dehydration develops. Insulin deficiency also causes lipolysis with the production of excess free fatty acids and ketone bodies (3-hydroxybutyrate and acetoacetate) leading to ketonuria. The accumulation of ketoacids in the blood causes a metabolic acidosis which results in compensatory rapid, deep breathing (Kussmaul respiration). Acetone, formed from acetoacetate, is responsible for the sweet smell of the breath. Furthermore, there is an increase in stress hormone (glucagon, adrenaline, cortisol and growth hormone) production which, because of their effects on metabolism, leads to a further rise in blood

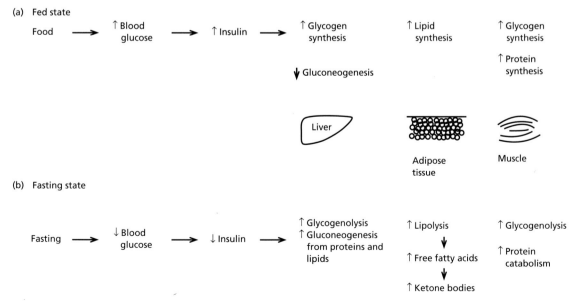

Fig. 1.1 Glucose homeostasis — a comparison of fed and fasting states.

glucose and other intermediary metabolite concentrations. Progressive dehydration, acidosis and hyperosmolality cause decreased consciousness and, if untreated, can lead to coma and death.

Clinical presentation

History
At diagnosis, the following symptoms may have been present from 1 week to 6 months:
- polyuria (may cause nocturnal enuresis);
- polydipsia;
- weight loss;
- anorexia or hyperphagia;
- lethargy;
- constipation;
- infection (especially candidal skin infections);
- blurred vision; and
- hypoglycaemia (rare, probably represents islet cell instability in the early stages of diabetes).

Although most school-aged children will report polyuria and polydipsia, these symptoms may be less obvious in the very young child who may be relatively asymptomatic (e.g. polyuria will be less obvious in an infant in nappies) and in whom the other less characteristic symptoms may predominate.

Patients with diabetic ketoacidosis (DKA) may also have:
- vomiting;
- abdominal pain; and
- symptoms of systemic infection.

Examination
At diagnosis, most (approximately 75%) patients will not have DKA. These individuals may have evidence of only weight loss or, possibly, a candidal skin infection. Patients with DKA may demonstrate the following:
- dehydration:
  5%—dry mucous membranes, decreased skin turgor
  10%—sunken eyes, poor capillary return
  >10%—hypovolaemia, tachycardia with thready pulse, hypotension;
- sweet-smelling breath;
- Kussmaul breathing (tachypnoea with hyperventilation);
- depressed consciousness/coma;
- signs of sepsis (fever is not a feature of DKA and suggests sepsis);
- ileus; and

- signs of cerebral oedema (e.g. deteriorating level of consciousness).

Children less than 5 years old are more likely to present with DKA partly as a result of their clinical presentation not having been recognized by health professionals as being compatible with diabetes, leading to a delay in diagnosis and referral to hospital. Other factors that increase the risk of presenting with DKA include low socio-economic status, medication with high-dose steroids and the absence of a first-degree relative with type 1 diabetes.

Differential diagnosis
In the vast majority of cases the diagnosis of type 1 diabetes is obvious because of the presence of the classical symptoms of polyuria, polydipsia and weight loss, associated with a random blood glucose >11 mmol/L and glycosuria with or without ketonuria. Diabetes should be considered in the differential diagnosis of any child presenting with impaired consciousness and/or acidosis.

Tachypnoea and hyperventilation in DKA may lead to the erroneous diagnosis of pneumonia. However, the lack of a cough or wheeze and the absence of abnormal findings on auscultation and/or a normal chest radiograph should raise the possibility of an alternative diagnosis such as diabetes. Abdominal pain and tenderness in DKA may suggest a surgical emergency such as appendicitis. However, appropriate fluid, insulin and electrolyte therapy will usually ameliorate the abdominal symptoms within hours. Diabetes should also be considered as a possible diagnosis in children with secondary nocturnal enuresis.

Acute illnesses, for example severe sepsis or a prolonged convulsion, may occasionally cause hyperglycaemia, glycosuria and ketonuria. However, these features are almost always transient and are rarely associated with previous polydipsia and polyuria. If in doubt, a fasting blood glucose or oral glucose tolerance test (Table 1.1) should be performed.

A family doctor who suspects or has made a definitive diagnosis of diabetes should refer the child promptly to a paediatrician. Children should be assessed on the day of referral or, if not unwell and in the absence of signs of DKA, the following day.

Investigations

At diagnosis it is advisable to perform the following investigations:

- plasma glucose concentration;
- venous blood gas measurement;
- serum electrolytes, urea and creatinine concentrations;
- full blood count (leukocytosis is common in DKA and does not necessarily mean that infection is present, while an increased haematocrit will reflect the degree of extra-cellular fluid loss);
- a few children may have signs of sepsis and need appropriate investigations (e.g. blood culture, chest radiograph, urine microscopy and culture);
- thyroid function tests (TFTs) and coeliac antibodies (to monitor these associated conditions).

At diagnosis most patients have ketonuria but the presence of an abnormally low pH (i.e. venous pH <7.30) is suggestive of DKA.

Management of the child presenting without ketoacidosis

Hospitalization versus outpatient (home) treatment

Hospital admission is necessary if intravenous therapy is required to correct dehydration, electrolyte imbalance and ketoacidosis or if there are psychosocial difficulties. Whether a child with newly presenting diabetes who is clinically stable and does not fulfil the above criteria can be treated at home will depend primarily on the availability of diabetes nurses who will need to visit at least daily in the first few days and maintain regular telephone contact, often outside normal working hours. The size of the geographical area that needs to be covered is also a factor. The advantages of home treatment include giving the family more confidence in dealing with diabetes at home, a more comforting environment and less disruption and financial cost to the family. There is also some evidence that home treatment is cheaper, reduces subsequent re-admissions and improves glycaemic control. The disadvantages include the risk of complications such as hypoglycaemia which may occur before the family is sufficiently experienced to cope with them. To avoid this, home-managed children are often started on a dose of insulin of slightly less than 0.5 IU/kg/24 hours with the dose gradually being increased over the next few weeks according to the blood glucose concentrations. Some families also prefer the security of being in hospital.

Some centres offer the alternative of ambulatory care and provide diabetes education and training in day care units for several days following diagnosis.

Main topics for discussion following diagnosis

If several members of the 'diabetes team' are to be involved in educating the newly diagnosed child and his or her family, good communication between team members to ensure consistency in the information given to the family is important. The following topics should be discussed with the child and family following diagnosis:

- their pre-existing knowledge of diabetes;
- our current knowledge of the cause of diabetes;
- the consequences of having diabetes and its lifelong implications;
- the concept of the 'diabetes team' of professionals who will be involved in their care;
- the role of insulin in type 1 diabetes management;
- practical details of insulin injections;
- practical details regarding when and how to monitor and interpret blood glucose concentrations;
- appropriate dietetic advice (see below);
- the effect of exercise on carbohydrate and insulin requirements;
- the causes and consequences of hypoglycaemia and how to treat it;
- when and how to measure urinary or blood ketone concentrations;
- management of diabetes during intercurrent illness;
- the 'honeymoon period' of relatively reduced insulin requirements following diagnosis;
- long-term microvascular complications;
- who to contact in an emergency (including phone numbers);
- details of outpatient follow up;
- the importance of carrying identification (e.g. medical bracelets etc.) indicating that the individual has diabetes;
- additional sources of information about diabetes;
- availability of support groups;
- sources and entitlement to financial aid; and
- future developments.

Diet

In view of the important effects of diet on glycaemic control and other longer term adverse effects of diabetes, a newly diagnosed patient and family should be referred to a dietitian who specializes in childhood diabetes within days of diagnosis. Several education sessions with the dietitian, preferably as part of the family's visit to the diabetes outpatient clinic, are usually required in the first weeks following diagnosis.

Principles of diet

Children should be encouraged to eat regular meals containing complex carbohydrates (e.g. potatoes and cereals), to reduce their intake of refined sugars, fats and salt and to increase their dietary fibre content. Very-high-fibre diets in young children are not recommended as they may be unpalatable and provide inadequate energy content. The advice should be tailored to the patient's lifestyle and, where possible, should avoid drastic changes. No particular food should be considered forbidden as this may lead to disturbed attitudes to food. Furthermore, to deprive children of some foods such as sweets, which their friends consume regularly, may be psychologically damaging. Foods with a high carbohydrate content can be taken before exercise, incorporated into a main meal or used as a source of energy during illness when children have a poor appetite.

Dietary compliance may be improved if the whole family can make similar dietary modifications and the concept of a 'healthy' diet should be encouraged. Families should also be educated about the dietary treatment of the child experiencing hypoglycaemia or intercurrent illness and dietary management during parties and holidays.

Timing of meals and snacks

Children receiving twice-daily injections of combined short- and intermediate-acting insulins require three main meals and three snacks (mid-morning, mid-afternoon and prior to bed). Occasionally, extra snacks are required if there are significant delays with meal times or if the child has eaten only a small proportion of a main meal. Children of pre-school age may have unpredictable eating habits and may require frequent, small meals.

Children receiving a basal bolus insulin regimen with rapidly acting insulin analogues and isophane [intermediate-acting insulin] do not require snacks between main meals but those on a regimen of short-acting insulin and isophane do require snacks between main meals. With both regimens an evening snack is advisable as a precaution against nocturnal hypoglycaemia. Those on a basal bolus regimen with a long-acting insulin analogue such as glargine or detemir should not require an evening snack although one may wish to continue the evening snack for the first few weeks following the commencement of this regimen. Children on a basal bolus regimen need to have the ability to adjust the dose of their bolus insulin according to their carbohydrate intake. The diet of patients on a basal bolus regimen needs to be particularly closely supervised as there is an increased risk of weight gain in this group.

Dietary composition

Caloric intake does not need to be calculated or altered unless the child is over- or underweight. It is recommended that approximately 35% of dietary energy intake should be derived from fat (mainly mono- and poly-unsaturated fats), 15% from protein and 50% from carbohydrate. Carbohydrates should always provide at least 40% of the total energy intake.

There are several approaches to the dietetic management of diabetes.

1 Children can be encouraged to choose a certain number of carbohydrate-containing foods ('portions') from a list of such foods, at each meal and snack time.

2 Food intake is based on the principles of a normal healthy diet.

3 Families are taught about the carbohydrate exchange system in which 10 g of carbohydrate is equivalent to one exchange and meals are calculated on the basis of the number of 'exchanges' required. Because of the uncertainties about the precise carbohydrate content of food and its physiological effects, dietary education on the basis of the carbohydrate exchange system was to a large extent abandoned in the 1990s. However, recently there has been renewed interest in a quantitative rather than a qualitative approach to diet in diabetes management. A dietary regimen called Dose Adjustment For Normal Eating (DAFNE) has been introduced in some centres for the management of adults with diabetes. Detailed education is given on the carbohydrate content of food and a very liberal diet is allowed with multiple insulin boluses being given in line with the carbohydrate intake. Good control has been achieved with these regimens but whether this is due to the dietary management or the additional education involved when commencing this regimen is difficult to say. An improved quality of life has also been associated with this regimen.

The numerous commercially available 'diabetic foods' are not generally recommended for children with diabetes as such foods tend to be expensive and have no particular advantages over a healthy diet based on normal foods. Non-alcoholic drinks containing sugar should be replaced with those containing artificial sweeteners.

Insulin therapy

A number of different insulin regimens are available. It is important to be flexible when choosing an insulin regimen and to bear in mind the family's needs and wishes. The initial insulin regimen may require changing if glycaemic control is poor or if there are practical difficulties. Following diagnosis, most children will require approximately 0.5 units of insulin per kilogram body weight daily, although this may decrease substantially during the first few months of therapy (occasionally to the point where patients may be transiently completely weaned off insulin) during the so-called 'honeymoon period'. This period, which represents partial recovery of the existing β-cell mass, may last from a few months up to 2 years. Parents should be warned that insulin requirements will increase significantly at the end of the 'honeymoon period'.

Children of pre-school age (≤4 years) can be very sensitive to rapid/short-acting insulin. Possible regimens in this age group include once-daily isophane before breakfast, once-daily isophane before breakfast with rapid/short-acting insulin prior to the evening meal (the rapid/short-acting insulin is sometimes best administered on a sliding scale depending on the pre-evening meal reading), twice-daily isophane, twice-daily mixed insulins with approximately 70% of the total daily dose being given at breakfast time, a basal bolus regimen (see below) or a continuous subcutaneous insulin infusion. It may be that a once-daily injection of a long-acting insulin analogue will also be suitable in this group of children but currently there is insufficient evidence to recommend such a regimen.

In many older children, the use of twice-daily injections using a mixture of rapid/short-acting and intermediate-acting insulins—most commonly in a ratio of 25–30% : 70–75% with approximately 70% of the total daily dose being given at breakfast time, is suitable and provides good control, especially in the first year of treatment during the honeymoon period.

For appropriately motivated children and families, and particularly in adolescents, the use of a basal bolus regimen may be most appropriate. Basal bolus regimens comprise injections of rapid/short-acting insulin prior to each main meal with an injection of isophane or a long-acting insulin analogue prior to bedtime. The advantage of the latter is a basal 'peakless' level of insulin for up to 24 hours (Table 1.9). There is also some evidence that nocturnal hypoglycaemia is less common with the long-acting insulin analogues. Normally, 30–40% of the total daily dose of insulin is given at bedtime as isophane or as a long-acting insulin analogue. The remaining insulin is given as rapid/short-acting insulin and is split between the pre-breakfast, lunch and evening meal injections. If there are marked discrepancies in the size of the meals then the dose of insulin should reflect this.

Basal bolus regimens allow greater variation in meal times and in the size of the meal compared to twice-daily injections of mixed insulins and are particularly popular with teenagers as they lead to greater independence.

Children and/or their parents need to be able to alter the dose of rapid/short-acting insulin in line with the planned dietary intake and any anticipated exercise.

In children reluctant to administer a pre-lunch injection at school, or in whom there are difficulties with a full basal bolus regimen, an intermediate solution is to give a mixed insulin before breakfast, rapid/short-acting insulin prior to the evening meal and isophane prior to bedtime.

Although hypoglycaemic episodes are unusual in newly diagnosed patients, care should be taken to avoid these in children treated at home until the family has had adequate training to respond appropriately. Children initially treated in hospital are less active than at home and most will experience a fall in their blood glucose following discharge.

Once on insulin therapy there is often concern about high blood glucose concentrations and the need for extra injections of insulin. If the child is well, and in the absence of ketones, the risk of developing DKA is minimal and extra injections of rapid/short-acting insulin are not required. If glucose concentrations remain high, additional insulin can be given with the next scheduled injection (e.g. 1 or 2 units of rapid/short-acting insulin if blood glucose is 15–20 mmol/L [270–300 mg/dL] or 3 or 4 units if blood glucose is >20 mmol/L) and the preceding scheduled dose of insulin should be increased by 1 or 2 units the following day.

It has been suggested that aggressive insulin therapy to achieve early onset of normoglycaemia may help to maintain residual β-cell function and lead to a prolonged 'honeymoon period'. However, there is insufficient evidence to prove this and the possible benefits of tight glycaemic control may be outweighed by the risks of hypoglycaemia.

Psychological support

The diagnosis of diabetes is invariably a shock to the child and family. Psychological or psychiatric problems may arise, particularly at diagnosis or during adolescence (see page 20). Psychological support can be provided by a psychologist or psychiatrist as well as by diabetes nurses, other parents and local and national support groups.

Requirements on discharge from hospital

The family doctor should be informed of the child's diagnosis on discharge from hospital and the school or nursery should be visited by the diabetes nurse and dietitian to ensure that suitable information and arrangements are in

Table 1.4 Equipment required on discharge.

Lancets or other finger-pricking devices
Blood glucose testing strips
Blood glucose meter
Oral glucose gel
Glucagon kit
Urinary or blood ketone testing sticks
Sharps bin
Literature on diabetes and how to obtain medical bracelets/
   necklaces
Pen-delivery system, disposable pre-filled pens or syringes with
   needles for insulin injections
Insulin cartridges for pen-delivery system or insulin vials
Short- or preferably rapid-acting insulin
Alcohol swabs
Needle clipper

place. The equipment that a child will need on discharge is shown in Table 1.4.

Management of the child presenting with ketoacidosis

Approximately 25% of new patients with diabetes will present with DKA. In children with established diabetes the risk of DKA is increased in those with poor metabolic control and previous episodes of DKA, adolescent girls, children with psychiatric disorders including eating disorders and those with psychosocial difficulties. Inappropriate interruption of insulin pump therapy may also lead to DKA. Seventy-five per cent of DKA episodes are associated with insulin omission or treatment error. The majority of the remainder are due to inadequate insulin treatment during intercurrent illness.

The diagnosis can be made on clinical and biochemical grounds. The biochemical criteria for the diagnosis of DKA include hyperglycaemia (glucose >11 mmol/L) [200 mg/dL] with a venous pH < 7.30 and/or bicarbonate <15 mmol/L. The blood glucose concentration is usually elevated but in 8% of cases may be <15 mmol/L [270 mg/dL] and there is ketonuria. DKA can be further classified by its severity: mild (venous pH < 7.30 and/or bicarbonate <15 mmol/L), moderate (pH < 7.2 and/or bicarbonate <10 mmol/L) and severe (pH < 7.1 and/or bicarbonate <5 mmol/L).

The mortality rate from DKA is approximately 0.2%. Death is usually caused by cerebral oedema but may also be caused by hypokalaemia-induced dysrhythmias, sepsis and aspiration pneumonia.

Resuscitation

DKA is a medical emergency and, in common with all emergencies, resuscitation should follow the 'ABC' pattern. The protocol which follows for the treatment of DKA is largely based on that published by the European Society of Paediatric Endocrinology and the Lawson Wilkins Paediatric Endocrine Society (Dunger et al 2004) and by the British Society of Paediatric Endocrinology and Diabetes (2004).

• Airway—if the child is comatose an airway should be inserted and if the conscious level is depressed or the child is vomiting, a nasogastric tube should be passed, aspirated and left on free drainage.

• Breathing—if there is evidence of hypoxia give 100% oxygen and consider the need for intubation and ventilation. However, airway and breathing problems are rare.

• Circulation—an intravenous cannula should be sited and blood samples (including a venous blood gas measurement) taken for investigations (see above). In cases of circulatory impairment (suggested by the presence of poor capillary refill, tachycardia or hypotension) give 10 mL/kg body weight of 0.9% saline intravenously as quickly as possible. This can be repeated, with further boluses to a maximum of 30 ml/kg being given more slowly until the circulation is restored.

If at presentation the child is too ill to weigh, for the purposes of calculating fluid requirements, weight can be estimated from a recent clinic weight, a centile chart or from the equation:

$$\text{weight (kg)} = 2 \times (\text{age in years} + 4).$$

Antibiotics should be given if sepsis is thought likely after appropriate samples for culture have been taken.

Initial monitoring

The child should be nursed in either a high dependency or intensive care unit. If the child is under 3 years of age, comatose or more than 10% dehydrated with circulatory impairment then transfer to a paediatric intensive care unit is advised. The following should be documented:

• Hourly *BP and basic observations*.

• *Weight* should be measured once or twice a day, using a weigh bed if available.

• A strict *fluid balance* chart should be kept which should include fluid losses from vomiting and diarrhoea.

• Urine samples should be tested for *ketones* (capillary

Table 1.5 Maintenance fluid requirements.

Age (years)	Maintenance fluid requirements (ml/kg body weight/day)
0–2	80
3–5	70
6–9	60
10–14	50
Adults > 15	30

Table 1.6 Example of fluid volume calculation.

An 8-year-old boy weighing 27 kg who is 10% dehydrated and who required 10 mL/kg 0.9% saline during resuscitation will need:

Daily maintenance = 27 kg × 60 mL = 1620 mL
Deficit = 27 kg × 10% = 2700 mL
Resuscitation fluid = 270 mL
Total requirements over 48 hours = (2 × 1620) + 2700 − 270 = 5670 mL
Hourly rate = 5670/48 = 118 mL/hour

blood ketone levels may be available and may be a more sensitive measure of suppression of ketogenesis following treatment).

• Hourly capillary *blood glucose* measurements should be performed. These may be inaccurate with severe dehydration/acidosis but are useful in documenting trends (ideally, an additional cannula should be inserted for blood sampling to prevent recurrent, painful finger pricks and to obtain more accurate results).

• *Blood gases, electrolyte and urea concentrations.* These should be re-evaluated 2 hours after the start of treatment or sooner if there are clinical concerns.

• A *cardiac monitor* should be used to monitor abnormal serum potassium concentrations (hypokalaemia is suggested by flat T-waves, prominent U-waves and dysrhythmias, whereas hyperkalaemia is indicated by the presence of tall, peaked T-waves with dysrhythmias).

• All patients with DKA should have at least hourly *neurological observations* and if comatose the Glasgow Coma Score should be recorded. The development of a headache or change in behaviour should be reported immediately to medical staff as this may be the first sign of cerebral oedema.

• If the patient is comatose or there is difficulty monitoring fluid losses, a *urinary catheter* should be passed.

Fluid therapy

Calculation of fluid requirements

Once the circulating fluid volume has been restored, ongoing fluid requirements can be calculated as follows:

fluid requirement = (fluid maintenance + fluid deficit) − fluid used for resuscitation.

The fluid deficit should be replaced over 48 hours and can be calculated from:

fluid deficit (L) = % dehydration × body weight (kg).

The extent of dehydration is usually 5–10%. It is often overestimated and, for the purposes of calculating fluid requirements, the fluid deficit used should not exceed 10% of body weight. The fluid used during initial resuscitation to restore the circulation should be taken into account when calculating fluid requirements and deducted from the total. Maintenance fluid requirements can be estimated from Table 1.5.

The hourly infusion rate is calculated using the following formula:

hourly rate = 48 hours maintenance + deficit − resuscitation fluid already given/48.

Significant ongoing fluid losses, such as those caused by vomiting or excess diuresis, should also be replaced. An example of calculations to estimate fluid requirements for a child with DKA is shown in Table 1.6. It is always important to double check these calculations.

Ongoing fluid prescription

At presentation in DKA, the serum sodium concentration is usually low. This is mainly caused by a deficit in body sodium. Hypernatraemia may be present if water loss has been severe and has exceeded sodium losses. Initially 0.9% saline should be used but once the plasma glucose concentration has fallen to 14–17 mmol/L glucose should be added to the fluid. If this occurs within the first 6 hours, the child may still be sodium depleted. This situation may necessitate continued use of 0.9% saline and added dextrose. If this occurs after the first 6 hours, and the child's plasma sodium is stable, the fluid may be changed to 0.45% saline with 5% dextrose.

In the early stages of DKA patients often experience marked thirst and request oral fluids. In severe dehydration with impaired consciousness no fluids should be allowed by mouth. Oral fluids should be allowed only after a significant clinical improvement with no vomiting. If a substantial clinical improvement has occurred prior to the 48 hours of rehydration oral intake can proceed and the intravenous infusions can be reduced to take account of the oral intake.

Potassium administration

Potassium is mainly an intracellular ion and at presentation in DKA there is invariably a large depletion of total body potassium even though initial serum potassium concentrations may be normal or even high. Early addition of potassium to the fluid regimen (40 mmol/L) is essential even if the serum concentration is normal as insulin will drive glucose and potassium into the cells, producing a rapid fall in serum potassium concentrations and increased potassium requirements.

Potassium should be added to intravenous fluids as soon as ongoing urine output has been established. In the rare cases where there is doubt about the urine output, the patient should be catheterized. Early potassium therapy should be avoided if anuria is present as a result of acute tubular necrosis. The serum potassium concentration should be maintained between 4 and 5 mmol/L.

Phosphate

Depletion of intracellular phosphate also occurs. The fall in plasma phosphate levels is exacerbated by insulin therapy as phosphate re-enters the cells. Phosphate depletion may last for several days after the DKA has resolved. Prospective studies have failed to show any significant benefit from phosphate replacement and phosphate administration may lead to hypocalcaemia.

Insulin therapy

Although rehydration alone will lead to a fall in plasma glucose and ketone concentrations, insulin is required to reverse the underlying metabolic abnormalities by further reductions in glucose concentrations and by prevention of ketone body formation.

The insulin infusion should be prepared by adding 50 units of short-acting insulin to 49.5 mL of 0.9% saline in a 50-mL syringe pump to produce an insulin concentration of 1 unit/mL. This may be connected to the fluid infusion through a Y-connector and prescribed as follows.

- The insulin solution should run initially at 0.1 mL/kg/hour at least until resolution of the ketoacidosis (pH >7.30, HCO_3 >15 mmol/L).
- If plasma glucose concentrations fall by more than 5 mmol/L/hour [90 mg/dL/hour] add dextrose (5–10%) to the intravenous fluids.
- When the blood glucose has fallen to 14–17 mmol/L [250–300 mg/dL], intravenous fluid with dextrose should be prescribed (usually a 5% dextrose/0.45% saline mixture is used, but dextrose concentrations of up to 10% may be necessary to maintain plasma glucose concentrations).
- The insulin infusion should not be stopped before the acidosis is corrected as insulin is required to switch off ketone production. If the blood glucose falls <4 mmol/L, [<72 mg/dL] a bolus of 2 ml/kg of 10% dextrose should be given and the dextrose concentration in the fluid increased.
- When the pH is >7.30, the blood glucose concentration has been reduced to 14–17 mmol/L [250–300 mg/dL], and a dextrose infusion has been started, the insulin infusion rate can be reduced—but not to less than 0.05 units/kg/hour.

Acidosis and bicarbonate therapy

Adequate hydration and insulin therapy will reverse even a severe acidosis. Appropriate hydration will also reverse any lactic acidosis, which may account for 25% of the acidaemia, due to poor tissue perfusion and renal function. Continuing acidosis usually reflects inadequate fluid resuscitation or insulin therapy. The use of bicarbonate therapy is very rarely required. Several small trials have failed to show any clinical benefit following bicarbonate administration. Bicarbonate should only be considered to improve cardiac contractility in patients who are severely acidotic (arterial pH < 6.9) with circulatory failure despite adequate fluid replacement. **Bicarbonate should never be given without prior discussion with a senior doctor.**

Subsequent management

Although plasma glucose concentrations may fall to near normal levels within 4–6 hours of treatment of DKA, the metabolic acidosis may take 24 hours or longer to resolve. Subsequent management should include the following:

- Blood gases and electrolyte and urea concentrations should be re-evaluated 2 hours after the start of treatment and 4-hourly thereafter, or more frequently if there are clinical concerns, until the child has recovered.
- The ongoing intravenous fluid prescription should be reviewed every 4 hours and adjusted according to the electrolyte results and fluid balance.
- If there is continuing massive polyuria, the rate of infusion of intravenous fluids may need to be increased and large gastric aspirates will need replacing with 0.45% saline with 10 mmol/L potassium chloride.

- Once the blood gases and electrolyte concentrations normalize, the frequency of blood sampling can be decreased and discontinued once the child is tolerating oral fluids and food.
- The frequency of bedside capillary blood glucose measurements may be reduced to 2- to 4-hourly if plasma glucose concentrations are relatively stable while the child is receiving intravenous dextrose.
- If the acidosis or hyperglycaemia do not improve after 4–6 hours the patient should be reassessed by a senior doctor. Insulin errors, inadequate rehydration or sepsis may be the cause. More insulin, 0.9% saline or antibiotics may be required.
- Intravenous fluids should be continued until the child is drinking well and able to tolerate snacks.
- The insulin infusion should be continued until significant ketonuria (+++) is no longer present. However, it is not necessary to wait for complete resolution of ketonuria before changing to subcutaneous insulin.
- When the patient is started on a conventional subcutaneous insulin regimen (see above), the insulin infusion should be discontinued 30 minutes (if using a short- or long-acting insulin) or 10 minutes (if using a rapidly acting insulin analogue) after the first subcutaneous injection to avoid rebound hyperglycaemia.

Cerebral oedema

Cerebral oedema has a mortality of approximately 25%. Significant neurological morbidity is present in 10–26% of survivors. It occurs in approximately 0.3–1% of cases of DKA.

Aetiology

The aetiology of cerebral oedema is poorly understood and even with optimum management of DKA, cases still occur. It is more common in children under 5 years of age and in newly diagnosed cases of diabetes. A fall in sodium concentration following treatment, a severe acidosis, the use of bicarbonate, marked hypocapnia and a high urea at presentation have all been implicated as risk factors. Much of the treatment is aimed at minimizing these possible contributory factors.

Clinical features

Cerebral oedema usually occurs 4–12 hours after the start of treatment and often follows an initial period of clinical and biochemical improvement. However, in some cases the patient's state of consciousness may decline from admission onwards, whereas in others cerebral oedema may occur after 48 hours. Typical symptoms and signs of cerebral oedema include:
- onset or worsening of headache (this is often present initially in DKA and should improve with treatment);
- confusion;
- irritability;
- reducing conscious level (patients are often drowsy at presentation but this should improve with treatment);
- convulsions;
- pupillary abnormalities;
- hypertension and bradycardia;
- decerebrate or decorticate posturing;
- papilloedema (late sign); and
- respiratory impairment or arrest.

Treatment

Only about 50% of patients have a period of neurological deterioration during which intervention may be effective prior to a respiratory arrest. If cerebral oedema is suspected senior staff should be informed immediately and the following measures should be taken as soon as possible:
- hypoglycaemia should be excluded;
- mannitol 1 g/kg (= 5 mL/kg of 20% mannitol over 20 minutes) or hypertonic saline (3%) 5–10 ml/kg over 30 minutes should be given as soon as possible;
- fluids should be restricted to two-thirds of maintenance with the deficit replaced over 72 hours rather than 48 hours;
- the child should be transferred to a paediatric intensive care unit;
- the child should be discussed with an intensive care consultant. If assisted ventilation is required the $P\text{co}_2$ should be maintained above 3.5 kPa;
- once the child is stable an urgent computed tomography scan should be performed to exclude other problems such as cerebral thrombosis, haemorrhage or infarction;
- a repeat dose of mannitol should be given after 2 hours if there is no initial response.

Other complications

- Infections—antibiotics are not required unless a significant bacterial infection is suspected.
- Abdominal pain—this is common and may be due to liver swelling, gastritis, bladder retention or ileus. However, surgical conditions such as appendicitis rarely occur and a surgical opinion may be required

once DKA is stable. A raised amylase is common in DKA.

The diabetes clinic

General principles

Children with diabetes should be seen in a designated diabetic clinic supervised by a senior paediatrician trained in the care of diabetes. It has been recommended that, within a clinical service, there be a specialist nurse for every 70 children with diabetes. Where possible, the clinical service should provide care for a minimum of 40 patients with diabetes to allow the necessary accumulation of expertise. Age banding of the clinic may help to bring families with similarly aged children together and facilitates group teaching of age-appropriate topics. The clinic should be held in a paediatric environment with facilities for auxology. Separate arrangements should be made for clinics for adolescents, which are described later in this chapter. Educational literature, videos and information about holidays for children with diabetes should be available.

The clinic visit

The following staff should ideally be available at each clinic:
- paediatrician with expertise in diabetes;
- diabetes nurse specialist with paediatric training or expertise;
- dietitian with paediatric experience;
- psychologist; and
- social worker to provide financial and other advice to the family.

Any child with diabetes attending the diabetes clinic should undergo the following.

1 Documentation of general health and life events (e.g. changing school), recent hospital admissions, insulin regimen, details of hypoglycaemic episodes and school absences.

2 Review of practical aspects of blood glucose monitoring and insulin injections.

3 If necessary, provision of advice on adjustments to the insulin regimen in the light of the results of blood glucose monitoring.

4 Measurement of height and weight.

5 Examination of injection sites.

6 Three-monthly measurement of glycosylated haemoglobin.

7 An annual review of all patients aged 11 years or older who have had diabetes for ≥2 years, which should include:

Table 1.7 Points to note on clinical examination of patients with diabetes at annual review.

System	Points to note
Height	Growth failure
Weight	Poor or excessive weight gain
Puberty	Delayed puberty / menarche
Skin	Lipohypertrophy at injection sites; necrobiosis lipoidica
Mouth	Presence of caries or other signs of poor dental hygiene
Eyes (through dilated pupils)	Presence of retinopathy / cataracts
Feet	Signs of poor foot care (e.g. calluses from poorly fitting shoes) verrucae
Hands	Finger-prick sites; limited joint mobility ('prayer sign')
Cardiovascular	Hypertension (if present, re-check at the end of the clinic visit)
Endocrine	Goitre or other signs of hypothyroidism or hyperthyroidism
	Increased pigmentation suggestive of Addison's disease
Neurological	Impaired vibration or pinprick sense; loss of ankle reflexes

- a physical examination for microvascular and other complications of diabetes (Table 1.7);
- thyroid function tests;
- random cholesterol measurement;
- screening for microalbuminuria by measurement of the albumin : creatinine ratio in an early morning urine sample;
- some centres perform retinal photography in addition to a clinical examination of the fundi (if the latter is abnormal then retinal photography is recommended to delineate the degree of retinopathy);
- screening for coeliac disease by measurement of coeliac antibodies—the anti-endomysium and anti-transglutaminase antibodies are the most specific (some centres screen annually, others screen every 3 years).

Details of the consultation (and non-attendance) should be documented using either paper records or computer software to enable future audit. Given the multidisciplinary nature of a diabetes clinic, it is helpful to have a team meeting at the end of the clinic to share information about patients who have attended clinic.

Insulin treatment

Insulin delivery systems

Insulin has an effective shelf-life of at least 2 years if kept in a refrigerator at 4°C and can be kept at room temperature for up to 1 month. However, if kept in tropical climates, car interiors or freezer compartments insulin may degrade more rapidly. Insulin is most commonly administered by a pen-delivery system or using syringes and needles. In general, vials of insulin are cheaper than insulin in pen cartridges which, in turn, are cheaper than insulin-filled disposable pens. For children with needle phobia, spring-loaded automatic injection devices in which the needle is not visible, or transjector systems in which a jet of insulin is delivered at sufficiently high pressure that it penetrates the skin without the need for a needle may be helpful.

Insulin pens

Using a pen-delivery system, insulin may be administered using either a pre-loaded disposable device or cartridges fitted into a re-usable pen device. Pen-delivery systems are generally preferred by children as they are quicker and easier to use than syringes and needles and lead to greater independence.

Syringes and needles

Insulin for injection may be drawn up from a vial and injected using a syringe and needle system. A choice is available between using pre-mixed insulin preparations or mixing separate supplies of short/rapid- and intermediate-acting insulins within the syringe by the patient.

When mixing insulins, the short/rapid-acting *clear* insulin should be drawn up into the syringe prior to the intermediate-acting (isophane) *cloudy* insulin. Any preparation containing intermediate-acting insulin should be gently inverted several times prior to use. Although mixing of separate insulins allows, in theory, greater flexibility, there is little evidence that in routine clinical practice this leads to better glycaemic control than that which can be achieved using pre-mixed insulins. Furthermore, mixing separate insulins is time-consuming and requires greater manual dexterity than other systems.

Injections

Depending on the maturity and confidence of the individual patient, children as young as 5 years can be taught to administer their own injections of insulin. However, the age at which children start to give their own injections is very variable. Peer pressure such as that which may be experienced by a child attending a diabetic camp where children may see their peers, or even younger children, administering injections may help a child to learn to self-inject.

Appropriate injection sites are demonstrated in Fig. 1.2. The use of different injection sites and rotation of these sites should be encouraged to avoid the development of lipohypertrophy (Fig. 1.3) which may be unsightly and lead to erratic absorption of insulin. If patients avoid injecting into these areas, lipohypertrophy will resolve, typically within 3 months.

Clinically significant variations in the amount of insulin absorbed from each injection can occur as a result of the factors listed in Table 1.8.

Injection technique

It is unnecessary to clean the skin prior to a subcutaneous insulin injection. It is recommended that patients be taught to give the injection at a 45° angle to the surface of the skin. When using the very short (e.g. 5 mm) needles the injection can be given vertically without pinching the skin unless the patient is very thin. In those who find injections painful, distraction techniques can be used or the skin rubbed with an ice cube prior to the injection. Pen needles should be changed after each injection. More frequent use will lead to blunting and painful injections.

Insulin requirements

Suggested starting dosages of insulin are outlined on pages 6–7. In established patients, it is unusual for prepubertal children to require more than 1 unit of insulin/kg body weight/day. By contrast, children in puberty may

Table 1.8 Factors affecting insulin absorption.

Slower insulin absorption	Faster insulin absorption
Leg or arm injection sites	Abdominal injection site
Subcutaneous injection	Intramuscular injection
Lipohypertrophy	Exercise
Cold skin	Peripherally vasodilated
Obese subjects	Thin subjects

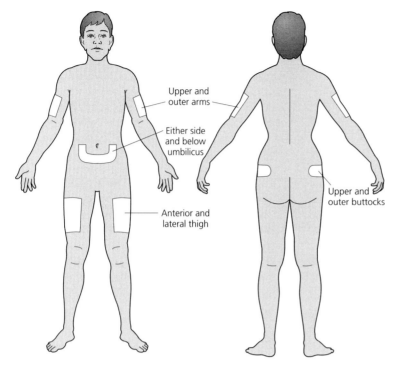

Upper and outer arms

Either side and below umbilicus

Upper and outer buttocks

Anterior and lateral thigh

Fig. 1.2 Appropriate insulin injection sites.

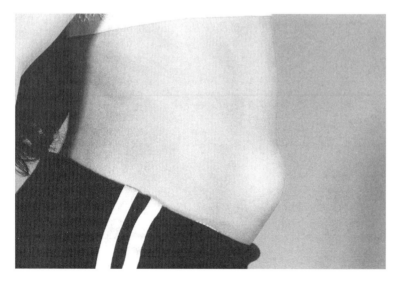

Fig. 1.3 Lipohypertrophy.

require 1–2 units/kg/day. Obese patients may be insulin-resistant and require relatively higher dosages. In children receiving twice-daily injections, most require approximately two-thirds of their total daily insulin dosage prior to breakfast with approximately two-thirds of their total dosage in the form of intermediate-acting insulin.

Altering insulin dosage

In children under 10 years insulin dosage can be altered by 1–2 units/day and in children over 10 years by 2–4 units/day, depending on the results of blood glucose testing. Following any change in insulin dosage, blood glucose concentrations should be monitored carefully for 5–7 days to assess the effect.

Injecting small doses

In infants, the injection of doses of insulin as small as 1 unit can result in significant inaccuracies, with actual doses delivered ranging from 0.89 to 1.23 units. In these circumstances, it is recommended to use pen-delivery systems available from the manufacturers of insulin which allows injections of insulin in increments of 0.5 units.

Insulin preparations

In solution, human insulin forms hexamers (six-molecule units) which are slowly absorbed across endothelial barriers when insulin is injected subcutaneously. The rate of absorption is mainly determined by how quickly these hexamers dissociate into monomers (single molecules), which are rapidly absorbed at the injection site. Children with diabetes should be treated with human sequence or human insulin analogues. In the UK, this is usually available in a concentration of 100 units/mL (U100) although more dilute forms may be necessary for the treatment of infants receiving very small doses of insulin. Table 1.9 outlines the different preparations of insulin available to treat children in the UK and their duration of action.

Most children who are treated with twice-daily injections of a pre-mixed insulin, use a biphasic mixture of 25–30% rapid/short-acting and 70–75% intermediate-acting insulin. However, individual patients may require other biphasic ratios of rapid/short- to intermediate-acting insulin ranging from 10:90 to 50:50. Several insulins are very similar in their duration of action (e.g. Human Actrapid, Humulin S and Human Velosulin). To simplify matters and to avoid confusion it is therefore recommended that a diabetes team limit the number of insulins they use.

Insulin analogues

Rapidly acting insulin analogues incorporate amino acid substitutions which make them quickly dissociate into monomers and dimers following injection and therefore lead to rapid absorption. They can be given just prior to a meal or, in very young children in whom there is concern about food refusal, within 15 minutes of starting a meal. Compared with short-acting insulin, they produce lower post-prandial glucose excursions but higher fasting and pre-prandial glucose concentrations. They may therefore be helpful in children who become hypoglycaemic prior to lunch. They do not lead to a decrease in the overall incidence of hypoglycaemia but there is some evidence that they lead to a decrease in the incidence of severe hypoglycaemia. Compared with conventional insulin these analogues are associated with a very small decrease in HbA1c of approximately 0.1%.

Rapidly acting analogues are also available in a pre-mixed form with intermediate-acting insulin. They decrease post-prandial glucose concentrations but when compared to similar mixtures of conventional insulin have similar effects on HbA1c and the incidence of hypoglycaemia.

Recently two long-acting insulin analogues have been developed. They both lead to a consistent and prolonged release of insulin with no peaks. Insulin glargine has glycine instead of asparagine at position 21 on the A chain and has two arginines added to the carboxyl terminal of the B chain at positions 31 and 32. These changes result in a low solubility at neutral pH but total solubility at the pH of its injection solution (pH 4). Following injection, the pH of the insulin solution increases, leading to the formation of micro-precipitates, from which small amounts of glargine are gradually absorbed into the circulation. This leads to a prolonged duration of action (about 24 hours). Insulin glargine is licensed in the UK for patients aged 6 years and above but has been used in younger children. It can be injected at any time but is usually given in the evening. There is some evidence that there is a decreased incidence of nocturnal hypoglycaemia when it is given at breakfast.

Insulin detemir has the terminal amino acid (B30) in the B-chain deleted and a 14 carbon fatty acid attached at position B29. This leads to a prolonged duration of action (up to 24 hours) as a result of two mechanisms: albumin binding via a fatty acid side-chain retains insulin in the subcutaneous depot and there is also strong self-association of insulin detemir hexamers at the injection site. It is administered once or occasionally twice daily. Detemir has recently been licensed in children aged 6 and above in the

Table 1.9 Insulin preparations recommended for the treatment of children in the UK.

Preparation	Manufacturer	Formulations	Approximate time course of action		
			Onset	Peak	Duration
1 *Very rapidly acting insulin*					
Humalog (insulin lispro)	Lilly	vial, cart, pen	15 min	30–70 min	2–5 h
Novorapid (insulin aspart)	NovoNordisk	vial, cart, pen	15 min	60–180 min	3–5 h
2 *Short-acting insulins (soluble, neutral)*					
Human Actrapid	NovoNordisk	vial, cart, pen	30 min	1–2 h	6–8 h
Humulin S	Lilly	vial, cart, pen	30 min	1–2 h	6–8 h
Human Velosulin	NovoNordisk	vial	30 min	1–2 h	6–8 h
3 *Intermediate-acting insulins (isophane)*					
Human Insulatard	NovoNordisk	vial, cart, pen	2 h	4–6 h	8–12 h
Humulin I	Lilly	vial, cart, pen	2 h	4–6 h	8–12 h
4 *Biphasic insulins ('fixed mixtures')*					
Human mixtard 30 (30% Actrapid /70% Insulatard)	NovoNordisk	vial, cart, pen	30 min	2–6 h	8–12 h
Humulin M3 (30% Humulin S /70% Humulin I)	Lilly	vial, cart, pen	30 min	2–6 h	8–12 h
Human mixtard 10, 20, 40, 50	NovoNordisk	vial, cart, pen	Mixtures containing respectively 10, 20, 40 and 50% soluble insulin. Less used than the 30 /70 mixtures. Have the same time course but differing intensity of early action according to the proportion of soluble insulin.		
Humalog mix 25	Lilly	cart, pen	15 min	1 h	8–12 h
Humalog mix 50	Lilly	pen	Same time course as Humalog Mix 25 but increased intensity of early action		
Novomix 30	NovoNordisk	cart, pen	15 min	60–240 min	8–12 h
5 *Long acting insulins*					
Insulin glargine	Aventis Pharma	vial, cart, pen	1–2 h	peakless	24 h
Insulin detemir*	NovoNordisk	cart, pen	1–2 h	peakless	24 h

Vial: Standard 10-mL bottle for use with syringes. Cart: 3-mL cartridges for reusable pen. Pen: disposable 3-mL pens.
*In practice, detemir may act for less than 24 hours and may be required twice daily.

European Union but to date has been used mainly in adolescents. There is currently little data on its use in children and adolescents.

Insulin glargine and detemir provide new opportunities to optimize glycaemic control. Both result in glycaemic control that is at least comparable to that using isophane insulin.

Some studies comparing basal bolus regimes with isophane or glargine have shown that the use of glargine leads to a small (0.1–0.4%) decrease in HbA1c, but other studies have shown no difference. There is some evidence that both glargine and detemir lead to a decrease in the incidence of hypoglycaemia, including nocturnal hypoglycaemia. Weight gain with both of these insulins may be less than that with isophane insulin.

In conclusion, insulin analogues may be a useful option in children and adolescents with diabetes who have frequent severe hypoglycaemia, especially at night. However, at present there is no convincing evidence to justify changing a patient from conventional therapy to analogues if they demonstrate satisfactory glycaemic control without troublesome hypoglycaemia. Also, there are insufficient data at present on the long-term efficacy and safety of the insulin analogues.

Basal bolus regimen

This regimen is discussed on page 7. When converting from twice daily insulin injections to a basal bolus regimen the total number of units is often decreased by 10% to reduce the risk of hypoglycaemia. Normally, 30–40% of the total daily dose of insulin is given at bedtime as an intermediate-acting insulin or a longacting insulin analogue with the remaining insulin being given prior to breakfast, lunch and the evening meal in the form of rapid/short-acting insulin. If there are marked discrepancies in the size of the meals then the pre-meal dose of insulin should reflect this. When converting from a basal bolus regimen containing isophane to one with a long-acting insulin analogue the same number of units of the analogue is usually given. In such cases the dose of rapid/short-acting insulin prior to each meal may need to be lowered by approximately 2 units if there is good glycaemic control. If day-time blood glucose levels are generally high then the doses of rapid/short-acting insulin can be left unaltered. As with any significant change in insulin regimen, blood glucose levels should be tested frequently to see what effect the change has had. It can take up to 2 weeks for the full effects of a change to a regimen incorporating glargine to become apparent (there is little experience of detemir in children and adolescents).

Example of how to convert a patient from twice-daily insulin to a basal bolus regimen

- Patient received 44 units of a 30:70 pre-mixed insulin in the morning and 22 units in the evening. He or she eats a small breakfast, an average-sized lunch and a large evening meal.
- Decrease total daily dosage of insulin from 66 to 60 units.
- Initially try 24 units (40%) of isophane or a long-acting insulin analogue prior to bedtime.
- Try rapid/short-acting insulin 10 units before breakfast, 12 units before lunch and 14 units before the evening meal.
- Adjust doses of insulin in the light of blood glucose test results.

Once on this regimen the bedtime dose should be slowly adjusted to achieve an average morning fasting glucose concentration of 6 mmol/L [108 mg/dL]. Further adjustments can then be made to the pre-prandial doses. Typical pre-meal doses in adolescents vary from 6 units for a small breakfast to 20 units for a large meal.

Continuous subcutaneous insulin infusions

These are used in about 1% and 25% of children and adolescents in the UK and USA respectively. They may be used as part of an intensive regimen to improve glycaemic control and were used in 42% of patients in the intensive treatment group in the Diabetes Control and Complications Trial (DCCT). The devices consist of a programmable pump (which may be as small as a match box) containing insulin which is connected by an infusion line to a small plastic cannula inserted subcutaneously, usually in the abdomen, and fixed by self-adhesive tape. The cannula is usually left in place for 2–4 days. The pump delivers short- or rapidly-acting insulin continuously at a constant or variable basal rate with additional boluses delivered at meal time. It is possible, for instance, to alter the overnight basal rate to try to prevent the dawn phenomenon (see below). The bolus dose delivered will depend on the carbohydrate content of the meal. Boluses may also be given to correct high blood glucose concentrations. Frequent testing, four or more times per day, is required. Modern pumps include occlusion detection devices and a remaining insulin counter and they can be programmed to limit the maximum basal and bolus rates to avoid overdosage.

Pump therapy is said to provide the best and most consistent glycaemic control. There is evidence, when compared to multiple daily injections, that it leads to a fall in HbA1c of approximately 0.5%. It can also lead to a reduction in the incidence of hypoglycaemia and in BMI. The incidence of DKA is no different when compared to multiple daily injections (although there may be a slightly increased risk of DKA during the early days of pump use). The pump enables a flexible life style and eating patterns and is associated with high satisfaction in appropriately motivated patients.

Complications include occlusion of the line or of the cannula and cannula dislodgement which, if undetected, can lead relatively rapidly to DKA as there is no subcutaneous reservoir of insulin. Infection at the cannula site is a further problem. Some patients resent being attached to a machine for 24 hours a day as this provides a constant reminder of their diabetes. Pump therapy is also expensive.

There are a number of guidelines available for the calculation of basal and bolus rates from the pump manufacturers. The vast majority of patients experience a significant reduction in their total daily insulin dose of up to 50% when converting to a pump from intermittent subcutaneous injections of insulin. In the UK insulin pump therapy is recommended as an option in patients with type 1 diabetes provided that multiple-dose insulin therapy (including the use of a long-acting insulin analogue) has failed to reduce the HbA1c to less than 7.5% (or below 6.5% in the presence of microalbuminuria or other complications) without disabling hypoglycaemia and that the patient and their family have the commitment and competence to use the pump effectively.

Continuous subcutaneous insulin infusion therapy should be administered only by a team experienced and trained in pump therapy. Patients and their families should be trained in its use, which also necessitates a detailed knowledge of the carbohydrate content of food to allow calculation of meal-related insulin bolus sizes. Frequent contact should be maintained with the diabetic team so that appropriate changes in the insulin dose and regimen can be made in accordance with the patient's diet, exercise regime and lifestyle.

Potential problems with insulin therapy

The dawn phenomenon
The dawn phenomenon describes the rise in insulin requirements and blood glucose concentrations in the latter part of the night, at approximately 05.00–08.00 hours. It occurs mainly in puberty and is thought to be caused by the insulin resistance produced by nocturnal growth hormone secretion. This is a difficult problem to resolve on conventional insulin regimens. Possible benefit may be derived in those using the twice-daily insulin regimen by dividing the evening injection so that short/rapid-acting insulin is given prior to the evening meal and intermediate-acting insulin prior to bedtime. Alternatively, in patients on a basal bolus regimen the pre-bedtime dose of intermediate-acting insulin or long-acting insulin analogue can be increased.

The Somogyi phenomenon
This is said to be the 'rebound' morning hyperglycaemia which may occur following nocturnal hypoglycaemia caused by the release of counter-regulatory hormones such as glucagon, adrenaline and cortisol. Whether this phenomenon exists is open to debate and it is more likely to be the consequence of excessive ingestion of refined carbohydrates used to treat the episode of nocturnal hypoglycaemia.

Monitoring glycaemic control

Blood glucose testing
A number of studies have shown that greater frequency of blood glucose monitoring improves metabolic control. The following principles for home blood glucose monitoring are recommended.
- Children should be encouraged to perform their own finger-prick blood glucose testing at as young an age as they feel able to do so (sometimes as young as 5 years old).
- Finger pricks should be performed at the sides of the finger tips.
- Finger-pricking devices with variable depth settings can make testing less painful.
- Forearm blood glucose testing is an acceptable and accurate alternative to finger prick testing.
- Electronic blood glucose meters with a memory which may allow data to be downloaded onto a computer for discussion in clinic are useful for recording results but need regular calibration.
- Date-expired blood glucose testing strips should be avoided as their use may lead to inaccurate blood glucose estimations.
- The child should be encouraged to monitor blood glucose concentrations regularly prior to each main meal and at bedtime; on rare occasions, it may be helpful to monitor values 2 hours after a main meal.
- More frequent blood glucose testing may be indicated if the child is unwell, partaking in unusual amounts of physical activity or feels hypoglycaemic.

Table 1.10 Interpreting glycosylated haemoglobin values.

HbA1c (%) value	Comment
5.0–5.9	Within non-diabetic reference range, possibility of frequent hypoglycaemia
6.0–6.9	Ideal glycaemic control
7.0–7.5	Very good glycaemic control in the absence of complications
7.6–8.9	Associated with increased risk of microvascular complications; advise to improve glycaemic control
9.0–10.9	Compliance likely to be a problem; associated with high risk of microvascular complications
>11.0	Poor compliance, probably associated with omission of insulin injections and unrestricted diet

• Devices that regularly monitor blood glucose readings, in some cases at 10-minute intervals for 12 hours, have recently become available (e.g. GlucoWatch biographer). These devices have been shown to detect hypoglycaemia more frequently than conventional monitoring and may also have hypoglycaemia alarms. Conventional blood glucose testing is still required to calibrate the device. Whether such a device can help to improve metabolic control in the long term is not known.

• The child should aim for pre-meal blood glucose concentrations of approximately 4–8 mmol/L [78–144 mg/dL], pre-bedtime values of 7–10 mmol/L [126–180 mg/dL] and <10 mmol/L [180 mg/dL] 1–2 hours after meals.

• In children under 5 years of age acceptance of slightly higher blood glucose concentrations may be necessary to avoid hypoglycaemia which may be a consequence of variable feeding patterns.

Urinary ketone testing

Urine should be tested for ketones during illness or when blood glucose concentrations are unusually high, particularly when associated with symptoms of polyuria, polydipsia, nausea or abdominal pain. The presence of hyperglycaemia and substantial (+++) ketonuria indicates that DKA may be present or that urgent increases to the dosage of insulin are required to avoid this happening.

Glycosylated haemoglobin measurement

HbA1c is formed by the adduction of glucose to adult haemoglobin and reflects average blood glucose values during the previous 6–8 weeks. Traditionally, many different assays have been used in different laboratories with differing normal ranges. It is now recommended that, to assist audit, laboratories should report their results adjusted to give comparable values to the assays used in the Diabetes Control and Complications Trial (DCCT). The DCCT-adjusted normal, non-diabetic range is 4–6%.

For clinics, bench-top machines for the measurement of blood HbA1c concentrations are now available and have the advantage of providing results for discussion with the patient while they are attending clinic. Such machines, however, require careful maintenance and quality control.

Haemoglobin variants may interfere with the glycosylated haemoglobin assays. Increased proportions of HbF, which may occur in β-thalassaemia, may cause an artefactual increase in HbA1c concentrations whereas HbS and HbC may produce artefactually low values.

For most patients the goal is an HbA1c of less than 7.5%. The clinical interpretation of HbA1c measurements is shown in Table 1.10. Depending on glycaemic control, HbA1c concentrations should be measured every 3–6 months.

Alternative methods for monitoring longer term glycaemia include the measurement of blood HbA1 concentrations which are approximately 2% higher than HbA1c levels, or fructosamine, which can be of value if the patient has increased proportions of haemoglobin variants but which provides a measure of glycaemia only in the previous 2 weeks and may be less accurate than HbA1c values.

Diabetes Control and Complications Trial (DCCT)

This trial, published in 1993, is arguably the most important publication on diabetes in the last 12 years. A total of 1441 subjects with diabetes aged 13–39 years were randomized either: (i) to continue with their conventional treatment, or (ii) to receive intensive therapy with increased support from the diabetes team and insulin administered either by a pump or by three or more injections daily. After a mean time interval of 6.5 years, compared with conventional therapy, intensive treatment resulted in a reduction in:

• mean HbA1c concentration of approximately 2%;
• the risk of retinopathy by 76%;
• the occurrence of microalbuminuria by 39%; and
• the occurrence of neuropathy by 60%.

Table 1.11 Characteristics of children of pre-school age with diabetes.

Atypical symptoms at diagnosis
Increased insulin sensitivity
Practical difficulties administering insulin injections
Prolonged night-time fast
Frequent bottle feeds in infancy
Food refusal
Inability to communicate symptoms of impending
  hypoglycaemia
Frequent infective illnesses often associated with vomiting
Rapid growth and neurodevelopment
Complete dependency on others to supervise their diabetes

The trial found that for every 10% reduction in HbA1c (e.g. 8 versus 7.2%) there was a 44% reduction in the risk of microvascular complications.

The disadvantages of intensive treatment included a two- to threefold increase in severe hypoglycaemia and a mean weight gain of 4.6 kg when compared with conventional treatment. This study clearly demonstrated the reduction in risk of the microvascular complications of diabetes which can result from improved glycaemic control. Furthermore, for a given mean HbA1c there was a significantly lower incidence of complications in the intensively treated group suggesting that this form of therapy produces less glycaemic excursion, thereby lowering the risk of complications. The challenge for clinicians, however, is to discover how to apply an intensive therapeutic regimen in conventional clinical practice in a manner that will be acceptable to children and adolescents.

Effect of exercise on blood glucose control

Exercise is beneficial to children with diabetes as it results in:
• reduced blood glucose concentrations;
• increased insulin sensitivity;
• reduced serum lipid concentrations; and
• reduced risks of hypertension and heart disease.
  Ideally, blood glucose monitoring should occur before and after exercise. Hypoglycaemia can be avoided by taking complex carbohydrate in the form of a snack before exercise and/or by decreasing the dose of insulin by approximately 10–20%. In school, the teacher should be aware that the child has diabetes and carbohydrate (e.g. glucose tablets or drinks) should be available for the treatment of hypoglycaemia. Exercise can also lead to delayed hypoglycaemia (e.g. during the night) and in such circumstances extra complex carbohydrate should be taken with the bedtime snack. Occasionally, short-duration exercise can cause hyperglycaemia because of the increased secretion of counter-regulatory hormones (e.g. adrenaline).

Diabetes in children of pre-school age

There are a number of factors which are pertinent to the management of very young children with diabetes, as shown in Table 1.11.

Diabetes in adolescence

Adolescence is accompanied by a rapid increase in linear growth, by the hormonal changes of puberty and by increasing maturity and independence. These changes can make diabetes difficult to manage during adolescence and metabolic control often deteriorates.

Adolescent clinics
Patients aged 14–18 years should be seen in a separate clinic. Ideally, the patient should be managed jointly by the paediatric and adult physicians in an environment appropriate to their age. It is not inappropriate for such clinics to include young adults. With increasing independence, the adolescent should be encouraged to attend the consultation on his or her own, or with a friend, rather than with parents. On occasions though, with the agreement of the patient, it may still prove necessary for the clinical staff to maintain a dialogue over certain issues with the parents. Group sessions where adolescents can exchange views about diabetes and their ways of coping with it can be useful. These meetings can be organized by the psychologist or diabetes nurse.

Insulin requirements
Insulin requirements increase in puberty partly because of the rapid increase in size and appetite but also because of increasing growth hormone secretion which increases resistance to insulin-stimulated glucose metabolism. This results in increased difficulty in maintaining good glycaemic control (including the dawn phenomenon) and, par-

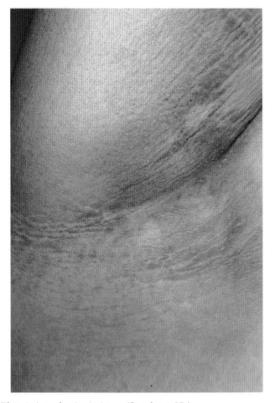

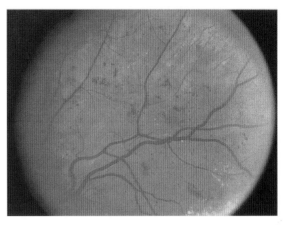

Plate 2 Background retinopathy showing scattered 'dots and blots' (microaneurysms and haemorrhages) and exudates. (See also p. 26.)

Plate 1 Acanthosis nigricans. (See also p. 25.)

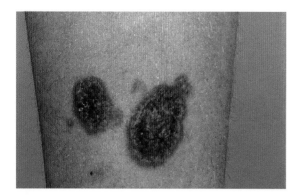

Plate 3 Necrobiosis lipoidica diabeticorum on the shin. (See also p. 28.)

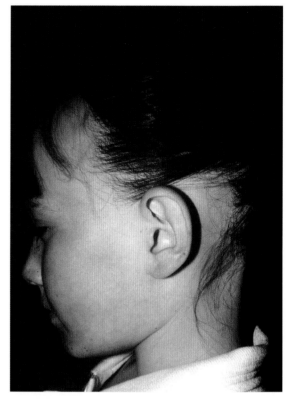

Plate 4 Pigmentation and alopecia areata in a 10-year-old girl with nail dystrophy caused by *Candida*. Investigations showed both Addison's disease and hypoparathyroidism. Genetic studies showed a homozygous 13-bp deletion in exon 8 of the autoimmune regulator gene on chromosome 21q 22.3. (See also p. 136.)

ticularly for girls, an increased tendency to be overweight. Insulin requirements may be greater than 1.3 units/kg body weight/day and on occasion may be as great as 2 units/kg/day. Inadequate insulin therapy may cause delayed puberty and impaired growth.

Insulin regimens

The results of the DCCT suggest that the basal bolus regimen should be considered in children over 13 years. However, a change to such a regimen may not be appropriate if there is good glycaemic control with twice-daily injections of insulin or if the patient is not keen on having four injections of insulin daily. For some adolescents, giving an injection before lunch at school may not be practical. In others, a three-injection regimen, dividing the evening injection into rapid/short-acting insulin prior to the evening meal and isophane prior to bedtime, may provide a useful compromise. Adolescents may be more concerned with short-term problems such as an increased risk of hypoglycaemia, which may lead to loss of a driving licence, than with decreasing the risk of longer term complications.

Psychological and psychiatric problems

Psychological problems are common during puberty. The presence of a psychologist or psychiatrist in clinic is particularly valuable in this age group. It is important to differentiate between the normal psychological changes of adolescence and a pathological response to a chronic disease. The latter may lead to depression and require skilled psychiatric care.

Many patients will not comply with the diet and some may binge. A higher than average number of diabetic children, particularly girls, have eating disorders. Abnormal eating patterns may develop as a means of manipulating their parents. Most eating disorders are mild and do not require formal intervention. However, occasionally a patient will develop anorexia nervosa or bulimia. These conditions can be very difficult to treat in a patient with diabetes and often necessitate a prolonged admission to an adolescent psychiatric unit.

Not infrequently, adolescents fail to comply with their insulin treatment, experimenting with omission and/or reduction of their insulin doses, sometimes in an effort to manipulate their weight. Poor compliance may also occur in their failure to monitor blood glucose concentrations. Results in the record book can also be fabricated. Recordings which for many days have been documented in the same pen, a significant discrepancy between these results and the HbA1c value, apparently excessively large

insulin requirements (>1.75 U/kg/day) and poor clinic attendance are suggestive of poor compliance. Negotiating appropriate solutions to these difficult problems may take considerable patience and skill and clinical psychological support may be particularly helpful. There is some evidence that motivational interviewing, a counselling approach to behaviour change, may improve wellbeing and glycaemic control in adolescents with diabetes.

The problems listed above can lead to an increased incidence of DKA and hypoglycaemia. Furthermore, puberty is the time when the early signs of microvascular complications, such as background diabetic retinopathy, may become evident.

Miscellaneous problems

There is an increased incidence of polycystic ovary syndrome and menstrual irregularities in girls with diabetes. The menstrual cycle may also effect blood glucose control with rising values in the 2–3 days prior to the start of the period. In those in whom this occurs regularly, insulin dosage can be increased during this time.

Hypoglycaemia

In children with diabetes, hypoglycaemia may be defined as a blood glucose concentration less than 4 mmol/L. However, children whose glycaemic control is poor may experience hypoglycaemic symptoms at concentrations above 4 mmol/L if a rapid fall in blood glucose has occurred.

Causes of hypoglycaemia

Although in up to half of cases there may be no obvious cause, hypoglycaemia may be caused by:
- a missed or delayed snack or meal;
- exercise (may also cause delayed hypoglycaemia);
- alcohol;
- an overdose of insulin;
- impaired food absorption as a result of gastroenteritis or coeliac disease; or
- Addison's disease.

Symptoms and signs of hypoglycaemia

Symptoms of hypoglycaemia are unusual with blood glucose concentrations above 3 mmol/L [54 mg/dL] and a surprising number of children, particularly those with very good glycaemic control or those with recurrent blood glucose values below 4 mmol/L [72 mg/dL], will have no symptoms even with glucose values below 2 mmol/L [36 mg/dL] (so-called 'hypoglycaemia unawareness'). The inability to respond to the usual warning signs of hypoglycaemia can lead to severe hypoglycaemia.

Fortunately, most school-aged children are quickly able to recognize the symptoms of hypoglycaemia (see Table 2.1). In young children symptoms are less obvious and may result in more severe hypoglycaemia. Chronic mild hypoglycaemia may affect concentration, school performance and intellectual function. Recurrent hypoglycaemic seizures may lead to deficits in perceptual, motor, memory and attention tasks.

Nocturnal hypoglycaemia

Nocturnal hypoglycaemia is common. Blood glucose concentrations fall to their lowest levels between 03.00 and 04.00 hours. Severe hypoglycaemia is more common at night. This may be because the patient is asleep and unaware of symptoms of impending hypoglycaemia or because of an impaired response from the counter-regulatory hormones. Nocturnal hypoglycaemia may be suggested by disturbed sleep and excessive sweating, morning headaches, difficulty waking from sleep or convulsions. Continuous glucose monitoring systems (e.g. Gluco-Watch biographer) may be helpful in monitoring nocturnal blood glucose concentrations in patients with suspected or confirmed nocturnal hypoglycaemia. Parents may be afraid that their child will die in the middle of the night from hypoglycaemia: the so called 'dead in bed' syndrome. This syndrome, thought to be caused by hypoglycaemia, is extremely rare (no recorded cases under 7 years of age) and parents should be reassured that it is very unlikely because of the effect of the counter-regulatory hormones.

Treatment of hypoglycaemia

Good glycaemic control is likely to be associated with occasional hypoglycaemic episodes which, if mild, may be acceptable. Avoidance of recurrent blood glucose concentrations below 4 mmol/L [72 mg/dL] may prevent the development of hypoglycaemia unawareness. Hypoglycaemia may be treated by:
• the ingestion of short-acting carbohydrate (e.g. glucose tablets or drinks or a snack-size chocolate bar) followed by complex carbohydrate (bread, cereal or pasta) to prevent a recurrence;
• application of a glucose gel (e.g. hypostop) to the side of the mouth and massage into the buccal mucosa or gums in a child who refuses or is unable to take any food or drink;

• intramuscular glucagon (0.5 mg should be administered to children under 8 years and 1 mg to those over 8 years) in unconscious or fitting patients who have been placed in the 'recovery position', the dose being repeated if there is no response after 10 minutes (side-effects of glucagon include nausea, vomiting, diarrhoea and hypokalaemia); glucagon can also be administered subcutaneously, although this route is probably slightly less efficacious than the intramuscular route;
• in hospital, with 2 mL/kg of 10% dextrose given intravenously.

A hypoglycaemic convulsion may be accompanied by a normal blood glucose concentration because of the effect of the counter-regulatory hormones. In patients with neurological signs and in those who remain in a coma following treatment, other disorders (e.g. epilepsy or meningitis) should be considered.

Nocturnal hypoglycaemia may be prevented by:
• decreasing the evening/bedtime insulin dose;
• increasing the evening snack or adding cornstarch;
• the use of rapid-acting human insulin analogues;
• the use of long-acting human insulin analogues;
• ensuring that young children going to bed at 19.00 hours have a blood glucose concentration >10 mmol/L [180 mg/dL] and older children going to bed at 22.00 hours a value >7 mmol/L [126 mg/dL]. If the blood glucose concentration is below these levels a larger than usual snack or, if a snack has already been eaten, a second snack should be consumed.

Recurrent diabetic ketoacidosis

Recurrent DKA is a particular problem in adolescents and may be fatal. It may be precipitated by:
• poor compliance with insulin therapy or diet (when responsible adults administer insulin a 10-fold reduction in episodes of DKA has been reported);
• infection;
• stress;
• alcohol; or
• psychosocial problems.

Management of diabetes during intercurrent illness

Acute febrile illness often leads to a rise in blood glucose due to raised levels of stress hormones and gluconeogenesis which, in turn, may progress to DKA. Conversely, diseases associated with diarrhoea and/or vomiting such

Table 1.12 Suggested insulin infusion rates during surgery (the same sliding scale can be used in cases of diarrhoea and vomiting).

Blood glucose concentration (mmol/L) [mg/dL]	Suggested insulin infusion rate (units/kg/hour)
<7.0 [<126]	0.01
7.0–11.0 [126–198]	0.04
11.1–17.0 [198–306]	0.06
17.1–22.0 [307–396]	0.08
>22.0 [>396]	0.10

as gastroenteritis may lead to a fall in blood glucose and hypoglycaemia. Families should have clear guidelines on the management of diabetes during intercurrent illness ('sick day rules').

The important principles for the management of diabetes during such illnesses are:
• Do not stop insulin therapy.
• Monitor blood glucose concentrations frequently, at least prior to each meal and prior to bedtime. Sometimes much more frequent monitoring, e.g. hourly, is required.
• Eat carbohydrate regularly. If the child has a poor appetite this may take the form of regular small snacks and/or sugary drinks, rather than large meals.
• Drink plenty of water and/or reduced sugar fluids to counteract the potential dehydration that may be associated with glycosuria, polyuria and a febrile illness.
• Test urine regularly for ketones.
• Adjust the dosage of insulin, increasing as necessary to treat hyperglycaemia and ketonuria. For example, in cases where the blood glucose is >13.0 mmol/L [234 mg/dL] (with or without ketonuria) an additional 2 units of short-, or preferably rapid-acting insulin, can be given prior to each meal and at bedtime (or at the equivalent times if the child is not eating regularly, roughly 4-hourly). If the blood glucose is >22.0 mmol/L [396 mg/dL] then an additional 4 units of short- or rapidly acting insulin can be given at those times. If the child is on a total insulin dose of <20 units/day the additional insulin doses stated above should be halved. This scheme is easiest to implement in children on a basal bolus regimen. In those on a twice-daily mixed insulin regimen it will entail an additional injection of short- or rapid-acting insulin at the time of the standard insulin injection as well as additional short- or rapid-acting insulin injections during the day. Blood glucose should be measured frequently when additional insulin is administered.

• If hypoglycaemia occurs, particularly in association with gastroenteritis and mild ketonuria, ensure that the child takes regular, frequent amounts of carbohydrate snacks and/or sugary drinks. Oral rehydration solutions are sometimes necessary. Occasionally hypostop or glucagon are required to treat hypoglycaemia and to help re-establish oral feeds. Vomiting may be treated with a single injection of an anti-emetic to try to improve carbohydrate intake. The insulin dosage may need to be reduced to two-thirds or a half of the regular dose.
• In cases of severe gastroenteritis and in those with severe or persistent vomiting, intravenous fluids may be necessary (e.g. 5% dextrose/0.45% saline with maintenance potassium). In such cases it is often best to also administer intravenous insulin. Insulin infusion rates such as those outlined in Table 1.12 may be used, initially with hourly blood glucose measurements.
• To treat the underlying illness, antibiotics may be required for some infections and anti-pyretics are also often required. Sugar-free medicines are preferable if available.
• If, despite these measures, the child has persistent vomiting and/or diarrhoea, severe hypoglycaemia, abdominal pain, drowsiness, tachypnoea, there is failure of blood glucose or urinary ketone concentrations to respond to changes in insulin treatment, the child is under 5 years old or the parents remain concerned, then they should contact the diabetes nurse, doctor or hospital for further advice.

Management of diabetes when travelling

When travelling, the following principles are recommended for the management of the diabetes.
• At least twice as much insulin and equipment as would normally be required should be taken with one set of supplies taken as hand luggage. Supplies should include hypostop and glucagon.
• Take a letter for Customs stating the diagnosis and outlining the equipment required.
• Appropriate insurance must be arranged.
• In very hot climates, insulin should be kept refrigerated.
• Snacks should be kept with the hand luggage in case the child does not like the food on the plane or the meals contain inadequate carbohydrate.
• With short flights or where the time zone between departure and arrival changes by less than 4 hours, no major changes to the insulin regimen are required.

• With long-haul flights crossing time zones, the most straightforward approach is to give 15–20% of the total daily dose of insulin as short/rapid-acting insulin before main meals on the plane and to revert to the usual regime on arrival at the new destination.

When on holiday, especially those involving physical activities, children with diabetes often require less insulin than usual to avoid hypoglycaemia. At the start of the holiday, the child should be advised to monitor blood glucose concentrations regularly to help decide what changes in insulin treatment are required.

Psychological aspects of diabetes management

Ideally, a psychologist should meet the family in clinic and be involved in the patient's care from the time of diagnosis. Additional support for the family can be gained by introducing them to other families with children with diabetes, local support groups or national diabetes associations. The child may benefit from meeting other children with diabetes by going on clinic 'away-day' trips, adventure weekends or holidays for children and families with diabetes. Whenever possible, positive encouragement should be given to the patient as constant negative criticism by clinical staff and/or family is unlikely to encourage compliance.

Needle phobia occasionally occurs in younger children. This problem may be helped by the child watching the parents performing blood tests or giving injections to themselves or to a teddy bear or doll. Spring loaded and jet injectors can also help (see page 13). Various blood testing devices allow the depth of penetration of the needle into the skin to be altered. Behaviour therapy under the supervision of a clinical psychologist can also help.

Psychological problems which are common in adolescence are described on page 21. In addition to these, severe stress, obsessive behaviour in relation to monitoring and occasionally problems from overprotective parenting may be encountered.

Management of diabetes during surgery

There are many protocols for the perioperative management of children with diabetes. These need to be agreed by the diabetes, anaesthetic and surgical team in the hospital. The main goals of the management of diabetes during surgery are to avoid hypoglycaemia, hyperglycaemia and DKA. Blood glucose control should be optimized in the weeks preceding elective surgery. Surgery should be performed in the morning with the patient first on the list whenever possible.

Evening prior to elective surgery

The day prior to elective surgery blood glucose should be measured before each meal and before bedtime. Urinary ketones should also be measured. The standard evening and/or bedtime insulin should be given. Severe hyperglycaemia or ketosis will require correction, ideally by overnight maintenance intravenous fluids and intravenous insulin and may result in delay or postponement of the surgery.

Morning operations

• No solid food from midnight.
• Clear fluids may be taken up to 4 hours pre-operatively.
• Omit morning insulin dose.
• Measure urea and electrolytes and urinary ketones pre-operatively.
• Start intravenous fluids, 5% dextrose/0.45% saline with 20 mmol of potassium chloride/litre, at a maintenance rate (Table 1.5) between 6 and 8 a.m.
• Simultaneously start an insulin infusion. Insulin should be administered as a continuous infusion, using a syringe pump (1 unit of short-acting insulin/mL) and the rate adjusted according to the sliding scale shown in Table 1.12 aiming for a blood glucose concentration of 6–12 mmol/L (108–216 mg/dL).
• Hourly blood glucose monitoring pre-operatively and half-hourly monitoring peri-operatively.
• Hourly blood glucose monitoring 4 hours post-operatively.
• Measure urea and electrolytes post-operatively.
• Continue intravenous fluids and insulin until the patient tolerates oral fluids and snacks (this may not be until 24–48 hours after major surgery).
• Change to the usual subcutaneous insulin regimen before the first meal is taken. The insulin infusion can be stopped 30 minutes after administering subcutaneous insulin containing short-acting insulin and 15 minutes after administering subcutaneous insulin containing a rapidly acting insulin analogue.
• Following minor operations it may be possible to discharge the patient after the evening meal if the child has fully recovered.

Afternoon operations

• Give a third of the usual morning insulin dose as short-acting insulin.

- Patient can have a light breakfast.
- Can have clear fluids up to 4 hours pre-operatively.
- Measure urea and electrolytes and urinary ketones pre-operatively.
- Start intravenous fluids and an insulin infusion at midday (see above).
- Then follow protocol for morning operations.

Emergency surgery

- Remember that diabetic ketoacidosis may present with severe abdominal pain which may be mistaken for a 'surgical abdomen'.
- Keep patient nil by mouth.
- Obtain intravenous access.
- Check weight, urea and electrolytes, blood glucose, a venous gas and urinary ketones pre-operatively.
- If ketoacidosis is present follow the diabetic ketoacidosis protocol and delay surgery until the circulating volume has been restored and any electrolyte imbalances have been corrected.
- In the absence of ketoacidosis, start intravenous fluids and an insulin infusion as for elective surgery.

Minor procedures requiring fasting (e.g. endoscopy, grommets)

- For short procedures (with or without sedation or anaesthesia) where a rapid recovery is anticipated, a simplified protocol can be followed by the diabetic/anaesthetic team. For instance, for an early morning procedure (between 8 and 9 a.m.) insulin and breakfast can be delayed and given immediately after completion. Alternatively, the normal pre-breakfast dose of subcutaneous insulin can be given, breakfast omitted, and the child can be administered intravenous 10% dextrose at a maintenance rate (Table 1.5) to provide approximately the usual morning calorie requirements.
- Blood glucose concentrations should be checked frequently and the rate or glucose concentration of the intravenous fluids adjusted accordingly.
- Following the procedure if the child is awake and hungry, a light lunch should be given or the intravenous fluids continued until the child is able to tolerate a light diet.
- If the child is well, the usual evening dose of insulin can be given and the patient can go home after their evening meal if eating normally.
- If the blood glucose concentration rises or the patient starts vomiting then blood samples should be taken for the measurement of electrolytes and gases and consideration given to treatment following the elective surgery or DKA guidelines.

Type 2 diabetes mellitus

Type 2 diabetes is most common over the age of 40 years but is becoming more frequent in childhood. In the UK at present, approximately 1% of children under 16 years of age with diabetes have type 2 diabetes. By contrast, data from the USA shows that 33% of newly diagnosed patients with diabetes aged 10–19 years have type 2 diabetes. Prevalence rates in the USA suggest that 0.41% of teenagers have type 2 diabetes. More specifically, in obese children and adolescents in the USA, the prevalence of impaired glucose tolerance was 25% and of silent type 2 diabetes 0.4%, independent of ethnicity. Many of these patients had risk factors for type 2 diabetes, including a positive family history, a sedentary lifestyle predisposing to obesity, and African, Hispanic or Asian ancestry. Type 2 diabetes is also more common in females and in infants born small for gestational age who have remained short.

Type 2 diabetes is characterized by diminished pancreatic insulin secretion and insulin resistance. Islet cell antibodies are absent. Children with type 2 diabetes may be asymptomatic and therefore those at high risk (primarily children who are obese and have a family history of type 2 diabetes) should be screened. Most children with type 2 diabetes are overweight at diagnosis and present with absent or mild polyuria and polydipsia, little or no weight loss, hyperglycaemia and glycosuria without ketonuria. However, up to one-third have ketonuria at diagnosis and 5–25% of patients who are subsequently classified as having type 2 diabetes have ketoacidosis at presentation. It can therefore be difficult, initially, to distinguish between type 1 and type 2 diabetes. Acanthosis nigricans (see Plate 1, facing page 20), polycystic ovary syndrome, hypertension and lipid disorders may also be present. In a small proportion of cases microvascular complications may be present at diagnosis.

As with type 1 diabetes, the aims of treatment are the normalization of blood glucose measurements and HbA1c, to decrease the incidence of long-term microvascular complications. The mainstay of treatment of type 2 diabetes involves restriction of dietary carbohydrate (see page 5), increased physical activity and weight reduction if obese. These measures may lead to good glycaemic control but most patients eventually require drug therapy. The following medications can be considered:

- biguanides (e.g. metformin) which, in the presence of residual endogenous insulin secretion, increase muscle glucose uptake and metabolism and decrease hepatic gluconeogenesis;

- sulphonylureas (e.g. gliclazide), which augment insulin secretion and therefore require residual β-cell activity to be effective;
- acarbose, which inhibits intestinal α-glucosidase and delays the digestion and absorption of starch and sucrose; or
- insulin therapy.

Metformin is the only biguanide therapy available. With metformin treatment, hypoglycaemia is extremely rare and less common than with the sulphonylureas. Oral treatment with metformin can be started with a dosage of 250 mg twice daily and increased, depending on the response, to 500 mg three times daily. The tablets should be taken with meals as they can cause nausea, abdominal discomfort and diarrhoea. Acarbose has a small effect on lowering blood glucose concentrations and can be used on its own or in addition to sulphonylurea or biguanide treatment. Side-effects of acarbose include flatulence. If monotherapy with metformin is unsuccessful after 3–6 months then a sulphonylurea or insulin can be added. Insulin is required at diagnosis if the patient is hyperglycaemic with significant ketonuria. At a later stage insulin may be required if blood glucose control is poor with an HbA1c >7% in spite of intensive oral medication and appropriate diet and exercise. About 10% of patients with type 2 diabetes eventually require insulin. It is often useful to discuss treatment with an adult diabetologist as they have greater experience than paediatricians of this disorder.

Long-term complications of diabetes

Long-term complications may be microvascular (retinopathy, nephropathy, neuropathy) or macrovascular (ischaemic heart disease, peripheral vascular disease). Microvascular complications may develop in puberty or early adulthood whereas macrovascular complications affect older adults. The longer the duration of diabetes, the greater the risk of complications which increase significantly following puberty. The risk of complications may also be increased by genetic factors, poor glycaemic control and behaviour such as smoking.

Nephropathy

The cumulative incidence of nephropathy after 40 years of diabetes is at least 40%. Nephropathy may lead to chronic renal failure and necessitate dialysis or renal transplantation. Risk factors include poor glycaemic control, long-standing diabetes, smoking and a family history of diabetic nephropathy and hypertension.

Nephropathy is preceded by the development of persistent microalbuminuria which affects approximately 10% of children and adolescents. In adults microalbuminuria is defined as an albumin excretion rate of 30–300 mg/24 hours (20–200 µg/minute) in two out of three timed collections. Timed collections may be difficult to collect in children and an alternative screening tool is the measurement of the albumin:creatinine ratio in the first voided morning urine sample which has been shown to correlate closely with the timed overnight albumin excretion rate. An albumin:creatinine ratio of 3.5 mg/mmol equates to an albumin excretion rate of 30 µg/minute.

The upper limit of the normal reference range for the albumin:creatinine ratio in an early morning urine is 1.5 mg/mmol. When values rise to between 1.5 and 3.5 mg/mmol patients should have their albumin:creatinine ratio checked annually. In the case of values above 3.5 mg/mmol a timed collection (overnight or ideally 24 hours) should be performed to confirm the diagnosis and the albumin:creatinine ratio should be repeated every 4–6 months. Repeated values >3.5 mg/mmol identify those who require treatment. Intermittent microalbuminuria precedes the onset of persistent microalbuminuria, although in some cases intermittent microalbuminuria will resolve. The significance of this type of protein leak is unknown.

Patients with persistent microalbuminuria should have their blood pressure and their serum urea, electrolytes and creatinine concentrations measured and a renal ultrasound performed. Attempts should be made to improve glycaemic control, ideally lowering the HbA1c to <6.5%, and this may lead to regression of the micro albuminuria. If microalbuminuria persists treatment with angiotensin-converting enzyme (ACE) inhibitors (e.g. captopril) should be considered, even in the absence of hypertension. This treatment should not be prescribed until the possibility of non-diabetic renal disease has been excluded. The first dose should be given to the patient under hospital supervision with the patient supine and the blood pressure monitored every 15 minutes for 2 hours after the medication has been given. It is advisable to discuss these cases with an adult diabetologist or a nephrologist.

Eye disease

The prevalence of retinopathy in adolescents varies from

18 to 47%. More than 90% of patients with type 1 diabetes will eventually develop some degree of retinopathy. Risk factors include poor glycaemic control, increased duration of diabetes, hypertension, hyperlipidaemia and smoking.

The earliest sign of diabetic eye disease is the development of background retinopathy which consists of microaneurysms and haemorrhages with exudates which do not involve the macula (Plate 2, facing page 20). This stage is asymptomatic and does not damage vision. It may stabilize, regress with improved glycaemic control or progress if poor control continues.

Background diabetic retinopathy may, rarely in childhood, progress to proliferative retinopathy. This can be successfully treated in its early stages with laser photocoagulation therapy. All patients with retinopathy should be referred to an ophthalmologist.

Cataracts may affect patients with diabetes but is very rare under the age of 20 years.

Neuropathy
The earliest symptoms include numbness and paraesthesia of the feet or hands with evidence of decreased vibration sense, loss of ankle jerk reflexes and a diminution in sensation to pinprick on clinical examination. However, clinically significant neuropathy in adolescence is very rare, although subclinical neuropathy demonstrated by abnormalities of motor nerve conduction velocity have been reported in 20–57% of children with diabetes.

Mortality
Mortality in young adults with diabetes is increased primarily as a result of poor glycaemic control resulting in DKA or hypoglycaemia. Mortality in older individuals is raised mainly as a result of circulatory disorders, especially myocardial infarction. A reduction in life expectancy of 5–10 years has been reported. However, because of improvements in treatment, the prognosis in diabetes is constantly improving.

Miscellaneous practical matters

Driving
Patients with diabetes have a 1.23-fold increased relative risk of accidents compared with those without diabetes, which is the same order of risk as for those with epilepsy. If a teenager with diabetes wishes to drive, the following measures are required:

- The patient's doctor needs to inform the driving authorities (in the UK: the Driving and Vehicle Licensing Authority). In the UK, assuming that the patient has satisfactory health, is not affected by recurrent hypoglycaemia or hypoglycaemia unawareness and has visual acuity greater than 6/9, a licence for 3 years may be granted.
- Prior to driving, blood glucose concentrations should be checked and a long journey broken by frequent rests and meals with blood glucose concentrations remeasured as required.
- If the patient feels hypoglycaemic, the car should be stopped, the engine turned off, the keys removed from the ignition and carbohydrate consumed.
- Stores of carbohydrate should always be kept in the car in case of unexpected delays.

School examinations
The stress of examinations can lead to impaired blood glucose control with adverse effects on academic performance. Glycaemic control should be optimized prior to examinations to try to ensure optimal performance.

Employment
Patients with diabetes should be aware that they are ineligible for certain careers. In the UK these include the armed forces and driving heavy goods or public service vehicles.

Alcohol
Ingestion of alcohol may cause a number of problems, including an increased risk of hypoglycaemia and DKA with symptoms that may make it difficult for the patient or others to distinguish between drunkenness and hypoglycaemia. The following guidelines are advised:

- the importance of avoiding drinking alcohol and driving should be stressed;
- not to drink alcohol on an empty stomach;
- to eat while drinking or shortly afterwards;
- if drinking in the evening, to take a snack prior to bedtime;
- not to substitute the carbohydrate content of alcohol for that contained in meals and snacks when estimating dietary carbohydrate requirements;
- to avoid beers with low sugar content as these tend to contain higher alcohol concentrations and may predispose to hypoglycaemia;
- to limit the consumption of low-alcohol beers with increased sugar content;

- to consume dry or medium wines in preference to sweet wines; and
- to use sugar-free mixers when drinking spirits.

Drug abuse

Cigarettes and recreational drugs are widely available to adolescents and their use should be strongly discouraged. Little is known about the effects of recreational drugs on diabetes. Marijuana may stimulate the appetite and lead to binge eating with a rise in the blood glucose concentration. Drug addiction may lead to neglect of the management of diabetes with adverse effects on glycaemic control. As with alcohol, it may be difficult for a patient with diabetes and others to distinguish between the effect of drugs and hypoglycaemia.

Contraception and pregnancy

To avoid unwanted pregnancies, most teenagers with diabetes should be advised to choose between using a condom or the combined oral contraceptive pill. Using a condom has the advantage of protection against sexually transmitted diseases. Adolescents with good glycaemic control and without microvascular complications can safely use a low-dose combined oral contraceptive pill containing ≤35 μg ethinyloestradiol. The same contraindications as in women without diabetes apply, namely, smoking, hypertension, hyperlipidaemia, a positive family history of coronary artery disease or venous thromboembolism and migraine. Patients with microvascular disease or risk factors for coronary artery disease can safely use the progesterone-only 'mini-pill' which is marginally less effective than the combined oral contraceptive. Further advice can be sought from a gynaecology or family planning clinic.

Poor glycaemic control in pregnancy may increase the risk of congenital abnormalities and stillbirth. There is also an increased risk of macrosomia, preterm birth and neonatal hyperinsulinism with hypoglycaemia. To reduce the risk of adverse effects of maternal diabetes on the fetus, pre-pregnancy clinics have been developed to provide advice to women with diabetes in advance of conception. Topics discussed at these clinics include the optimization of control (including basal bolus regimes if the patient is not already on one), diet, cessation of smoking and alcohol, possible changes in other medications (e.g. angiotension-converting enzyme inhibitors), folate therapy and assessment of retinal, renal and thyroid status. Should a teenager with diabetes become pregnant, then their medical supervision should be shared with an adult physician and an obstetrician with experience of managing pregnant women with diabetes.

Endocrine and other disorders associated with diabetes

Thyroid disease

This is the most common autoimmune endocrinopathy associated with diabetes. The possibility of occult thyroid disease should be considered at diagnosis and when a patient is assessed at the annual review. Thyroid microsomal antibody titres are abnormally elevated in 7–24% of children with diabetes although their predictive value for the development of clinically significant thyroid disease is poor. Hypothyroidism affects approximately 3.9% of children with diabetes. Hypothyroidism may be asymptomatic and significant changes in glycaemic control are not usually observed, although hypothyroidism may on occasion lead to a decrease in insulin requirements and to hypoglycaemia.

Hyperthyroidism affects 1% of children with diabetes and may also be relatively asymptomatic. However, hyperthyroidism may also be associated with increasing insulin requirements. Further details of the investigation and treatment of thyroid disease can be found in Chapter 6.

Addison's disease

Addison's disease is a potentially life-threatening autoimmune disorder which affects 0.03% of individuals with diabetes. It commonly presents with evidence of recurrent hypoglycaemia and unexpectedly falling insulin requirements. Other classical symptoms include fatigue, hyperpigmentation of the skin and mucous membranes, weight loss, abdominal pain or presentation with an adrenal crisis during an intercurrent illness.

The diagnosis of Addison's disease should be confirmed by the presence of adrenal autoantibodies and inappropriately low circulating serum cortisol concentrations. Further details of other relevant investigations and of treatment with glucocorticoids and mineralocorticoids can be found in Chapter 8.

Coeliac disease

Coeliac disease affects 3–5% of the diabetic population and may be present prior to the onset of diabetes. It is usually asymptomatic although it may present with diarrhoea, abdominal distension, anaemia or poor weight gain and linear growth. Malabsorption may lead to a fall in insulin requirements and to a predisposition to hypoglycaemia. The possibility of coeliac disease can be further investigated by the measurement of coeliac antibodies (the anti-endomysium and anti-transglutaminase anti-bodies are the most specific) and the diagnosis confirmed by the demonstration of the classical histological findings on a jejunal biopsy.

Treatment of coeliac disease requires a gluten-free diet. The combination of the dietary implications of a gluten-free diet and the appropriate diet for a child with diabetes can pose particular difficulties for the family and special-ist dietetic advice is needed as compliance may be poor.

Necrobiosis lipoidica diabeticorum

Necrobiosis lipoidica diabeticorum affects 0.3% of the population with diabetes. In childhood, it is most likely to occur in teenagers but is more common in adults. The aetiology is unknown. The lesions consist of slowly growing round or irregular non-scaling plaques with atrophic yellow centres, surface telangiecta-sia and livid, sometimes raised erythematous borders (Plate 3, facing page 21). They usually occur on the shins but may also affect the feet, arms, hands or face. The development of necrobiosis lipoidica diabeticorum is not influenced by glycaemic control. Complications include infection and ulceration of the lesions.

Approximately 20% of lesions resolve spontaneously. Treatment is difficult and consists mainly of a cosmetic approach using camouflage skin creams. Limited success has been achieved from the use of topical and systemic steroids and in extreme cases skin grafts may be necessary.

Unusual causes of diabetes in childhood

Maturity onset diabetes of the young (MODY)

MODY is a rare form of autosomal dominant diabetes mellitus developing before the age of 25 years. Patients have a strong family history of diabetes in two or more consecutive generations. It results from β-cell dysfunc-tion, with the severity of dysfunction depending on the underlying gene mutation. To date, six mutations have been shown to cause MODY and these account for ap-proximately 80% of patients.

MODY2 is caused by a mutation of the glucokinase gene on chromosome 7p. This leads to mild hypergly-caemia that develops in childhood and rarely requires specific treatment or results in complications.

MODY1 is caused by a mutation of the hepatic nuclear factor 4 alpha gene on chromosome 20q and MODY3 by a mutation of the hepatic nuclear factor 1 alpha gene on chromosome 12q. These forms of MODY lead to diabetes in adolescence which, unlike MODY2, require treatment with sulphonylureas or occasionally insulin and may lead to microvascular complications. The identification of the gene mutation in a child with MODY confirms whether or not treatment is necessary, predicts the risk of future complications and allows specific genetic counselling.

Neonatal diabetes mellitus

Transient neonatal diabetes is rare, with an incidence of 1 in 400 000 births. Some of these patients have been shown to have paternal uniparental isodisomy of chromosome 6. Transient neonatal diabetes is thought to be caused by a delay in the maturation of the β-cells leading to hypoinsu-linaemia. Permanent neonatal diabetes is even rarer and may be associated with neurological abnormalities. A proportion of these patients have activating mutations in the gene encoding the ATP-sensitive potassium channel subunit Kir6.2.

The condition presents in the first few days or weeks of life with polydipsia, polyuria, marked weight loss, severe dehydration and vomiting. Hyperglycaemia and glycos-uria are present but ketonuria is unusual.

Initial treatment consists of rehydration and a continuous intravenous infusion of insulin. Thereafter, once-daily subcutaneous injections of long-acting insulin can be introduced although some patients are best managed by subcutaneous insulin pump therapy. Treat-ment in transient neonatal diabetes may be needed for a few days to 18 months (median 3 months). However, some of these patients may develop type 2 diabetes in later life.

Diabetes following pancreatectomy for persistent hyperinsulinaemic hypoglycaemia of infancy

Severe persistent hyperinsulinaemic hypoglycaemia of infancy may require treatment with a 95% pancreatectomy in early life (see Chapter 2). A proportion of these patients will progress to develop diabetes several months or years following surgery. It is usually relatively easy to achieve satisfactory glycaemic control in these patients, possibly because of residual pancreatic insulin secretion and reduced glucagon secretion.

Diabetes secondary to cystic fibrosis

Diabetes can develop in 5–10% of adolescents and young

adults with cystic fibrosis and is thought to be caused by islet cell damage from chronic pancreatic inflammation. As with diabetes following pancreatic resection, glucagon secretion is reduced and DKA is rare although these patients are at greater risk of hypoglycaemia than those with type 1 diabetes.

The diagnosis may be made on clinical grounds or by measuring the fasting glucose or the HbA1c. The most sensitive test is the oral glucose tolerance test.

Treatment consists of insulin therapy although the dosage of insulin required varies widely. These patients require close liaison between the paediatric diabetes and cystic fibrosis teams. The dietary management of these children may be rather different to that of type 1 diabetes because of difficulties with malabsorption and their frequently poor nutritional state. The adequacy of management of the diabetic aspects of these cases includes monitoring of both glycaemic control and weight gain.

Miscellaneous disorders

Diabetes is also associated with a number of other disorders such as Down's syndrome, Turner's syndrome, Klinefelter's syndrome, Prader–Willi syndrome, DID-MOAD syndrome, asparaginase and steroid treatment, thalassaemia and the autoimmune polyendocrine syndromes.

Audit

Auditing practice against agreed regional, national or international standards is an essential part of running a diabetes service. A register of all patients is essential to allow audit to take place. Increasingly these registers are computer-based. Several aspects of diabetes care can be audited, including:
- HbA1c concentrations;
- evidence of normal growth, weight gain and puberty;
- the adequacy of management of newly diagnosed patients, DKA, hypoglycaemia or diabetes during surgery;
- the completeness of the annual review process;
- the incidence of complications;

- patient education; and
- the patients' satisfaction with the service.

Information gained from audit can be used to promote service developments.

Future developments

- Prophylactic therapy or earlier diagnosis through genetic and immunological screening of high-risk children.
- Non-invasive methods of glucose monitoring.
- Improved versions of an artificial pancreas.
- The development of new and improved insulins.
- Administration of insulin by alternative routes (e.g. oral, nasal, inhalation and transdermal).
- Improvements in the management and outcome of pancreatic and islet cell transplantation.
- The development of stem cell therapy to generate a potentially limitless source of genetically modified, artificially cultured pancreatic β-cells suitable for transplantation.

Controversial points

- Should the initial insulin infusion rate for DKA be 0.05 or 0.1 units/kg/hour in young children?
- Why does cerebral oedema occur? Should mannitol or hypertonic saline be used in the treatment of cerebral oedema?
- Should a new patient with diabetes, but without DKA, be treated in hospital or at home?
- From what age and at what stage is an annual review necessary?
- What should the annual review comprise of?
- What are the indications for changing a patient to a basal bolus regimen or an insulin pump?
- How should human insulin analogues be prescribed to achieve the optimum outcome?
- How much of a risk factor for future complications is poor glycaemic control before puberty?
- How can the implications of the results of the DCCT study be applied in routine clinical practice?

Potential pitfalls

- Failure to realize that the blood glucose readings in the patient's book are fictitious (may all be written

with the same pen, may not be in keeping with the HbA1c result).
- Recommending insulin doses in excess of 1.5 units/kg/day to help lower a high HbA1c when the most

likely explanation is poor compliance and omission of injections.

- Recommending multiple injection regimens in patients on twice-daily injections with poor HbA1c values when the most likely cause is omission of insulin or anxiety about injections.
- Failure to diagnose psychological/psychiatric problems, especially in adolescents, which may also be having an impact on glycaemic control.
- Errors in fluid calculations during therapy of diabetic ketoacidosis.
- Stopping the insulin infusion during therapy for diabetic ketoacidosis when hypoglycaemia occurs.

- Omitting to perform annual reviews.
- Failure to identify the early signs of retinopathy when using direct ophthalmoscopy.
- Loosing track of patients, frequently adolescents, who often repeatedly fail to attend clinic.
- Failure to consider Addison's disease as a possible cause for decreasing insulin requirements when the patient is beyond the honeymoon period.
- Failure to distinguish between type 1 and type 2 diabetes resulting in inappropriate therapy.
- Failure to diagnose MODY in a patient with only mild abnormalities of glucose homeostasis and a relevant family history.

CASE HISTORIES

Case 1

A 14-year-old girl had recurrent severe hypoglycaemia with two episodes leading to a convulsion and hospital admission. She was diagnosed with type 1 diabetes at 9 years of age and was treated with twice-daily injections of a pre-mixed insulin with a ratio of short- to intermediate-acting insulin of 30:70, 30 units before breakfast and 18 units before the evening meal (0.9 units/kg/day). There had not been any recent changes in her diet or levels of physical activity.

Questions

1 What investigations would you consider doing?
2 If the results of these investigations proved normal, what further explanation could account for her recurrent hypoglycaemia?

Answers

1 Measurement of HbA1c concentration to assess overall glycaemic control, thyroid function tests to exclude hypothyroidism and anti-endomysial or anti-transglutaminase antibody titres to exclude coeliac disease. Measurement of adrenal autoantibody titres and a Synacthen stimulation test may also be required to rule out Addison's disease.
2 Self-administration of high doses of insulin. This adolescent girl was not coping with her diabetes and the recurrent hypoglycaemic episodes were 'a cry for help'. The episodes stopped following a referral and advice from the child psychiatry service.

Case 2

A 15-year-old boy who had had type 1 diabetes for 5 years and who was a frequent non-attender at clinic presented with short stature and delayed puberty. He was receiving a pre-mixed insulin with a ratio of short- to intermediate-acting insulin of 30:70, 24 units in the morning and 12 units in the evening (0.7 units/kg/day). His height had fallen from the 25th to the 2nd centile since diagnosis and his weight was on the 2nd centile. His testes were 4 mL in volume with Tanner stage 2 pubic hair. His HbA1c concentration was 11.4%.

Questions

1 How would you investigate this patient?
2 How would you manage this patient?

Answers

1 Dietary assessment and measurement of thyroid function tests and anti-endomysial or anti-transglutaminase antibody.
2 The patient appears to have delay in the onset of puberty which is likely to have contributed to his poor growth velocity in recent years. The dietary assessment revealed a poor calorie intake and the results of his tests for hypothyroidism and coeliac disease were normal. There had been little change in his diet or insulin dosage since diagnosis. Poor glycaemic control because of an inadequate dosage of insulin with an inadequate dietary intake is the most likely cause for his delayed puberty and short stature. Therefore he should be advised to increase his dietary intake and significantly increase his daily dosage of insulin in an effort to improve glycaemic control. If this proves

successful, this is likely to stimulate further progression of puberty and the pubertal growth spurt.

Case 3

A 15-year-old boy presented with a 6-week history of polyuria and polydipsia. His father had developed type 2 diabetes at the age of 35 years which was controlled by diet. His paternal grandfather had developed type 2 diabetes at 48 years of age, controlled by diet and gliclazide. On examination his body mass index was 22.4 kg/m^2 and he was well and not dehydrated. His blood glucose was 19 mmol/L [342 mg/dL]. He had glycosuria but no ketonuria.

Questions

1 What is the likely diagnosis?
2 How would you investigate this boy?
3 Why is it important to establish a precise diagnosis?

Answers

1 The most likely diagnosis is MODY. As hyperglycaemia in MODY may be mild and asymptomatic, the age of diagnosis can be considerably later than the age of onset, which is the likely explanation for the late age of diagnosis in the father and grandfather.
2 Screening of genes, mutations of which are known to cause MODY. This patient was demonstrated to have a mutation of the glucokinase gene (MODY2).
3 The patient can be reassured that he is most unlikely to experience complications from his MODY and he and his family can be counselled about the autosomal dominant inheritance of MODY.

When to involve a specialist centre

- Neonatal diabetes mellitus.
- Diabetes associated with hyperthyroidism or Addison's disease.
- Diabetes associated with cystic fibrosis or following pancreatic resection.
- If proliferative retinopathy or deteriorating renal function is present.

References and further reading

American Diabetes Association (2000) Type 2 diabetes in children and adolescents. *Paediatrics* **105**, 671–680.

British Society of Paediatric Endocrinology and Diabetes (BSPED) Recommended DKA guidelines (2004). www.bsped.org.uk

Campbell, F.M. (1995) Microalbuminuria and nephropathy in insulin dependent diabetes mellitus. *Archives of Disease in Childhood* **73**, 4–7.

Court, S. & Lamb, B. (eds) (1997) *Childhood and Adolescent Diabetes.* Wiley, Chichester.

Deary, I.J. & Frier, B.M. (1996) Severe hypoglycaemia and cognitive impairment in diabetes. *British Medical Journal* **313**, 767–768.

Diabetes Control and Complications Trial Research Group (1993) The effect of intensive treatment of diabetes on the development and progression of long-term complications in insulin dependent diabetes mellitus. *New England Journal of Medicine* **329**, 977–986.

Dunger, D.B., Sperling, M.A. & Acerini, C.L. et al ESPE/LWPES (2004) Consensus statement on diabetic ketoacidosis in children and adolescents. *Archives of Disease in Childhood* **89**, 934–937.

Edge, J.A., Ford-Adams, M.E. & Dunger, D.B. (1999) Causes of death in children with insulin dependent diabetes 1990–96. *Archives of Disease in Childhood* **81**, 318–323.

Hanas, R. (2004) *Type 1 Diabetes in Children, Adolescents and Adults*, 2nd edition. Class Publishing, London.

Lowes, L. & Gregory, J.W. (2004) Management of newly diagnosed diabetes: home or hospital? *Archives of Disease in Childhood* **89**, 934–937.

National Institute for Clinical Excellence (NICE). Type 1 Diabetes — Diagnosis and Management of Type 1 Diabetes in Children and Young People (Sept 2004). www.nice.org.uk

Shield, J.P.H. (1997) Relevance of the diabetes control and complications trial to paediatric practice. *Current Paediatrics* **7**, 85–87.

Swift, P.G.F (ed.) (2000) ISPAD *Guidelines 2000.* Medforum, Zeist, The Netherlands.

Torrance, T., Franklyn, V. & Greene, S. (2003) Insulin pumps. *Archives of Disease in Childhood* **88**, 949–953.

Update on Insulin Analogues (2004) *Drug and Therapeutics Bulletin* **42** (10).

2 Hypoglycaemia

Physiology

Blood glucose is the main fuel for brain function and the brain is the main consumer of blood glucose. Important differences exist between children and adults in the mechanisms which maintain blood glucose concentrations within a relatively narrow normal range and which protect the infant and child from the adverse consequences that may occur when blood glucose concentrations fall to below 2.6 mmol/L [46.8 mg/dL]. The infant and small child have relatively limited glycogen stores with larger brain:body ratios than adults and are therefore at greater risk of hypoglycaemia during prolonged starvation. However, in younger children, increased production of ketone bodies provides an alternative fuel source for cerebral metabolism when glucose supplies are restricted.

In response to feeding, blood glucose concentrations increase, stimulating insulin and suppressing glucagon secretion with the result that blood glucose concentrations are usually maintained below 9 mmol/L [162 mg/dL]. During prolonged fasting, blood glucose concentrations fall. To prevent hypoglycaemia, a counter-regulatory endocrine response occurs. The main counter-regulatory hormones are glucagon, adrenaline, noradrenaline, cortisol and growth hormone. The endocrine responses to the fed and fasted states are summarized in Figure 2.1.

During progressively severe hypoglycaemia, a hierarchy of physiological responses occur with adrenaline-induced autonomic symptoms developing at higher blood glucose concentrations than symptoms resulting from neuroglycopaenia (Table 2.1). These symptoms are relatively non-specific and are particularly difficult to identify in the premature neonate and the newborn who is small for gestational age, who are at greatest risk of developing hypoglycaemia.

Definition

There is considerable debate about the definition of hypoglycaemia. Blood glucose concentrations are influenced by the circumstances in which the sample is being taken (i.e. length of time since last meal) and to a lesser extent by the source of blood (e.g. arterial, capillary or venous) and whether measurements are to be made on whole blood, serum or plasma samples.

Hypoglycaemia can be defined in the following ways:
- statistically (from the blood glucose responses of large samples of subjects);
- by the presence of physiological counter-regulatory hormone responses;
- by the presence of acute symptoms; or
- in relation to evidence that a particular blood glucose concentration was associated with longer term neurodevelopmental sequelae.

When investigations into the cause of hypoglycaemia are being considered, blood glucose concentrations less than 2.6 mmol/L should be taken as evidence of hypoglycaemia although it should not be assumed that such values are necessarily dangerous or that investigations are inevitably required (e.g. an asymptomatic term infant may utilize ketones for cerebral metabolism).

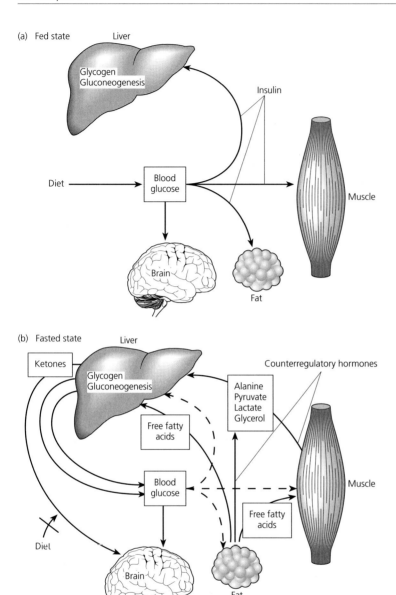

(a) Fed state

Liver

Glycogen
Gluconeogenesis

Insulin

Diet

Blood
glucose

Muscle

Brain

Fat

(b) Fasted state

Liver

Ketones

Glycogen
Gluconeogenesis

Counterregulatory hormones

Alanine
Pyruvate
Lactate
Glycerol

Free fatty
acids

Blood
glucose

Muscle

Free fatty
acids

Diet

Brain

Fat

Fig. 2.1 The control of blood glucose in the fed state and the fasted state.

Aetiology

Hypoglycaemia occurs when blood glucose utilization exceeds supply and most commonly presents during prolonged fasting or at times of intercurrent illness, particularly when associated with anorexia or vomiting.

Hypoglycaemia may also result when blood glucose production is limited by an impaired counter-regulatory response resulting from hormone insufficiency or an inborn error of metabolism or when excess blood glucose utilization occurs (e.g. hyperinsulinism). The main causes of hypoglycaemia are listed in Table 2.2.

Table 2.1 Symptoms of hypoglycaemia.

Neonate	Older infant or child
Autonomic	
Pallor	Anxiety
Sweating	Palpitations
Tachypnoea	Tremor
Neuroglycopaenic	
Jitteriness	Hunger and abdominal pain
Apnoea	Nausea and vomiting
Hypotonia	Pins and needles
Feeding problems	Headache
Irritability	Weakness
Abnormal cry	Dizziness
Convulsions	Blurred vision
Coma	Irritability
	Mental confusion
	Unusual behaviour
	Fainting
	Convulsions
	Coma

Table 2.2 Causes of hypoglycaemia.

Reduced glucose availability	Increased glucose consumption
Intrauterine growth retardation	Hyperinsulinism
Prematurity	Transient neonatal hyperinsulinism
Hypopituitarism	Infant of a diabetic mother
Adrenal insufficiency	Persistent hyperinsulinaemic hypoglycaemia of infancy
Growth hormone deficiency	Insulinoma
Hypothyroidism	Rhesus haemolytic disease
Glucagon deficiency	
Accelerated starvation (ketotic hypoglycaemia)	Beckwith–Wiedemann syndrome
Inborn errors of metabolism	Perinatal asphyxia
Drugs (alcohol, aspirin, β-blocker)	Malaria
Liver dysfunction	
Congenital heart disease	

Preliminary examination and investigation

History and examination

When hypoglycaemia occurs in the neonate, the following details should be obtained:
• pregnancy (duration, maternal symptoms suggestive of diabetes);
• mode of delivery (breech delivery is said to occur more often in infants with hypopituitarism);
• birth weight (may be increased in the infant whose mother has experienced gestational diabetes or may be consistent with intrauterine growth retardation); and
• relationship between hypoglycaemia and feeding (evidence of hypoglycaemia related to excessive calorie intake is strongly suggestive of hyperinsulinism).

In the older child, clarify the following details:
• the maximum length of time that fasting has been tolerated without symptoms suggestive of hypoglycaemia;
• any symptoms suggestive of hypopituitarism (e.g. prolonged jaundice in the neonatal period);
• consider the possibility of accidental ingestion or factitious symptoms following administration to the child of oral hypoglycaemic agents or insulin;
• a careful family history, as parental consanguinity or unexplained infant death may be suggestive of an inborn error of metabolism; and
• hypoglycaemic or other symptoms, such as vomiting, diarrhoea, jaundice, hepatomegaly or failure to thrive following consumption of lactose or fructose and sucrose-containing foods, suggests galactosaemia or disorders of fructose metabolism, respectively.

Most individuals presenting with hypoglycaemia will have no abnormalities on clinical examination. However, careful examination is required to identify abnormalities which may be associated with hypoglycaemia. Table 2.3 lists the most common signs and associated disorders.

Investigations

Although hypoglycaemia is a clinical emergency requiring prompt therapy, wherever possible, a blood sample for investigations should be drawn *prior to the administration of glucose*. Urine should be collected at the earliest opportunity and stored together with blood samples at −20°C or below. The processing of these samples should be discussed with the local biochemistry department to

Table 2.3 Clinical signs on examination.

Clinical sign	Possible diagnosis
Optic atrophy	Septo-optic dysplasia
Cranial midline defects	Growth hormone deficiency
Short stature or decreased height velocity	
Microgenitalia	
Increased skin or buccal pigmentation	Addison's disease
Hypotension	
Underweight or malnutrition	Accelerated starvation
Tall stature or increased height velocity	Hyperinsulinism
Excess weight	
Abnormal ear lobe creases (Fig. 2.2)	Beckwith–Wiedemann syndrome
Macroglossia	
Umbilical hernia	
Hemihypertrophy	
Hepatosplenomegaly	Glycogen storage disorder

Table 2.4 Investigation of hypoglycaemia at time of presentation.

Sample	Investigation
Blood sample	Glucose
	Urea and electrolytes
	Bicarbonate or pH
	Liver function tests
	Ammonia
	Insulin and C peptide
	Cortisol and ACTH
	Growth hormone
	Free fatty acids and β-hydroxy butyrate
	Lactate
	Alanine
Administer glucose	
Next urine sample	Ketones
	Reducing sugars
	Dicarboxylic acids
	Glycine conjugates
	Carnitine derivatives
	Toxicology screen

Abbreviation: ACTH, adrenocorticotrophic hormone.

ensure proper storage of samples. Such samples may produce clear biochemical evidence of the cause of the hypoglycaemic episode thus avoiding having to subject the child to further potentially hazardous investigations.

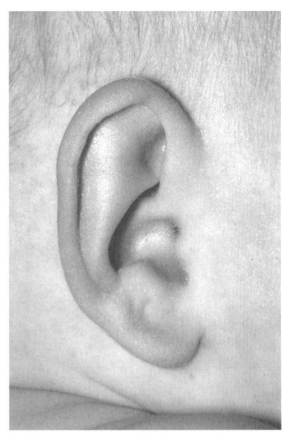

Fig. 2.2 Ear lobe creases in a child with Beckwith–Wiedemann syndrome.

A protocol for the preliminary investigation of hypoglycaemia is shown in Table 2.4.

If the blood and urine samples taken at the time of the initial episode of hypoglycaemia do not demonstrate the cause of the hypoglycaemia, then, depending on the level of clinical concern, additional investigations may need to be considered. These may include the measurement of intermediary metabolites before and after meals and the investigations listed in Table 2.4 following a prolonged fast. In addition to these, a blood sample may need to be taken for the measurement of pyruvate, glycerol, glucagon, lipids, urate, free and acyl carnitine.

It is most important to remember that any investigation, such as a prolonged fast which may render a child hypoglycaemic, is potentially dangerous. Such tests should therefore be discussed in advance with a specialist centre. The length of the fast will be determined by the age

Table 2.5 Length of fasts for children undergoing investigation of possible hypoglycaemia.

Age	Duration (hours)
<6 months	8
6–8 months	12
8–12 months	16
1–2 years	18
2–4 years	20
4–7 years	20
>7 years	24

of the child (Table 2.5). Children undergoing these investigations should be closely supervised by staff who are experienced in dealing with hypoglycaemia. Therefore, the timing of the latter stages of the fast when susceptible children are most likely to become hypoglycaemic should be planned to coincide with periods of the day when plenty of staff are available to monitor the patient and assist in any resuscitation which may be required. Intravenous glucose and hydrocortisone should be available at the bedside. All symptoms should be carefully documented, sample times clearly recorded and on no account should a patient be left unsupervised until the test has been completed and the patient treated with glucose and/or food such that they are no longer at risk of hypoglycaemia. Should hypoglycaemia occur during investigations, the treatment is described below.

Investigations frequently fail to identify a cause of hypoglycaemia which may occur in the context of a normal endocrine counter-regulatory response, associated with appropriately raised free fatty acids and ketone bodies. Plasma lactate and pyruvate concentrations may be normal but alanine low, suggesting a reduced supply of gluconeogenic precursors. This disorder of unknown aetiology is known as 'accelerated starvation' or 'ketotic hypoglycaemia'. It is more common in boys than girls, is often associated with a previous history of intrauterine growth retardation or a thin physique and usually resolves spontaneously by puberty. Accelerated starvation should only be diagnosed once other endocrine and metabolic causes of hypoglycaemia have been excluded.

Treatment

Acute treatment at initial presentation

Once the initial blood samples have been taken, the patient should be given 0.2–0.4 g glucose/kg body weight as an intravenous bolus (2–4 mL/kg of 10% dextrose) over 4–6 minutes followed by an infusion of intravenous 10% dextrose at an initial rate of 10 mg/kg body weight/minute (6 mL/kg/hour).

The response to treatment should be monitored and the infusion rate altered as necessary to maintain blood glucose concentrations in excess of 4 mmol/L [72 mg/dL]. The use of intermittent boluses of glucose in concentrations in excess of 25% should be avoided because of the risk of cerebral oedema.

If the patient remains unconscious despite normalization of the blood glucose concentrations, then 50–100 mg of hydrocortisone should be administered intravenously in case of undiagnosed adrenal insufficiency. If the patient does not respond to hydrocortisone, then the possibility of an intracranial disorder or an inborn error of metabolism should be considered.

In the newborn, small-for-gestational-age baby with hypoglycaemia who is asymptomatic and tolerating feeds, increasing feed volume and frequency and, if necessary, the use of high-calorie milk formulae or the addition of calorie supplements to feeds may be all that is necessary to prevent further episodes of hypoglycaemia. If this fails, then intravenous dextrose should be added, starting at the rate described above.

Hyperinsulinism

Medical

There are several causes of hyperinsulinism which are listed in Table 2.2 and which should be considered when glucose requirements to avoid hypoglycaemia exceed 10 mg/kg body weight/minute. Persistent hyperinsulinaemic hypoglycaemia is the commonest cause of persistent and recurrent hypoglycaemia in childhood and is heterogenous in its clinical manifestations. Mutations of five different genes (including those which encode the sulphonylurea receptor and the associated potassium inward rectifying channel) have been described which lead to dysregulated insulin secretion from the beta cells of the pancreas.

Infants with hyperinsulinism should not be allowed to fast for significant lengths of time. In the presence of significant hyperinsulinism, enteral feeds may not prevent further episodes of hypoglycaemia and, in these circumstances, additional intravenous glucose should be given. Glucose infusion rates may need to be increased up to 25 mg/kg body weight/minute and increased concentrations of glucose will need to be administered through a central venous line. Most cases of hyperinsulinism presenting in the neonatal period will resolve spontaneously

but, when the requirement for increased glucose infusion rates persist, the following specific treatments for hyperinsulinism should be considered:
• diazoxide 5–25 mg/kg/day (subdivided 8- to 12-hourly) and chlorothiazide 20 mg/kg/day (subdivided 12-hourly); or
• somatostatin analogue (Sandostatin) 6–40 μg/kg/day by subcutaneous injection (subdivided 4-hourly).

Side-effects of long-term diazoxide therapy include hypertrichosis of the lanugo type, fluid retention and tachyphylaxis.

Surgical
In patients who do not respond to medical therapy the only alternative is a partial pancreatectomy. Histological and biochemical differentiation between focal and diffuse forms has radically altered the surgical approach. Relatively modest degrees of pancreatic resection are appropriate for those with focal disease whereas a 95% subtotal pancreatectomy is required only for diffuse forms. The latter treatment is associated with a risk of postoperative insulin-dependent diabetes mellitus and pancreatic exocrine insufficiency. If hypoglycaemia recurs postoperatively then medical therapy should be restarted. If this is unsuccessful, further pancreatic tissue should be removed which may necessitate a total pancreatectomy.

Diabetes
See Chapter 1.

Hypopituitarism and adrenal insufficiency
Hypopituitarism in infancy may be associated with a recurrent predisposition to hypoglycaemia resulting from adrenal or growth hormone insufficiency. Hypoglycaemia should be prevented by the avoidance of prolonged periods of fasting and replacement of glucocorticoids (hydrocortisone 10–15 mg/m²/day) and growth hormone (0.17 mg/kg/week) as necessary. At times of intercurrent illness, the dosage of oral hydrocortisone may need to be increased two- to threefold or the equivalent dosage of hydrocortisone may have to be given parenterally if the patient is vomiting or has gastroenteritis.

Inborn errors of metabolism
A detailed review of the treatment of inborn errors of metabolism is beyond the scope of this book. The principles of therapy involve the prevention of a catabolic state in such children by the use of frequent high-carbohydrate-containing meals and the avoidance of prolonged periods of fasting. In common with children who suffer from accelerated starvation, the use of uncooked cornstarch (1–2 g/kg body weight) mixed with a drink or yoghurt at bedtime is useful in the prevention of nocturnal episodes of hypoglycaemia. For advice regarding the management of inborn errors of metabolism at times of intercurrent illness so as to avoid hypoglycaemia, the reader is referred to an excellent review by Dixon Leonard (1992).

Guidelines for follow-up

Infants who have experienced significant hypoglycaemia demonstrate electro-encephalographic abnormalities which persist for several hours after correction of the hypoglycaemia. There is also evidence to suggest that premature infants exposed to recurrent blood glucose concentrations below 2.6 mmol/L are at increased risk of neurodevelopmental abnormalities. It would therefore seem appropriate to undertake careful neurodevelopmental surveillance during childhood of all individuals who have experienced severe hypoglycaemia in early life so that appropriate support can be provided where necessary.

Individuals who have been demonstrated to be at risk of significant hypoglycaemia require continued follow-up so that their tolerance to fasting with treatment can be re-evaluated as they grow older. In general, the older the subject, the greater their tolerance to fasting.

When to involve a specialist centre

The management of infants and children with severe and potentially life-threatening hypoglycaemia, such as can occur with persistent hyperinsulinaemic hypoglycaemia of infancy, requires urgent referral to a specialist centre for rapid diagnosis and adequate treatment to ensure that the patient does not experience preventable, irreversible brain damage. Such patients require a multidisciplinary team approach involving:
• paediatricians with expertise in endocrinology and metabolism;
• access to laboratories with facilities for undertaking the relevant endocrine and metabolic assays; and
• paediatric surgical and intensive care expertise to ensure adequate venous access for the emergency administration of intravenous glucose which may require insertion of central lines, etc.

Cases which should be discussed with a specialist centre are outlined below.

When to involve a specialist centre

- Persistent hyperinsulinaemic hypoglycaemia of infancy.
- Panhypopituitarism.
- Addison's disease and other causes of adrenal insufficiency.
- Recurrent hypoglycaemia of unknown aetiology.
- Those whose planned investigations may include a prolonged fast.
- Inborn errors of metabolism.

Patients who are identified as having hypoglycaemia secondary to an underlying endocrine abnormality should be followed-up in clinics in which specialist paediatric endocrine expertise is available to ensure optimization of therapy and to prevent further episodes of hypoglycaemia.

Future developments

- Clinical studies are required to clarify uncertainties which relate to the definition of hypoglycaemia and the relationship between severity of hypoglycaemia in the neonatal period and its inter-relationship with other complications of prematurity which may affect neurological morbidity.
- New techniques, such as magnetic resonance spectroscopy, will allow sophisticated *in vivo* neurological studies to take place to assess further the acute adverse effect of hypoglycaemia and to evaluate mechanisms which may protect against these pathophysiological consequences.
- Persistent hyperinsulinaemic hypoglycaemia is known to be a consequence of a mutation of a gene encoding the sulphonylurea receptor which is a regulatory subunit of the pancreatic β-cell ATP-sensitive K^+ channel. This defect leads to closure of this channel which results in membrane depolarization, uncontrolled calcium influx and subsequent stimulation of insulin secretion. Knowledge of the pathophysiological basis of this disorder has led to interest in possible novel therapeutic approaches, including calcium-channel blockers such as nifedipine.

Controversial points

- How should hypoglycaemia be defined — symptomatically, physiologically or biochemically?
- Should clinically significant hypoglycaemia be defined by different blood glucose concentrations at different ages?
- Should hypoglycaemia be as aggressively managed in the neonate as in the older child?
- How extensively should a child with hypoglycaemia be investigated when initial tests fail to provide a diagnosis?
- What is the pathophysiological basis of 'accelerated starvation'?
- Why do some cases of persistent hyperinsulinaemic hypoglycaemia of infancy resolve spontaneously whereas others do not?

Potential pitfalls

- Failure to obtain blood samples for relevant investigations before treating a child to reverse hypoglycaemia.
- Failure to treat hypoglycaemia aggressively enough (e.g. with intravenous dextrose if necessary) to prevent further unnecessary episodes.
- Failure to refer infants with severe early-onset hypoglycaemia which is proving difficult to manage early enough to a specialist centre where adequate venous access can be secured surgically to prevent further unnecessary episodes of hypoglycaemia and results of investigations can be obtained relatively quickly.
- When subjecting children to a planned fast for further investigations into the cause of hypoglycaemia, inadequate skilled supervision, failure to extend the fast long enough to achieve hypoglycaemia, obtaining blood samples for measurement of hormones and intermediary metabolites before hypoglycaemia has occurred or failure to note time of blood sample on either the biochemistry request form or blood sample container.
- In children known to be at risk of hypoglycaemia, failure to make appropriate arrangements (e.g. planned use of intravenous dextrose and monitoring of blood glucose concentrations) to avoid hypoglycaemia while subjecting them to elective procedures requiring fasting.
- Failure to recognize the diagnostic significance of an excess glucose demand to avoid hypoglycaemia (implies hyperinsulinism) and the ineffective use of glucocorticoid treatment in these circumstances to prevent further episodes of hypoglycaemia.

CASE HISTORIES

Case 1

A 2-day-old boy presented with sleepiness, jitteriness and hypoglycaemic convulsions. He required 20 mg glucose/kg body weight/minute to avoid further episodes of hypoglycaemia. When intravenous glucose was temporarily discontinued, the following results were obtained from a blood sample drawn at the time of hypoglycaemia:

glucose 1.8 mmol/L [32 mg/dL]
cortisol 141 nmol/L [5.1 micrograms/dL]
growth hormone 29.6 mU/L [9.9 ng/ml]
insulin 72.4 mU/L
C peptide 4.0 pmol/mL (fasting reference range 0.14–1.39)
nonesterified fatty acids 0.13 mmol/L (fasting reference range 0.1–0.6)
3β-hydroxy butyrate 0.45 mmol/L (fasting reference range 0.03–0.3).

Questions

1 What do the above results demonstrate?
2 Are further investigations indicated?
3 Is additional therapy indicated and, if so, what?

Answers

1 Hyperinsulinaemic hypoglycaemia with an inadequate cortisol response. With a blood glucose of 1.8 mmol/L [32 mg/dL], serum concentrations of cortisol should be >550 nmol/L [>20 mg/dL], growth hormone >20 mU/L [>7 ng/ml] and insulin should be undetectable.
2 A poor cortisol response in hyperinsulinaemic hypoglycaemia is not uncommon and does not usually indicate adrenal insufficiency in this circumstance. Nevertheless, a short Synacthen test may be necessary to ensure that there is no associated adrenal disorder.
3 Given that glucose requirements are markedly elevated, this infant should be given a trial of diazoxide and, possibly, chlorothiazide treatment. If this is unsuccessful, Sandostatin [octreotide] should be tried before subtotal pancreatectomy is considered.

Case 2

A 9-year-old boy presented to a hospital casualty department with a 2-month history of recurrent abdominal pain, vomiting and increasing lethargy. On examination, he appeared ill, dehydrated and hypotensive. An initial blood sample demonstrated the following:

sodium 112 mmol/L
potassium 7.9 mmol/L
urea 28.4 mmol/L [30 g/dL]
glucose 2.6 mmol/L [47 mg/dL]
cortisol 290 nmol/L [11 mg/dL].

Questions

1 What additional investigations are necessary to confirm the diagnosis?
2 What emergency treatment is required?
3 What further clinical sign may help to establish the diagnosis?

Answers

1 Measurement of serum concentrations of adrenocorticotrophic hormone (ACTH), 17-hydroxyprogesterone, adrenal autoantibodies and urinary steroid metabolite analysis should distinguish primary from secondary adrenal failure and the various causes of congenital adrenal hyperplasia from Addison's disease.
2 Ensure an airway and adequate respiratory support as required. Parenteral hydrocortisone (approximately 60 mg/m^2/day, subdivided 6- to 8-hourly), intravenous glucose 200 mg/kg body weight given over 4–6 minutes and a bolus of 10–20 mL/kg body weight of intravenous saline (0.9%) should be given to restore the circulation. Thereafter, an infusion of 0.9% saline with dextrose (5–10% as required) should be continued. When able to take medication orally, fludrocortisone should be started.
3 Increased skin pigmentation, especially of the palmar creases, genitalia, nipples and areas exposed to sunlight, is a consequence of increased melanin production in primary adrenal failure.

Further reading

De Lonlay, P., Fournet, J.C., Touati, G. et al (2002) Heterogeneity of persistent hyperinsulinaemic hypoglycaemia. A series of 175 cases. *European Journal of Pediatrics* **161**, 37–48.

Dixon, M.A. & Leonard, J.V. (1992) Intercurrent illness in inborn errors of intermediary metabolism. *Archives of Disease in Childhood* **67**, 1387–1391.

Gregory, J.W. & Aynsley-Green, A. (eds) (1993) *Ballière's Clinical Endocrinology and Metabolism*: *Hypoglycaemia*. Ballière Tindall, London.

Matyka, K., Ford-Adams, M. & Dunger, D.B. (2002) Hypogly-caemia and counterregulation during childhood. *Hormone Research* **57(suppl 1)**, 85–90.

Mehta, A., Hawdon, J.M., Ward Platt, M.P. & Aynsley-Green, A. (1994) Prevention and management of neonatal hypoglycaemia. *Archives of Disease in Childhood* **70**, F54–F65.

Mitrakou, A., Ryan, C., Veneman, T. *et al.* (1991) Hierarchy of glycemic thresholds for counter-regulatory hormone secretion, symptoms and cerebral dysfunction. *American Journal of Physiology (Endocrinology and Metabolism)* **260**, E67–E74.

Morris, A.A.M., Thekekara, A., Wilks, Z., Clayton, P.T., Leonard, J.V. & Aynsley-Green, A. (1996) Evaluation of fasts for investigating hypoglycaemia or suspected metabolic disease. *Archives of Disease in Childhood* **75**, 115–119.

3 Short stature

Definition

Short stature can be broadly defined as a perceived or real impairment of linear growth which may result in the referral of a patient because of the presence of physical, psychological or social difficulties. In most patients the cause of short stature is a variation of normal physiology rather than a true pathological process. However, in order for the paediatrician to make a correct diagnosis in cases of short stature, a logical process of assessment, based on clinical and laboratory procedures, is required.

Assessment of short stature

Physiology of growth

Normal linear growth

Human linear growth can be divided into three phases, namely infancy, childhood and pubertal growth. These are not distinct entities as the process of growth is a continuum. However, during these periods of development distinct features of growth can be recognized, corresponding with subtly different regulatory mechanisms.

Infancy

During infancy, linear growth is initially rapid, i.e. approximately 25 cm in the first 12 months of life. This is a continuation of the fetal growth pattern. However, the growth rate (height velocity) shows a marked decrease during this period. The major regulating influence on growth in infancy is nutritional status.

Childhood

The childhood growth pattern starts to occur from approximately 6 months of age and predominates from the age of 3 years. During this interval nutrition becomes less important and hormonal influences, particularly the effect of the growth hormone (GH)–insulin-like growth factor (IGF) axis, become the principal regulating mechanisms for linear growth. Normal thyroid status is also a requisite for normal growth. During childhood height velocity ranges between 4 and 8 cm/year.

Puberty

During puberty, the pattern of human growth changes dramatically, but differs in important ways between females and males (Fig. 3.1). The adolescent growth spurt (AGS) is caused by increasing levels of androgen and oestrogen production in males and females, respectively, as a result of hypothalamic pituitary gonadal activation, which results in a significant increase in GH secretion.

In females, the AGS starts approximately 2 years earlier than in males. The onset of the AGS coincides with the start of clinical puberty, namely breast development. The fastest point of the AGS, i.e. peak height velocity (PHV), occurs on average at approximately 12 years of age and the onset of menstruation (menarche) follows PHV by a variable interval, being close in early developers and more distant in late developers. Consequently, menarche occurs when height velocity is falling and is followed by approximately 2 years of gradually diminishing growth. A further difference between females and males is the amplitude of PHV which, in females, reaches approximately 8 cm/year compared with 10 cm/year in males.

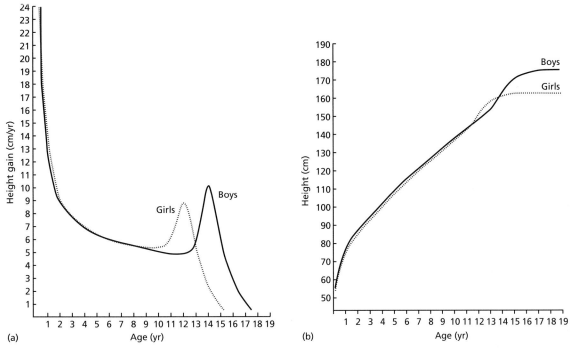

Fig. 3.1 (a) Height velocity and (b) typical individual height curves in girls and boys throughout childhood and adolescence. (From Tanner, 1986.)

In males, the AGS begins when puberty is already well established and coincides with a testicular volume of 10–12 mL. PHV is reached at an average age of approximately 14 years (15 mL testicular volume). The average difference in adult height between males and females is 13–13.5 cm, according to UK standards, being accounted for by two additional years of prepubertal growth, a greater amplitude of the AGS, and a larger prepubertal height in males.

Endocrine control of growth

Growth hormone secretion

Growth hormone is the major endocrine regulator of linear growth. GH is a single-chain polypeptide consisting of 191 amino acids which circulates in the blood bound to one or more binding proteins (GHBP). The predominant form (75%) of GH exists as a 22-kDa protein with 5–10% of pituitary GH release represented by a smaller 20-kDa form which lacks amino acids in positions 32–46. GH is secreted by somatotroph cells of the anterior pituitary gland under the dual regulation of two hypothalamic peptides: GH-releasing hormone (GHRH) is stimulatory and somatostatin is inhibitory to GH synthesis and release. These two peptides are in turn influenced by central neurotransmitters. GH is secreted in an episodic or pulsatile manner, reflecting the interaction of GHRH and somatostatin. Secretion of GH, mostly via its hypothalamic control, is influenced by a wide variety of environmental, genetic and physiological factors including nutrition, sleep, exercise and stress.

Growth hormone–insulin-like growth factor axis (Fig. 3.2)

The insulin-like growth factors (IGF-I, IGF-II) are related peptides which are thought to mediate many of the biological actions of GH. The IGFs were named as such because of their close structural relationship with proinsulin and their weak insulin-like metabolic effects.

IGF-I is a single-chain polypeptide of 70 amino acids which is encoded from a complex gene on chromosome 12. IGF-I is the product of the binding of GH to its receptor in the liver and other target organs. The concentration of IGF-I in the circulation is closely related to physiological secretion of GH, although this relationship may be disturbed in a number of pathological states. IGF-I interacts specifically with a number of soluble proteins called

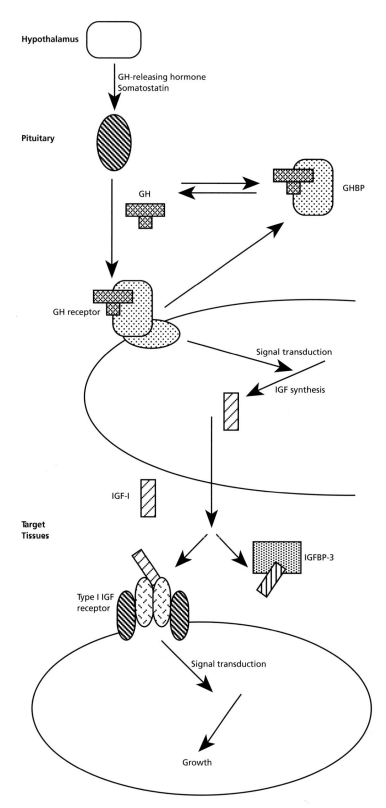

Fig. 3.2 The growth hormone–insulin-like growth factor axis.

IGF-binding proteins (IGFBPs). The principal carrier protein for IGF-I is IGFBP-3, the systemic levels of which depend on GH status. When IGFBP-3 has an IGF molecule bound to it, it can then associate with a further GH-dependent glycoprotein, known as acid-labile subunit (ALS), to form a ternary complex.

Consequently, unlike insulin, most IGF-I circulates in an inactive or bound form. The IGFBPs extend the half-life of the IGF peptides, transport them to target cells and modulate their interaction with their respective receptors. IGF-I binds to the type 1 IGF receptor in target tissues, such as the growth plate at the ends of long bones. Therefore the GH–IGF axis is, according to our current knowledge, the predominant endocrine axis relating to growth and its integrity directly influences linear growth during infancy, childhood and puberty.

Clinical assessment of growth

Procedures for growth assessment
Table 3.1 lists the procedures for the clinical assessment of growth. Most of these techniques are within the scope of all healthcare professionals who deal with children, including family practitioners, school nurses and health visitors.

Auxology
The term 'auxology' (Greek root, *'auxien'* — to increase) is used to describe the study of human growth using repeated measurements of the same individual over successive time periods. It was Professor James Tanner in the 1970s who established auxology as a scientific discipline and introduced its routine use as an essential part of clinical growth assessment. Growth charts are shown in Appendix 2.

Table 3.1 Procedures when a child with short stature is seen in an outpatient clinic.

---

 1 Height, weight, sitting height, height velocity (when available)
 2 Decimal age
 3 Height of parents
 4 Birth weight, gestation
 5 History of short stature, past medical history
 6 Family history, consanguinity, social history, school performance
 7 Systematic inquiry
 8 Examination for dysmorphic features (with patient standing)
 9 Systematic examination
10 Pubertal development staging

Techniques of measurement
Accurate measurement is essential for growth assessment. Errors may be the result of unreliable equipment, but more often measurement procedures are at fault. It is ideal that there should be a *single* trained measurer—or, at the most two, measuring children in a single clinic. The standardization of techniques aims to minimize errors of this type. The following techniques enable reliable data to be collected from the most commonly used measurements.

Weight
Weight should be taken with the subject wearing the minimum of clothing; nappies should be removed. Use of electronic bathroom-type scales, which can be set to zero, is recommended. In order to weigh a baby, the scale is zeroed while an adult stands on it. When they take the baby in their arms, it is the baby's weight which is displayed.

Measurement of children from birth to 2 years of age
Neonates and toddlers are notoriously difficult to measure accurately. The supine table and neonatometer, both consisting of a flat surface with a fixed headboard and moving baseplate, are two devices developed to reduce error in measuring babies and children too young to stand up (Fig. 3.3). Two people are necessary to obtain a reliable measurement. The assistant holds the child's head in firm contact with the headboard, so that the Frankfurt plane is vertical; with neonates it is also advisable to use the forefingers to pin the shoulders down. At the same time the legs are straightened and when the measurer is satisfied that the head is still in contact with the headboard, the measurement can be taken.

Height
The cost of equipment for measuring height varies considerably. The accuracy of the measurement depends on the skill of the measurer. The stadiometer is recommended for use with children from the age of 2 years. The subject stands with heels (without shoes and socks), buttocks and shoulder blades against the backplate and the measurer ensures that the imaginary line from the centre of the external auditory meatus to the lower border of the eye socket (the Frankfurt plane) is horizontal. The measurer then applies pressure on the mastoid processes and the reading is taken at maximum extension without the heels losing contact with the baseboard.

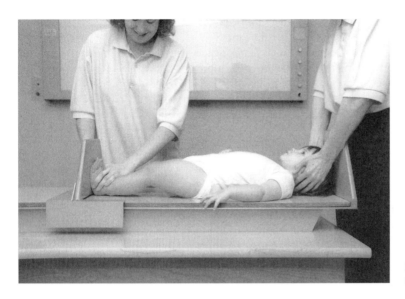

Fig. 3.3 A table used for measuring height (length) in the supine position.

Sitting height

It is technically more difficult to measure sitting height than standing height. Sitting height is required to derive subischial leg length, a means of assessing body proportion. A sitting height table is required and the subject sits on the table with the back of the knees resting on the edge, with the feet supported on a variable height step so that the upper surface of the thighs is horizontal. The subject is then asked to sit up straight. The headboard, with a suitable weight, is placed on the subject's head, upward pressure is then applied to the mastoid process and the measurement is taken.

Skinfold measurement

Skinfold measurements, traditionally using triceps and subscapular sites, are not essential in routine clinical paediatric endocrine practice. They are of value in research studies of nutritional status and of therapy such as growth hormone which influences subcutaneous fat.

Upper arm circumference

Upper arm circumference is also not used in routine clinical practice in the developed world. The site for measurement is mid-way between the acromion and the olecranon process.

Head circumference

Head circumference measurement is important and should be routine in children under the age of 2 years. The tape is slipped over the head and passed around the occipital prominence. The object is to measure maximal head circumference and accurate positioning of the tape is vital to ensure reliability.

Reliability

Any competent measurer should be aware of their error of measurement. The error of measurement (Smeas) is calculated by using a small sample of subjects, i.e. at least 10. These individuals are measured twice and the difference between the two can be used to calculate the error:

$$\text{Smeas} = \sqrt{\Sigma d^2 / 2n}$$

where d is the difference between measurements and n is the number of subjects measured.

Other practical procedures for growth assessment

Decimal age

Expression of age as a decimal makes calculations, particularly height velocity, much simpler. The Table of Decimals of Year, which normally accompanies clinical growth charts shows what decimal fraction of a year has elapsed by each day, for example 0.5 occurs near the beginning of July and 0.75 just after the end of September. So, on 2 July 1991 the year 1991 has passed 0.501 of the way to 1992 and that date can be expressed as 91.501.

To calculate the decimal age of a child seen at the clinic on 9 May 1986 and born on 26 August 1979, the decimal birthday (79.649) is subtracted from the decimal clinic appointment (86.351):

$$86.351 - 79.649 = 6.702$$

The decimal age is 6.702 years.

Calculation of height velocity
Height velocity should not be calculated from measurement intervals of less than 4 months. Intervals of 6 or 12 months are preferable. Height velocity is calculated by dividing the difference in height (cm) by the difference in interval (years). For example, a child born on 28 March 1972, measuring 132.6 cm on 3 February 1981 and 138.2 cm on 4 January 1982 will have decimal ages at the times of 8.854 and 9.772 so that the height velocity is:

$$\frac{1382 - 1326}{9.772 - 8.854} = \frac{5.6}{0.918} = 6.1 \text{ cm/year.}$$

An idea of height velocity can also be obtained by examining the growth curve constructed from a series of accurate measurements. If the height curve crosses the centile bands downwards, height velocity is abnormal and the child may require investigation.

Mid-parental height and target range
When a boy is seen in the clinic, the father's height centile should be indicated at the right-hand side of the growth chart. As the mother's height centile must be plotted on a male chart, this is done by adding 14.0 cm to her height. The mid-parental height (MPH) centile is the mid-point between these two centiles. The target range is calculated as the MPH $\pm$ 8.5 cm, representing two standard deviation confidence limits.

When a girl is seen in the clinic, 14.0 cm is subtracted from the father's height for the position of the father's height centile. The mother's true height is plotted. With normal parents and healthy children, the children's final heights will be normally distributed around the MPH, with only a 5% probability of falling outside the target range.

Pubertal staging
Staging of pubertal development using the criteria of Tanner and the Prader orchidometer in boys is *essential* in the clinical assessment of *all* patients irrespective of age. Details of the criteria for pubertal staging are given in Chapter 5.

Height and height velocity standard deviation score
Height for chronological age and bone age can be expressed as standard deviation scores (SDS) according to the following formula:

$$\text{Height SDS} = \frac{\text{child's height} - \text{mean height for age}}{\text{SD for height at that age}}$$

Height velocity SDS can be calculated according to the following formula:

$$\text{Height velocity SDS} = \frac{\begin{array}{c}\text{child's height velocity} - \text{mean} \\ \text{height velocity (for the mid age} \\ \text{over which height velocity was} \\ \text{measured)}\end{array}}{\text{SD for height velocity at that age}}$$

The SDS for height and height velocity at different ages can be obtained by consulting the original publications from which local growth standards have been derived.

The advantage of using SDS to express height and height velocity values is that data on groups of children of both sexes and different ages can be pooled and compared statistically. When SDS values are calculated for patients in puberty, adjustments must be made for the pubertal stage of the child and the age at which PHV occurred.

Body mass index
The relationship between weight and height of an individual can be expressed by calculation of body mass index (BMI). BMI can be alculated using the formula:

Body weight in kilograms/(height in metres)^2.

This method has been criticized for assessment of obesity in children because the average values for BMI vary considerably with age. Normal standards for BMI in British children have recently been published (see Chapter 11 and Appendix 2).

Assessment of skeletal maturity

Skeletal age
Several methods have been developed to assess the skeletal maturity of growing children from an X-ray of the left wrist, commonly known as 'bone age'. The two most commonly used methods are the 'atlas method' (e.g. Greulich and Pyle) and the 'bone-specific scoring system' (e.g. Tanner–Whitehouse).

Greulich and Pyle method. In this method there is a published atlas of standard or typical X-rays of the left hand and wrist of normal girls and boys at specific ages throughout childhood and adolescence. The overall standard that most closely resembles the film in question is chosen and this becomes the bone age. Critics of this method claim that a single radiograph may yield bone ages that are several years apart when assessed by different observers. The standards, which are derived from North American children, are also relatively advanced (6–9 months) compared with European children. However, this method is the most widely used throughout the world, with relatively little specialized training being required.

Tanner–Whitehouse method. In this method criteria have been established for set stages in skeletal maturation. The most commonly used system is the TW2 method, which also incorporates a methodology for predicting adult height. The system is a bone-by-bone, stage-by-stage method and the assessor assigns a score to each bone according to written criteria. The composite score is the bone age. This system is generally considered by connoisseurs in the field as being superior to the atlas method as subjectivity is almost eliminated. However, specific training of the assessor is required and use of this method outside the UK is relatively limited.

Baseline investigations for short stature

When a child is seen as an outpatient, certain clinical features will suggest that investigations are indicated. Clearly, clinical judgment is needed and not every indication can be listed below. Most children seen for short stature will have no clinical abnormalities. The management of these patients is a question of experience; however, Table 3.2 is given as a guide.

Laboratory investigations for short stature

Once the decision has been made to perform laboratory investigations on the child with short stature, it is extremely important that the doctor proceeds at this stage as a general paediatrician and not as a paediatric endocrinologist. If the approach is too specialized disorders such as anaemia, malabsorption, renal disease, Crohn's disease or even Turner's syndrome can easily be missed. Note that no investigations of GH status are included at this time. Baseline investigations for short stature are given in Table 3.3. Clearly, not every indication for investigation is listed. The management of patients with short stature is a question of experience; however, Table 3.3 is given as a guide.

The decision to investigate GH secretion in the patient is made only after the above investigations have been per-

Table 3.2 Clinical features suggesting that investigations for short stature are indicated.

Extreme short stature
Height significantly below target height
Subnormal height velocity
History of chronic disease
Obvious dysmorphic syndrome, e.g. Turner and Noonan syndromes
Precocious or abnormally delayed puberty
Extreme parental concern

Table 3.3 Baseline investigations for short stature.

Full blood count, ESR
Creatinine, urea, electrolytes
Calcium, phosphate, liver function tests
Ferritin, endomysial antibodies
Karyotype (in girls)
T4, TSH
Cortisol, prolactin
Skeletal survey in dysmorphic children
Bone age X-ray (this is not a diagnostic investigation)

Abbreviations: ESR, erythrocyte sedimentation rate; T4, thyroxine; TSH, thyroid-stimulating hormone.

formed and have been documented to be normal. At the second and third consultations additional auxological information, particularly on height velocity, will be available. A second stage in the investigation of the child is then embarked on. Indications and procedures for investigation of possible GH insufficiency are covered in the section on the diagnosis of GH deficiency, which discusses this disorder in detail.

Differential diagnosis of short stature

The differential diagnosis of short stature is broad and involves a range of different pathogenetic mechanisms which may also coexist. The paediatrician needs to have a working knowledge of this differential diagnosis when a child is referred with short stature. Above all, the doctor needs to take a broad view and to think laterally. A classification of the major aetiological categories is shown in Table 3.4. All patients with short stature can be fitted into one of these categories. Each category will be described briefly below.

Table 3.4 Classification of short stature.

Genetic short stature
Constitutional growth delay
Short stature following intrauterine growth retardation
Dysmorphic syndromes (including skeletal dysplasia)
Endocrine disorders
Chronic diseases
Psychosocial deprivation

Causes of short stature

Genetic short stature

This is probably the most common cause for referral of a child with short stature. Essentially the child is perfectly healthy but has inherited short stature genes from one or both parents or, occasionally, a more distant relative. There is no endocrine abnormality and the bone age is usually not delayed, unless there is also a component of growth delay. Some children with genetic short stature are extremely small and it may be frustrating for the paediatrician who cannot define a precise aetiology. As molecular genetic studies progress it is likely that new growth genes will be identified and that subtle new defects in the GH–IGF-I axis may come to light.

Constitutional growth delay

The diagnosis of constitutional growth delay can be made when other causes of short stature have been excluded and the child or adolescent has evidence of late maturation which is the cause of short stature. Slow physical maturation is the hallmark of this condition. It is said to be 'constitutional', i.e. part of the child's make-up. However, in most cases the actual cause of this delay is unknown. The condition is much more commonly seen in boys and in many cases there is a component of genetic short stature because it is the shorter children who, when in addition have slow maturation, present with short stature. A family history of delayed puberty is often present.

Frequently, the slow maturation starts in early childhood and the delay of physical development accumulates. Consequently, an 11-year-old boy could well have the physical maturity, bone age and height of an 8-year-old. Constitutional growth delay can cause great anxiety to parents and also psychological disturbance in the patient, particularly at the time of normal puberty. Consistent with the delay in physical maturity, pubertal development is late and as boys start their adolescent growth spurt only when they are well advanced in puberty with 10–12 mL testes, the combination of slow growth and lack of meaningful virilization can be very stressful. Fortunately, effective treatment is available (see below).

Important studies have been performed on the natural history of this condition. The final adult height usually falls short of the mid-parental centile and is almost always below the predicted final adult height, calculated on the basis of height and bone age. For this reason, such predictions may be misleading. Patients with constitutional growth delay and their parents require regular reassurance and should be followed in the clinic at least until the adolescent growth spurt is firmly established.

Short stature following birth size

Small for gestational age (SGA) can result from fetal, placental or maternal aetiologies. The fetal defects can be of chromosomal origin or related to structural malformations or genetic syndromes. Intrauterine infection may also impair fetal growth. Maternal causes include chronic illness, smoking and alcohol. The most common cause of SGA is impaired uteroplacental function which, depending on its severity, can cause fetal malnutrition, hypoxaemia and acidaemia.

Symmetrical fetal growth retardation consists of a reduction in weight, length and head circumference and is related to *early* growth failure. Asymmetrical growth failure, with preservation of head growth, occurs because of *late* deprivation of nutrients usually related to placental insufficiency. Potential for postnatal catch-up growth is reduced in the fetus with symmetrical compared to asymmetrical growth failure.

The definition of SGA is variable. A definition of 'birth weight less than the 10th centile' for gestation will include many small normal babies and if one of 'less that the 3rd centile' is used, a higher percentage of infants with long-term growth failure will be identified. Follow-up studies on non-dysmorphic SGA infants indicate that all but 10–15% show catch-up growth by the age of approximately 5 years. Consequently, a population of short SGA children exists who may present with short stature. The same rules apply as with other short children concerning the investigation of these patients. In broad terms, they are usually endocrinologically normal. Surveillance in a growth clinic, however, is recommended, as reassurance is needed and therapeutic intervention with growth hormone may be beneficial (see below).

Dysmorphic syndromes

The paediatrician seeing children with short stature needs to become experienced in recognizing physical features which may hold the key to the diagnosis of a dysmorphic syndrome of which short stature is a feature. The diagnosis of such a syndrome is important because: first, it provides a diagnosis for the short stature; secondly, it allows disease-specific growth charts to be used (e.g. for Down's and Turner syndromes); and, thirdly, it permits the discussion of prognosis and likely outcome in terms of final height with the patient and family. It should, however, be remembered that all dysmorphic syndromes are heterogeneous.

The recognition of dysmorphic features is largely a question of experience. Professor James Tanner used to teach that identification of dysmorphic features was easier with the patient standing opposite the doctor who is sitting. Every patient in Professor Tanner's clinic was photographed, which also accentuates unusual features. A child with a dysmorphic syndrome is not seen very frequently in a growth clinic; however, the examination of a patient with this in mind is an essential part of the consultation.

The most common syndromes are Turner and Noonan syndromes, with which all paediatricians should be familiar. Other syndromes which are seen occasionally, rather than extremely rarely, are Russell–Silver, Williams, and Aarskog syndromes. The diagnosis of Down's syndrome has almost always been made prior to referral for short stature.

Turner syndrome

Growth

This disorder, which is caused by complete or partial absence of one of the X chromosomes occurs in about 1 in 2500 liveborn girls. Turner syndrome is characterized by three main clinical features: abnormal external appearance and abnormality of certain internal organs, malformation of the ovaries and short stature. Short stature is always present, irrespective of the karyotype, and may be the only clinical feature. Ranke has divided growth in Turner syndrome into four phases:

1 intrauterine growth retardation;
2 subnormal growth during infancy and childhood;
3 loss of 15 cm in height compared with normal girls between the ages of 3 and 12 years; and
4 absence of the pubertal growth spurt with prolongation of the total growth phase.

Final adult height in Turner syndrome from white European populations ranges from 142 to 147 cm. There is a positive correlation between final adult height and parental height. The assessment of skeletal maturity in Turner syndrome is particularly difficult because of structural abnormalities of the bones.

Other features

Turner syndrome is a disorder characterized by the presence of recognizable abnormalities (Fig. 3.4). These are varied and are present with varying frequency. The principal phenotypic abnormalities are given in Table 3.5.

Diagnosis and follow-up

Because of the subtlety and variable incidence of many of these features, Turner syndrome cannot be diagnosed or excluded clinically. A karyotype analysis is therefore indicated in all girls presenting with short stature of unknown aetiology. The karyotype 45,X is present in approximately 50% of cases, with 46,X,i(Xq) and 45,X/46,XX the next

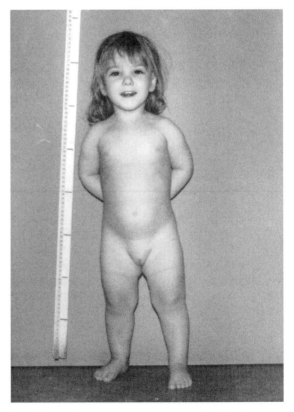

Fig. 3.4 Typical clinical features in a 3-year-old child with Turner's syndrome.

Table 3.5 Principal phenotypic features of Turner syndrome.

Short stature
Gonadal dysgenesis
Low hairline
Nail hyperconvexity
Neck webbing
Cubitus valgus
Broad chest (widely spaced nipples)
Abnormal body proportions (short legs)
Short 4th/5th metacarpals
Lymphoedema
Cutaneous naevi
High arched palate
Cardiac defect (e.g. coarctation of the aorta)
Renal anomaly

Table 3.6 Principal phenotypic features in Noonan syndrome.

Dominant or sporadic inheritance
Short stature
Characteristic facies
   ptosis
   hypertelorism
   low-set ears
Right-sided cardiac defect (usually pulmonary stenosis)
Low hairline
Neck webbing
Pectus carinatum
Cubitus valgus
Cryptorchidism
Delayed puberty
Mild intellectual impairment
Coagulation defect
Mutation in the PTPN11 gene in approximately 50%

Table 3.7 Principal clinical features of Russell–Silver, Williams, and Aarskog syndromes.

Russell-Silver syndrome
   Dominant, X-linked dominant or sporadic inheritance
   Intrauterine growth retardation
   Prominent forehead
   Triangular face
   Diminished subcutaneous fat
   Asymmetry of limbs
   Increased naevi

Williams syndrome
   Autosomal dominant or sporadic inheritance
   Seven q11.23 deletion
   Intrauterine growth retardation
   Elfin face
   Aortic stenosis
   Mental handicap
   Loquaciousness
   Hypercalcaemia

Aarskog syndrome
   X-linked dominant or sporadic inheritance
   Hypertelorism, ptosis
   Short nose
   Interdigital webbing
   Short, broad hands
   Brachydactyly
   Shawl scrotum

most frequent chromosomal anomalies. Late complications, such as autoimmune thyroiditis, middle ear disease, learning difficulties and hypertension, are important to exclude during follow-up. Evidence is growing for the value of specialist adolescent and adult clinics for Turner syndrome patients. Sex steroid replacement therapy is usually indicated to induce secondary sexual characteristics (see below), consequently follow-up is indicated throughout childhood and adolescence, followed preferably by hand-over to specialist adult care.

Noonan syndrome

Noonan syndrome is perhaps even more heterogeneous than Turner syndrome and for this reason must be care-fully considered in both boys and girls presenting with short stature. Its frequency in the general population is unknown; however, it may be as common as 1 in 1000. Noonan syndrome is a completely separate entity from Turner syndrome, existing equally in both sexes. There is no specific defect of gonadal development. Growth is usually affected with height velocity being subnormal. Ranke quotes final adult heights of approximately 162 cm in males and 152 cm in females. Puberty is usually delayed and the adolescent growth spurt is blunted. The principal phenotypic abnormalities in Noonan syndrome are given in Table 3.6.

Russell–Silver, Williams, and Aarskog syndromes

These three syndromes, associated with short stature, are all rare. However, it is helpful to have a grasp of their clinical features, which can then be confirmed in more detail in a dysmorphology textbook. The principal clinical features are given in Table 3.7.

Endocrine disorders

Growth hormone insufficiency

Clinical features

Growth hormone insufficiency is the most common endocrine disorder presenting with short stature. Its frequency in the general population has been estimated at 1 in 3500–4000. Consequently, most general paediatricians may see only a handful of cases. However, the fact that this condition can be safely and effectively treated means that it is of great importance. GH insufficiency can be severe or mild and the presentations of the two extremes are essentially different (Fig. 3.5). 'Severe' or 'mild' GH insufficiency cannot, unfortunately, be defined quantitatively—as no two paediatric endocrinologists would agree! However, it would be reasonable to suggest that severe GH insufficiency is associated with a maximum stimulated GH concentration of <5 mU/L. The features of these two ends of the spectrum are shown in Table 3.8.

Causes of GH insufficiency (Table 3.9)

Idiopathic isolated GH insufficiency. In the majority (>80%) of cases, GH insufficiency is 'isolated', i.e. not associated with other anterior pituitary hormone deficiencies. Most cases also come into the 'mild' rather than the 'severe' category described above. It is now known that the basic defect in this aetiological category is related to the synthesis or release of the hypothalamic peptide GHRH. The precise pathogenesis is unknown. However, these patients respond to administration of exogenous GHRH by secreting GH, indicating that the somatotroph cells are functional and that the primary defect is in the hypothalamus. These patients have been labelled as 'idiopathic' because no space-occupying lesion can be identified radiologically in the region of the pituitary or hypothalamus.

As imaging techniques have improved a radiological appearance known as *pituitary stalk interruption syndrome*

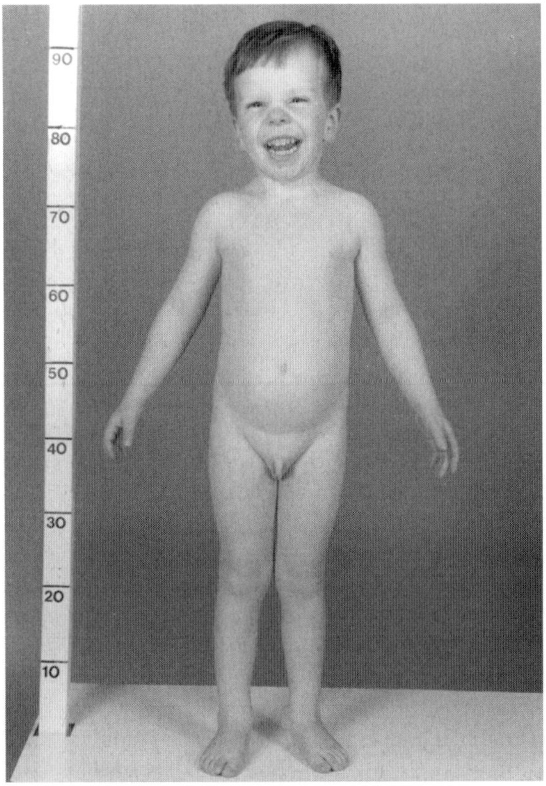

Fig. 3.5 Appearance of a 5-year-old child with severe growth hormone deficiency. Note the excess subcutaneous fat, immature appearance and small genitalia.

Table 3.8 Clinical features of severe and mild GH insufficiency.

Severe GH insufficiency
  Presents before age 3 years (unless acquired)
  Obvious short stature
  Subnormal height velocity from birth, becoming more
    abnormal with age
  Hypoglycaemia
  Micropenis
  Possible associated anterior pituitary hormone deficiencies
    (TSH, ACTH, LH, FSH)
  Excess subcutaneous fat, increasing with age
  Mid-facial hypoplasia (only in extreme cases)
  Possible features of septo-optic dysplasia
  Delayed skeletal maturation
  Maximum stimulated GH concentration <5 mU/L

Mild GH insufficiency
  Unlikely to present before school entry
  Less severe short stature
  Subnormal height velocity documented by careful auxology
    over minimum interval of 12 months
  Isolated GH insufficiency
  Normal subcutaneous fat
  Delayed skeletal maturation
  Delayed puberty

Abbreviations: ACTH, adrenocorticotrophic hormone; FSH, follicle-stimulating hormone; GH, growth hormone; LH, luteinizing hormone; TSH, thyroid-stimulating hormone.

Table 3.9 Principal causes of GH insufficiency.

Genetic
GH-1 mutations
GHRH receptor mutations
Pit-1, Prop-1 mutations

Congenital
GHRH deficiency
Structural defects
    septo-optic dysplasia
    agenesis of the corpus callosum
    single central incisor
    holoprosencephaly
Intrauterine infection

Acquired
CNS tumours
    craniopharyngioma
    germinoma
    optic glioma
Histiocytosis
Cranial irradiation
Head injury
Inflammatory/granulomatous diseases

Transient
Psychosocial deprivation
Prepubertal
Hypothyroidism

Abbreviations: CNS, central nervous system; GH, growth hormone; GHRH, GH-releasing hormone.

has now been described in some patients with severe GH deficiency. This is seen at the severe end of the spectrum of 'idiopathic' defects and is frequently associated with multiple pituitary deficiencies.

Idiopathic multiple anterior pituitary hormone deficiencies. Idiopathic GH deficiency may be associated with deficiency of other anterior pituitary hormones. Multiple pituitary hormone deficiency usually presents in infancy with hypoglycaemia, as a result of a combination of adrenocorticotrophic hormone (ACTH) deficiency, leading to hypocortisolaemia, and GH deficiency. Cholestatic jaundice related to low cortisol is also a well-recognized neonatal manifestation. The presence of micropenis—caused mainly by prenatal luteinizing hormone (LH) deficiency—with hypoglycaemia and jaundice is almost diagnostic of congenital hypopituitarism. Hypothyroidism of pituitary origin is likely to be present, becoming manifest later, but usually without intellectual impairment.

The treatment of congenital hypopituitarism is a neonatal emergency. It is crucial to give hydrocortisone to prevent persisting hypoglycaemia. If this is not effective, GH therapy may be added and thyroxine replacement will also be indicated. GH reserve should not be tested, as GH stimulation tests can induce serious and life-threatening hypoglycaemia. Low serum IGF-I and IGFBP-3 levels may be suggestive of GH deficiency.

GH deficiency of genetic origin. As molecular studies in patients with GH deficiency advance, a number of new genetic disorders resulting in severe GH deficiency have been described. Most of these defects have been reported in families with several affected siblings. It must be stressed that they are extremely rare in the general population.

Deletions of the GH-1 gene appear to result in four variants of hereditary GH (hGH) deficiency. These are:
• type IA (recessive, absent GH, antibodies to hGH therapy);
• type IB (recessive, low GH, response to hGH therapy);
• type II (dominant, low GH, response to hGH therapy); and
• type III (X-linked, low GH, response to GH therapy).

GHRH receptor gene mutations have now been described in several rural communities with high incidences of consanguinity. Severe isolated GH deficiency is the result.

Deficiencies of the pituitary transcription factors Pit-1 (deficiency of GH, ACTH, thyroid-stimulating hormone (TSH), prolactin) and *Prop-1* (deficiency of GH, ACTH, TSH, LH, follicle-stimulating hormone (FSH)) are now well documented in families with hereditary multiple pituitary hormone deficiencies.

Congenital structural CNS defects. Congenital CNS defects occurring in the mid-line may cause GH insufficiency, usually with multiple pituitary hormone deficiencies. However, these lesions cause considerable endocrine heterogeneity.

The most frequent is the syndrome of septo-optic dysplasia consisting of optic nerve hypoplasia, which may be associated with absence of the septum pellucidum and variable hypothalamic dysfunction leading to hypopituitarism. GH insufficiency may occur with deficiencies of ACTH, TSH, LH, FSH and, not infrequently, vasopressin. Presentation is usually in early infancy, when the visual abnormality becomes apparent. Defects in the HESX-1 gene have been described, mainly in familial cases.

Other congenital defects which can cause GH insufficiency are agenesis of the corpus callosum, holoprosencephaly and arachnoid cysts. These conditions can be diagnosed by magnetic resonance imaging (MRI) scan, although the risks of general anaesthetic in the hypopituitary infant must be carefully considered.

CNS tumours: craniopharyngioma. Although rare, this is the most common tumour in the hypothalamo–pituitary region to cause pituitary deficiency in childhood. The tumour usually arises in the region of the hypothalamus and, although histologically benign, is locally invasive, involving adjacent structures, which affect pituitary function. Clinical presentation is frequently as a result of raised intracranial pressure or visual disturbance because of the proximity of the optic chiasm. Biochemical endocrine abnormalities, of which GH deficiency is the most frequent, are often detectable at presentation. The management of craniopharyngioma is complex and controversial. Studies by Stanhope at Great Ormond Street Hospital, London, have emphasized the devastating endocrine and psychoneurological morbidity of radical surgery with removal of hypothalamic tissue.

CNS tumours: germinoma, optic nerve glioma. These two tumours frequently involve the hypothalamo–pituitary axis. Germinoma may present with diabetes insipidus alone for many years before the tumour itself and other pituitary deficiencies become manifest. Consequently, so-called 'idiopathic' diabetes insipidus must always be viewed with suspicion and investigated with regular CNS imaging. Pituitary stalk thickening may be the first radiological abnormality. Elevation of serum and possibly cerebrospinal fluid β-human chorionic gonadotrophin (hCG) levels can be used as a tumour marker.

Optic nerve glioma, which occurs more commonly in patients with neurofibromatosis, may also be associated with pituitary deficiency. Both of these tumours can be treated with targeted radiotherapy, which may cause GH insufficiency (see Chapter 12).

Histiocytosis. The infiltrative lesion of histiocytosis typically involves the hypothalamus and causes diabetes insipidus. In a proportion of cases this will be associated with GH insufficiency.

Cranial irradiation. The topic of endocrine disturbance related to treatment of childhood cancer is addressed in detail in Chapter 12. Suffice it to say that all children who have received CNS irradiation, whether for prophylaxis for leukaemia, for tumours distant from or adjacent to the hypothalamo–pituitary region or during total body irradiation are at some risk for the development of GH insufficiency. These patients therefore constitute an important group who require close endocrine monitoring and follow-up.

Diagnosis of GH insufficiency

Growth hormone insufficiency is, perhaps surprisingly, not an easy condition to diagnose. Of course, there are exceptions, where the young child clearly shows auxological evidence of growth failure and a diagnostic test for GH secretion shows unequivocal evidence of GH insufficiency. However, as indicated earlier, most children with GH insufficiency do not come into this category of 'severe' GH insufficiency (see Table 3.8). A combination of both auxological and biochemical criteria are required to make this diagnosis. GH therapy should not be prescribed without documentation of biochemical GH insufficiency.

Auxological criteria can be summarized as:
- short stature;
- height inappropriately low for target height; and
- subnormal height velocity (must be <25th centile for age).

Biochemical diagnosis

Physiological tests: GH profile. GH secretion is pulsatile, with peaks occurring approximately every 3 hours. A pattern of GH secretion, demonstrating physiological peaks and troughs can be obtained by continuous or 20-minute venous sampling for serum GH levels through an indwelling cannula. This so-called GH profile can be performed overnight or for 24 hours. The child must be acclimatized to the ward. GH insufficiency can be diagnosed or excluded by examining the peak GH level reached during sampling. GH insufficiency should be considered if the peak GH value is <15 mU/L.

A GH profile is a time-consuming, labour-intensive and expensive procedure and is not recommended for routine clinical practice. It is an important technique for research, when sophisticated analyses of GH secretory dynamics can be performed.

Physiological tests: urinary GH excretion. Determination of urinary GH concentration in an overnight or 24-hour urine collection can be used more as a screening test, to exclude GH insufficiency, than as a definitive test for its diagnosis. The method has been criticized because of poor reproducibility from day to day. Consequently, several sequential collections are recommended and each laboratory must establish its own normal range.

Serum markers of GH secretion or action. Serum IGF-I and IGFBP-3, as explained in the section on normal physiology, are two peptides which reflect the status of GH secretion, provided that the GH receptor is functioning normally. In severe GH deficiency IGF-I and IGFBP-3 levels are low, whereas in normally growing children they are normal. The problem is that there is a large overlap in both their ranges in normal children and children with less than severe GH deficiency, i.e. most GH-insufficient children. Consequently, IGF-I and IGFBP-3, for which the assays are difficult and expensive, are not of proven value in the diagnosis of most GH-insufficient children.

Pharmacological tests. GH stimulation tests. GH levels are low during much of a 24-hour period. Therefore GH insufficiency cannot be diagnosed by a random blood test. The GH stimulation test was established to assess the maximum serum GH level which can be released in response to a pharmacological stimulus. There are *many* pharmacological agents which will induce GH release. Those which also stimulate ACTH secretion, causing an increase in serum cortisol, have some theoretical advantage.

A particular test is usually adopted for routine use in a paediatric endocrine unit. Hindmarsh, at the Middlesex Hospital, London, has published widely on the relative advantages of the different tests. Five tests are described in Table 3.10, followed by brief comments on their merits.

Comments and interpretation

The two most commonly used tests in paediatric endocrine practice in the UK are the glucagon and clonidine tests. The glucagon test stimulates cortisol secretion, which can be an advantage if multiple pituitary hormone deficiencies are suspected. As indicated, the glucagon test can cause hypoglycaemia, particularly in young children. The insulin-tolerance test (ITT) is gradually going out of paediatric practice in the UK because of the risks of serious hypoglycaemia. The test should never be used for children under 5 years. In experienced hands, in an established paediatric endocrine unit, the ITT is safe and probably provides the best validated stimulus for GH secretion. It should not be performed in a general paediatric environment. The GHRH test stimulates the pituitary directly and in our experience the GH response may not differentiate the GH-insufficient child from the normal short child.

Table 3.10 Details of GH stimulation tests. Absolute requirements *before* all GH stimulation tests are to document normal serum thyroxine concentration and normal serum cortisol concentration (>100 nmol/L). Stilboestrol (priming 1 mg twice daily for 2 days) is performed in some centres before the test in patients with a bone age >10 years.

Glucagon test	
Dose	15 µg/kg intramuscularly
Sampling	GH, cortisol, glucose at 0, 30, 60, 90, 120, 150, 180 minutes
Complication	Hypoglycaemia, particularly in young children; nausea
Requirement	Doctor in attendance throughout test
Contraindication	Epilepsy in young children
Clonidine test	
Dose	0.15 mg/m^2 orally
Sampling	GH at 0, 30, 60, 90, 120, 150, 180 minutes
Complication	Potential hypotension
Requirement	BP monitoring
Insulin-tolerance test	
Dose	0.15 units/kg intravenously
Sampling	GH, cortisol, glucose at 0, 20, 30, 60, 90, 120 minutes
Complication	Hypoglycaemia
Requirement	Doctor at bedside throughout test, blood glucose <2.2 mmol/L
Contraindication	Age <5 years, epilepsy
Arginine test	
Dose	0.5 g/kg intravenously over 30 min
Sampling	GH at 0, 30, 60, 90, 120, 150 minutes
Complication	Nausea; irritation at i.v. site
GHRH test	
Dose	1 µg/kg intravenously
Sampling	GH at 0, 15, 30, 60, 90, 120 minutes
Complication	Mild facial flushing

Abbreviations: GH, growth hormone; GHRH, GH-releasing hormone.

How many GH stimulation tests are required to make a firm diagnosis of GH insufficiency? In the UK we usually take the view that one technically satisfactory test, if combined with valid auxological observations, is sufficient. This certainly is not the general view in the rest of Europe or the USA, where at least two tests are usually performed. Confidence in the value of high-quality auxology should remove the need for a second test. What constitutes a normal—or even an abnormal—GH stimulation test? If only paediatric endocrinologists could agree! At the risk of oversimplifying the interpretation of a stimulation test:

- a peak GH level during a satisfactorily performed test (with all samples collected) of <15 mU/L is suggestive of GH insufficiency;
- a peak GH level of 15–25 mU/L may be consistent with GH insufficiency if the auxological criteria are present; and
- a peak GH level of >25 mU/L is unlikely to be consistent with GH insufficiency.

An entity known as GH neurosecretory dysfunction was described by Bercu in the 1980s. This refers to the combination of:

- 'normal' GH secretion in response to pharmacological stimulation;
- clinical GH insufficiency with subnormal height velocity;
- subnormal spontaneous GH secretion examined on 24-hour GH profile; and
- response to GH therapy.

This entity has generally been accepted by the paediatric endocrine community and it is important to remember its existence. It can explain the apparently anomalous combination of normal GH response to stimulation and clinical GH insufficiency. If in doubt, trust the auxology!

Other endocrine causes of short stature

Hypothyroidism

If untreated, congenital hypothyroidism leads to severe stunting of growth. Since the introduction of neonatal screening, this cause of short stature has largely been eliminated. Acquired hypothyroidism caused by autoimmune thyroiditis may, however, present with short stature. Hence the need to assess thyroid function in all short children requiring investigation.

Cushing's syndrome

Hypercortisolaemia suppresses linear growth. Consequently, most patients with Cushing's syndrome, if present for more than several months, will develop subnormal growth. Exceptions are cases where excess adrenal androgens are secreted, which may counteract the growth-suppressive effect of high cortisol. In children and adolescents with Cushing's disease, height may be significantly discrepant with weight, being below the 3rd centile in approximately 50% of patients.

GH resistance

GH resistance accounts for a relatively small number of patients with short stature. In its severe form, it presents as Laron syndrome, an autosomal recessive disorder caused by a homozygous mutation of the GH receptor. These patients are very rare and the growth failure is extreme, with a final adult height of 120–130 cm. There is some evidence that milder forms of GH resistance may be a cause of short stature, but this has yet to be established.

Skeletal dysplasias

This is a varied group of disorders which combines genetics, dysmorphology, radiology, orthopaedics and endocrinology. These patients are referred because stature may be disproportionate and growth severely affected with grossly reduced adult height. The classification of skeletal dysplasias is highly complex and is beyond the scope of this chapter. However, the key features of three forms—achondroplasia, hypochondroplasia and cartilage hair hypoplasia—are given in Table 3.11.

Chronic paediatric diseases

It is now well recognized that chronic illness impairs linear growth in childhood and adolescence and may be an unsuspected cause of short stature. The degree of growth failure varies considerably from a relatively mild effect in, for example, asthma and sickle cell disease to potentially severe short stature in Crohn's disease and juvenile chronic arthritis. Decreased calorie intake and increased energy expenditure are probable contributing factors. The pathogenesis of growth suppression is poorly understood; however, certain mechanisms such as malnutrition (cystic fibrosis, Crohn's disease) (Fig. 3.6), systemic inflammation (chronic arthritis), hypoxia (cyanotic congenital heart disease) and metabolic disturbance (glycogen storage disease, renal failure) are likely to be influential. GH resistance may also be present (Crohn's disease, renal failure). Delays of maturation and puberty usually accompany impaired growth. Some of the more common causes of growth failure resulting from chronic illness are shown in Table 3.12.

Psychosocial deprivation

It is also well recognized that an adverse family and social environment can delay a child's physical development. There is an established relationship between socio-economic status and physical growth. Consequently, to exclude social status from an analysis of psychological deprivation is difficult. Blizzard & Bulatovic (1992) have

Table 3.11 Clinical features of achondroplasia, hypochondroplasia and cartilage hair hypoplasia.

Achondroplasia
FGF receptor 3 mutation
Autosomal dominant
Severe shortening of long bones
Large head
Hypoplastic mid-face
Lumbar lordosis
Childhood anaemia
Childhood height –5 to –6 SDS
Approximate adult height:
    male, 132 cm
    female 125 cm

Hypochondroplasia
  FGF receptor 3 mutation, genetically heterogeneous
Autosomal dominant
Marked variation in severity
Normal head and face
Short limbs
Radiological lack of lumbar interpedicular distance
Blunted pubertal growth
Approximate adult height:
    male, 155 cm
    female, 142 cm

Cartilage hair hypoplasia
Autosomal recessive
Intrafamilial phenotype heterogeneity
Short limbs
Sparse, fine hair
Hypertelorism
Defective cellular immunity
Blunted pubertal growth
Approximate adult height:
    male, 131 cm
    female, 123 cm

Abbreviations: FGF, fibroblast growth factor; SDS, standard deviation scores.

divided psychosocial deprivation into two types. Type 1 refers to children <3 years of age with non-organic failure to thrive, whereas type 2 describes older children with short stature and GH insufficiency. Skuse *et al* (1996) has reported a variant known as 'hyperphagic short stature', which describes children who demonstrate abnormal behaviour with hyperphagia, polydipsia, growth failure, GH insufficiency and resistance to exogenous GH therapy. The GH insufficiency is reversible on moving the child to a favourable environment.

Psychosocial deprivation should always be considered when a child is referred with short stature. However, this diagnosis is seldom made in the consulting room. It is more likely that a child, who is found to be at risk, is noticed to be short and often underweight. The crucial role of the endocrinologist is to insist that the child be carefully measured and that height be documented. Sequential heights (and weights) may provide the only quantitative evidence of neglect and may thus be of enormous benefit to the child's future care.

Treatment of short stature

A great deal of attention is paid in paediatric endocrinology to treatment of short stature with different hormone preparations. In fact, we have a poor choice of growth-promoting therapies that are available for clinical use. Growth hormone is licensed for treatment of GH insufficiency, Turner syndrome, Prader–Willi syndrome, short SGA children and short children with renal failure. Sex steroid therapy is available for stimulation of pubertal growth. Other therapies, such as GHRH and IGF-I, are used in research but are still far from being available for routine practice.

Consequently, the paediatrician is concerned not so much with which licensed preparation to use, but rather *when* to use it. In this section, guidelines will be discussed for safe and effective use of established hormone therapies.

Constitutional delay of growth and puberty

The physical and psychological well-being of a child or adolescent with delay of growth and puberty can be safely and effectively improved by hormone therapy. In fact, this is one of the most rewarding conditions to treat, for the patient, family and paediatrician. By far the majority of patients seen with this problem are boys. Society appears to favour tall individuals, at all ages, consequently to be short and physically immature may understandably create psychological stress, particularly during adolescence. The indications for consideration of therapy are summarized in Table 3.13.

Aims of treatment

Males

The aims of treatment depend on the age of the patient. In the boy aged 10–13 years, the aim is to induce growth acceleration. In the boy aged 14 years and over the aim is

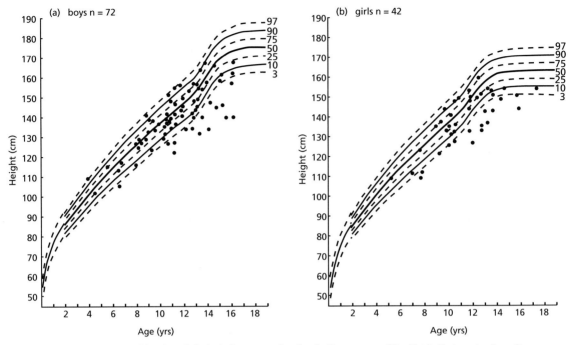

Fig. 3.6 Heights in (a) boys and (b) girls with Crohn's disease at referral to the Department of Paediatric Gastroenterology, St Bartholomew's Hospital, London.

Table 3.12 Chronic paediatric disorders causing impaired linear growth.

System	Disorder	Comments on pathogenesis
Gastrointestinal	Coeliac disease, Crohn's disease, gastro-oesophageal reflux, protein-losing enteropathy	Reduced energy intake, cytokines suppressing IGF-I production, malabsorption
Haematological	Leukaemia, sickle cell disease, thalassaemia	Intensive chemotherapy, iron deposition from transfusions
Cardiac	Large defects between ventricles or great arteries, cyanotic CHD, pulmonary hypertension	Reduced energy intake, increased expenditure, increased work of breathing, hypoxaemia
Respiratory	Asthma, cystic fibrosis, bronchopulmonary dysplasia	Increased energy expenditure, inhaled steroids, reduced calorie intake, pancreatic insufficiency
Renal	Chronic renal failure, post-transplantation	Protein-energy malnutrition acidosis, sodium loss, low IGF-I bioactivity, high IGFBPs, GH resistance, steroid therapy
Metabolic	Diabetes mellitus, inborn errors	Insulin and IGF-I deficiencies, reduced energy intake
Neurological	Cerebral palsy, hemiplegia, myelomeningocele	Reduced energy intake, increased expenditure, neurological damage, associated chronic illness

Abbreviations: CHD, congenital heart disease; IGF, insulin-like growth factor; IGFBP, IGF-binding protein.

to induce growth acceleration together with virilization. In both groups treatment should avoid excess advance of bone age. Treatment consists of short-term androgen therapy.

Oxandrolone
Oxandrolone is a non-aromatizable testosterone deriva-

tive with anabolic effects and weak androgen activity. It is not licensed in the UK, but can be prescribed on a named-patient basis.

In the younger age group mentioned above, growth acceleration can be induced by the use of oxandrolone 1.25–2.5 mg/day orally for 6–12 months. A useful guide to dosage is: 1.25 mg for <12 years, 2.5 mg for >12 years. This

Table 3.13 Indications for consideration of hormone therapy in the patient with constitutional delay of growth and puberty.

Short stature
Low height velocity
Delayed secondary sexual development
Abnormal body proportions (long legs, short trunk)
Reduced bone mineral density
Psychological disturbance related to
    poor self-image
        looking and feeling different or younger than peers
    lack of confidence
    depression
    school refusal
    aggressiveness, delinquency
    reduced employment opportunities
Parental concern

regimen will increase height velocity from approximately 4 cm/year to 7.5 cm/year during the first 6 months of therapy. There will be no virilization and bone age will not advance abnormally. If, at the end of the course of treatment, the patient shows evidence of testicular enlargement of >4 mL, linear growth can be expected to continue at greater than the prepubertal rate.

Testosterone

Testosterone therapy will induce growth acceleration and virilization. Its use is therefore indicated in the older age group mentioned above, where growth and secondary sexual development is required. Testosterone esters are licensed as replacement therapy.

Testosterone cypionate (Sustanon) or enanthate (Primoteston Depot) 25–50 mg 2-weekly to 100–125 mg 4-weekly by intramuscular injection for 3–6 months will induce growth acceleration and virilization. A course of 3- to 6-monthly injections must be terminated to allow re-evaluation of height, puberty stage and bone age. If necessary, particularly if testicular volume is <5–6 mL, a second course can be given at a later date. Final height is not affected, provided appropriate dosage is used.

Females

In girls with delay of growth and puberty, ethinylestradiol 2 μg/day orally for 6–12 months is likely to induce some growth acceleration, which may be associated with early breast development.

Growth hormone insufficiency

GH insufficiency can be effectively treated with recombi-
nant growth hormone. Successful treatment is potentially able to normalize height, but this is achieved at a significant economic cost and using invasive therapy in the form of daily subcutaneous injections. A fundamental biological principle needs to be accepted which is that the more severe the GH insufficiency the greater the benefit from replacement therapy.

Every child considered for GH therapy must be assessed in detail so that treatment is reserved for those who will unequivocally benefit by increase in final adult height. Currently in the UK, the diagnosis of GH insufficiency is made at an average age of approximately 9 years. This is really too late to achieve an optimal long-term result. Early diagnosis and initiation of therapy must be the goal of all those involved in growth assessment.

Guidelines for GH therapy

Before starting treatment, auxological assessment for 12 months is essential for several reasons.

1 Pubertal assessment and bone age must indicate that growth potential exists.

2 Height velocity must be subnormal before treatment is started.

3 Pre-treatment height velocity assessment, preferably for 12 months, is necessary to compare with the on-treatment height velocity after 1 year of treatment.

4 The family must be fully committed after a detailed discussion.

It is helpful to explain at the start of therapy that a formal assessment of response will take place after 1 year. At this time, an *increase* in height velocity of >2 cm/year compared with the pre-treatment value is needed to justify continuation of therapy. When no such increment exists, treatment should be stopped. If an unequivocal response occurs, treatment can be continued until final height is reached. Auxological monitoring with adjustment of dosage should be performed every 6 months.

Increasing the dosage of GH during puberty is controversial. Provided normal pubertal growth is occurring, we recommend leaving the dose regimen unchanged. After linear growth is complete, GH secretion should be retested. Many patients will now have a normal response. Those with a subnormal response should be handed over for adult endocrine follow-up.

Guidelines for GH therapy are summarized in Table 3.14.

Adverse events

Recombinant GH is remarkably free of side-effects. The complication of Creutzfeldt–Jakob disease associated

Table 3.14 Guidelines for GH therapy in children with GH insufficiency.

Early diagnosis and initiation of therapy
Dose: 0.025–0.05 mg/kg/day
Route of administration: subcutaneous
Time of administration: evening
Formal assessment after 1 year of therapy
6-monthly auxology
Close monitoring of pubertal growth
Discontinue GH at completion of growth (height velocity <2.0 cm/year)
Retest GH secretion prior to adult hand-over

Table 3.15 Summary of GH therapy in Turner syndrome.

GH therapy increases height velocity in Turner's syndrome
The effect is dosage dependent and supra-physiological doses are indicated
Long-term GH therapy statistically increases final height
The mean increase appears to be approximately 7–9 cm
A dosage of 0.05 mg/kg/day is recommended
The response to GH in individual patients is highly variable
The optimal age for starting therapy is not established

with pituitary-extracted GH has been widely publicized. For this reason, only biosynthetic GH should be used. Leukaemia has been reported in association with GH therapy. This caused great alarm, and recently a number of careful epidemiological studies demonstrated that the incidence of leukaemia, at least in Europe and the USA, in patients receiving growth hormone was no greater than in the general population nor is there any convincing evidence that GH therapy stimulates tumour regrowth in children with cancer.

Genetic short stature (the normal short child)
Evidence is accumulating that GH therapy does not significantly increase final height in most children with genetic short stature or those labelled as being 'short normal'. These children are not GH-insufficient and therefore would not be expected to be sensitive to GH therapy. GH therapy may increase height velocity in the short term but the apparent benefit is soon lost, because of simultaneous stimulation of bone maturation. The only situation where a trial of GH may be indicated is when GH neurosecretory dysfunction is suspected. If the clinical features of GH insufficiency are present—short stature and low height velocity, combined with apparently normal GH

secretion—a 1-year trial of standard dosage GH therapy may be indicated.

Growth hormone therapy in non-GH-deficient disorders
The availability of recombinant GH, although admittedly at very high cost, has led to its use in a number of non-GH-deficient disorders, where its pharmacological properties might benefit growth. Prominent among these are Turner and Noonan syndromes, short stature related to SGA, renal disease and skeletal dysplasias. Each of these categories will be discussed briefly.

Turner syndrome
As described above, the mean final height in Turner syndrome is approximately 145 cm. Consequently, if GH therapy could improve this height significantly, routine therapy may be justified. A summary of the current situation is shown in Table 3.15. It should be appreciated that new data are appearing continuously on this subject.

Turner's syndrome is currently a licensed indication for GH therapy, using a recommended dosage of 0.05 mg/kg/day. The addition of oestrogen does not appear to improve response. New information has suggested that addition of oxandrolone in a dosage of 0.0625 mg/kg/day may augment response.

Sex steroid replacement therapy in Turner syndrome
Oestrogen replacement therapy can be started at about 11 years of age using the following regimen; ethinylestradiol 2 µg/day for 1 year, then 4 µg/day for 1 year, then 6, 8, 10 µg increasing 4-monthly. Once a dosage of 10 µg/day has been given for approximately 6 months, norethisterone 5 mg/day can be added to be taken on days 1–14 of each calendar month. Transfer to a gynaecologist/adult endocrinologist should be arranged on completion of pubertal development.

Noonan syndrome
There are far fewer published data on the effect of GH therapy in Noonan syndrome. The group at St Bartholomew's Hospital, London, published the results of 1 year's treatment using a dosage of 0.05 mg/kg/day. There was sustained growth acceleration, with height velocity increasing from 3.8 to 10.5 cm/year. No deleterious effects on cardiac muscle thickness were detected. Long-term benefit of GH therapy is not yet established and Noonan's syndrome is not a licensed indication for GH therapy. Patients should be entered into official therapeutic trials,

rather than treated on an *ad hoc* basis. Further long-term data are awaited.

Short stature associated with SGA

A number of studies have shown that GH therapy causes a dose-dependent increase in height velocity in this group of patients. De Zegher et al (1998) reported that high-dose therapy for a period of 2 years induced catch-up growth which can be maintained after the treatment is stopped. Catch-down growth has since been reported to occur if treatment is discontinued in childhood. In 2003, a European license was granted for the treatment of short SGA children. This was based on data showing final adult height in the normal target range. The recommended dose is 0.033–0.066 mg/kg/day.

Renal disease

Children with chronic renal failure usually grow poorly and treatment with GH has been extensively studied. These patients usually have some degree of GH resistance and consequently require pharmacological doses of GH for a growth-promoting effect. GH therapy in a dosage of 0.05 mg/kg/day was able to increase height velocity significantly in pre-terminal chronic renal failure and also, but less impressively, in end-stage renal disease. GH may also be used post-transplantation to counteract the effect of steroid therapy. Again, supra-physiological doses are required. Optimization of electrolytes and nutritional aspects of management are also important to promote growth. The use of GH in renal disease should be monitored in a specialist renal department with experience of this treatment.

Skeletal dysplasias

Patients with skeletal dysplasia have normal GH secretion. It appears unlikely that long-term GH therapy will significantly increase final height. Data from the Middlesex Hospital, London, suggests that GH may be effective in stimulating pubertal growth, particularly in hypochondroplasia. Additional long-term data are awaited.

Treatment of short stature in chronic paediatric diseases

The short stature seen in chronic disease is usually the result of a combination of pathogenetic mechanisms. For example, in Crohn's disease there is both malnutrition and active inflammation. In cystic fibrosis there is reduced energy intake combined with increased energy expenditure and pancreatic insufficiency. It is not logical to expect treatment with a growth-promoting agent such as GH to overcome or eliminate these processes. The child with chronic disease may have a catabolic state which induces GH resistance, consequently GH therapy is unlikely to be effective.

As described above, most chronic diseases cause a delay in maturation. It is reasonable to attempt to treat the delayed puberty with sex steroids, although the disease process may result in some resistance to androgens and oestrogens. The most effective treatment of the short stature of chronic illness is the effective treatment of the primary illness itself. This has been dramatically demonstrated in Crohn's disease, where successful resection of the inflamed bowel results in spectacular catch-up growth (Fig. 3.7).

Psychosocial deprivation

Psychosocial deprivation may also be regarded as a chronic disease state. The best therapy for associated growth failure is to correct or reverse the disadvantageous home setting or, if this is not possible, to remove the child to a supportive environment. GH therapy is not indicated in this context.

IGF-I

Recombinant IGF-I was developed in the late 1980s and is the only therapy available for treatment of severe genetic GH resistance. It is effective in stimulating growth in Laron syndrome and has been shown to improve glycaemic control in adolescent diabetes mellitus. However, a major therapeutic indication for IGF-I has still to be found. A compound which complexes IGF-I with IGFBP-3 has also been developed. This physiological approach is logical; however, its clinical efficacy for treatment of growth disorders remains to be demonstrated.

Use of GnRH analogue therapy to improve growth

Gonadotrophin-releasing hormone (GnRH) analogues are now an established treatment for central precocious puberty (see Chapter 5). They can suppress gonadotrophin secretion and therefore arrest pubertal development. The possibility of their use in children with short stature has been studied as a way of delaying puberty and hence prolonging prepubertal growth, which might increase final height.

A wealth of literature has emerged on this topic, with the general consensus being that any benefit is marginal. However, there is one clinical situation where they are

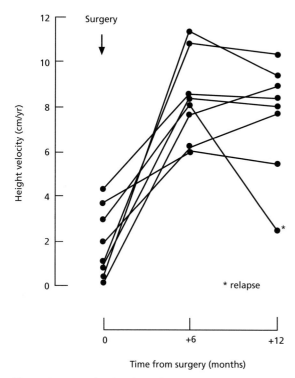

Fig. 3.7 Increase in height velocity following successful resection of inflamed bowel in prepubertal and early pubertal patients with Crohn's disease.

likely to be beneficial. The child with a *combination of early puberty and GH insufficiency*, for example after cranial irradiation, requires maximum treatment to enhance growth before epiphysial closure. In this situation, we would recommend a combination of GnRH analogue and GH therapy. Puberty can be allowed to continue at a more appropriate age.

When to involve a specialist centre

- Severe GH deficiency or GH resistance.
- CNS lesion causing GH deficiency.
- Dysmorphic syndromes associated with severe short stature.
- Management of Turner syndrome.
- Severe short stature associated with SGA.
- Cranial irradiation associated with GH deficiency.

Future developments

- Alternative methods of GH administration, including a long-acting preparation are being developed.

- Growth-promoting preparations, such as IGF-I and IGF-I/IGFBP-3, have been tried as an alternative to GH, but are not currently established as being superior, except in severe genetic GH resistance.
- The use of GnRH analogues to delay puberty and possibly increase final height has been tried but this treatment, except in patients with severe GH deficiency, has not been established to give a better long-term outcome.
- Genetic studies to identify the molecular basis of individual growth disorders will develop. The essential clinical component of these studies is to establish the precise clinical phenotype in combination with the genetic analysis.

Controversial points

- Treatment of non-GH-deficient children with hGH is an important controversial issue which relates to clinical benefit, risk of therapy and health economics.
- The optimum organization of growth screening in the community is controversial. In general, community paediatricians favour a smaller number of measurements, whereas paediatric endocrinologists and patient support groups, such as the Child Growth Foundation, favour multiple measurements throughout the pre-school period and during school years. The latter view is probably ideal; however, resources are not available for detailed and comprehensive growth screening.
- Genetic analysis of patients with short stature is growing in frequency. Although direct benefit to the patient may be difficult to prove, unlike in disorders such as multiple endocrine neoplasia, genetic analysis and identification of gene mutations does contribute to the characterization and understanding of the pathophysiology of growth disorders.

Potential pitfalls

- Over-diagnosis of GH deficiency by focusing on biochemical results rather than auxology.
- Over-reliance on bone age assessment, which is not a diagnostic investigation.
- Reluctance to use testosterone therapy for delayed puberty in males. In short courses, using the appropriate dose, there is no compromising effect on final height and the psychological benefits are great.

CASE HISTORIES

Case 1

A 4-year-old boy was being followed in a joint medical/surgical cryptorchidism clinic and was found to have short stature. He had subtle dysmorphic features with a small mid-face. He was apparently healthy. Both testes were palpable, but the penis was rather small. Height was below the 3rd centile, weight on the 10th centile and height velocity was 3.4 cm/year.

These findings indicated that he was abnormally short (mid-parental height was 75th centile) and that he needed investigation. The results were as follows. Full blood count, erythrocyte sedimentation rate (ESR), electrolytes, creatinine, liver function tests and endomysial antibodies were normal.

Total thyroxine (T4)	48 nmol/L [0.37 microg/dL, NR 4.6–10.5]	[NR 58–174]
TSH	1.8 mU/L	[NR 0.3–5.0]
Free T4	6.6 pmol/L [0.53 ng/dL, NR 0.8–2.4]	[NR 11–25]
Cortisol	255 nmol/L [9.3 microg/dL, NR 8.0–25.0]	[NR 09.00h, 300–700]
Prolactin	286 mU/L	[NR up to 360]

Question

1 What do these baseline results mean?

Answer

1 They show that he has hypothyroidism of pituitary origin because his TSH level is not elevated.

Question

2 What is the next step?

Answer

2 He needs a thyrotrophin-releasing hormone (TRH) stimulation test.

Results of the TRH test (200 μg i.v.)

0 min	TSH 1.1 mU/L
20 min	TSH 4.2 mU/L
60 min	TSH 4.8 mU/L

Questions

3 Is this test normal?
4 Should he now have assessment of his GH secretion?
5 Are any more investigations needed before he starts his GH therapy?
6 Are there any other pituitary hormone deficiencies?

Answers

3 No, because the rise in TSH is inadequate. In a normal TRH test the 20 min TSH level should be higher than the 60 min level.

4 No because, in a child with hypothyroidism, of any cause, GH secretion is suppressed. The next step is to treat his hypothyroidism with thyroxine 75 μg/day.

Once his thyroxine level is normal, one can proceed to a glucagon (15 μg/kg i.m.) stimulation test to assess his GH secretion. The results are shown in Table 3.16.

All GH values less than 10 mU/L indicate severe GH deficiency.

5 Yes, he needs an MRI scan of the pituitary and hypothalamus to exclude an organic cause of GH deficiency, such as craniopharyngioma. The MRI scan was reported as showing an extremely shallow pituitary fossa with no evidence of pituitary tissue. **The diagnosis is idiopathic hypopituitarism with deficiency of GH and TSH.**

6 He had cryptorchidism and a small penis. This could be caused by gonadotrophin deficiency, which will need investigating at the time of puberty.

He started GH therapy in a standard dosage of 0.025 mg/kg/day. His height velocity increased in 6 months from 4.9 to 19.2 cm/year. This was a record for the clinic. At the age of 9.5 years his

Table 3.16 Results of glucagon stimulation test.

Time (min)	GH (mU/L)
0	0.8
60	0.5
90	1.6
120	1.4
150	0.6
180	0.7

height was 139.6 cm, i.e. between the 75th and 90th centiles and within his height target range.

Case 2

A 6-year-old girl was referred with growth failure, poor appetite, recurrent abdominal pain, 'thick custard' stools and vomiting.

Question

1 What is the differential diagnosis of this child's short stature?

Answer

1 Look at Table 3.4 and remember that the paediatrician should always approach the problem of short stature as a generalist and not as an endocrinologist. On examination her height was below the 0.4th centile and her weight was on the 2nd centile. Her height velocity was 1.8 cm/year (normal is >4 cm/year).

This means that she needs baseline investigations for short stature (Table 3.3). The results of these investigations were as follows.

Hb	12.2 g/dL
Ferritin	8.0 µg/L [NR 15–300]
Anti-endomysial antibodies	Positive
ESR	24 mm/hour

Question

2 What is the next investigation needed?

Answer

2 Jejunal biopsy. This showed villous atrophy and lymphocytic infiltrate in the lamina propria with hyperplastic crypts. This confirmed a diagnosis of **coeliac disease**.

References and further reading

Blizzard, R.M. & Bulatovic, A. (1992) Psychosocial short stature: a syndrome with many variables. *Baillière's Clinics in Endocrinology and Metabolism* **6**, 687–712.

Borochowitz, Z.U. & Rimoin, D.I. (1998) Genetic and dysmorphic syndromes of short stature. In: *Growth Disorders: Pathophysiology and Treatment* (eds C.J.H. Kelnar, M.O. Savage, H.F. Stirling & P. Saenger), pp. 297–322. Chapman & Hall Medical, London.

Bourguignon, J.P. (1998) Constitutional delay of growth and puberty. In: *Growth Disorders: Pathophysiology and Treatment* (eds C.J.H. Kelnar, M.O. Savage, H.F. Stirling & P. Saenger), pp. 673–689. Chapman & Hall Medical, London.

Cowell, C.T. (1995) Short stature. In: *Clinical Paediatric Endocrinology* (ed. C.G.D. Brook), pp. 136–172. Blackwell Science, Oxford.

De Zegher, F., Francois, I., Van Helvoirt, M., Beckers, D., Ibanez, L. & Chatelain, P.G. (1998) Growth hormone treatment of short children born small for gestational age. *Trends in Endocrinology and Metabolism* **9**, 233–237.

Donaldson, M.D.C. & Paterson, W. (1998) Abnormal growth: definition, pathogenesis and practical assessment. In: *Growth Disorders: Pathophysiology and Treatment* (eds C.J.H. Kelnar, M.O. Savage, H.F. Stirling & P. Saenger), pp. 197–224. Chapman & Hall Medical, London.

Hagenäs, L. (1998) Skeletal dysplasias. In: *Growth Disorders: Pathophysiology and Treatment* (eds C.J.H. Kelnar, M.O. Savage, H.F. Stirling & P. Saenger), pp. 338–355. Chapman & Hall Medical, London.

Hindmarsh, P.C. (1998) Endocrine assessment of growth. In:

Growth Disorders: Pathophysiology and Treatment (eds C.J.H. Kelnar, M.O. Savage, H.F. Stirling & P. Saenger), pp. 237–250. Chapman & Hall Medical, London.

Hindmarsh, P.C. (1999) Evidence-based decisions in growth hormone therapy. In: *Current Indications for Growth Hormone Therapy* (ed. P.C. Hindmarsh), pp. 1–12. S. Karger, Basel.

Johnston, L.B. & Savage M.O. (2004) Should recombinant human growth hormone therapy be used in short small for gestational age children? *Archives of Disease in Childhood* **89**, 740–744.

Jones, K.L. (1997) *Smith's Recognizable Patterns of Human Malformation*. W.B. Saunders, Philadelphia.

Mullis, P.E. (1998) Genetic control of growth. In: *Growth Disorders: Pathophysiology and Treatment* (eds C.J.H. Kelnar, M.O. Savage, H.F. Stirling & P. Saenger), pp. 39–61. Chapman & Hall Medical, London.

Ranke, M.B. (1998) Turner and Noonan syndromes: disease specific growth and growth-promoting therapies. In: *Growth Disorders: Pathophysiology and Treatment* (eds C.J.H. Kelnar, M.O. Savage, H.F. Stirling & P. Saenger), pp. 623–639. Chapman & Hall Medical, London.

Skuse, D., Albanese, A., Stanhope, R., Gilmore, J. & Voss, L. (1996) A new stress-related syndrome of growth failure and hyperphagia in children, associated with reversibility of growth hormone insufficiency. *Lancet* **348**, 353–358.

Tanner, J.M. (1986) Normal growth and techniques of growth assessment. In: *Growth Disorders, Clinics in Endocrinology and Metabolism*, Vol. 3, pp. 411–451. W.B. Saunders, London.

Tonshoff, B. & Mehls, O. (1999) Growth retardation in children with chronic renal disease: pathophysiology and treatment. In: *Current Indications for Growth Hormone Therapy* (ed. P.C. Hindmarsh), pp. 118–127. S. Karger, Basel.

4 Tall stature

As tall stature becomes more prevalent and more acceptable, referrals, particularly of tall girls, appear to be decreasing. The referral of a child with tall stature is frequently the result of parental concern about actual or future final height. However, knowledge of the pathogenesis, clinical and biochemical associations and potential treatment of tall stature is clinically relevant.

Pathogenesis and differential diagnosis

Tall stature is usually associated with one of three aetiological categories. In order of frequency these are: familial advanced growth; a syndrome associated with tall stature, which has usually been present since infancy; and an abnormal increase in growth rate of endocrine origin. The differential diagnosis is shown in Table 4.1.

Assessment of the child or adolescent with tall stature

Repeated height measurements are essential for the assessment of tall stature. The combination of auxology, careful history-taking and physical examination will exclude the need for laboratory investigations in most cases. Procedures needed for the clinical assessment of a child or adolescent referred with tall stature are given in Table 4.2.

Investigations

Patients with intellectual delay may well have had previous investigations. If physical examination is completely normal and the child comes from a tall family, investigations are usually not indicated. Regular height measurements will be sufficient. If abnormalities are detected in the history or on examination, basal investigations are indicated, as shown in Table 4.3.

Further investigations will be dictated by the results of the baseline tests. If the diagnosis of excess growth hormone (GH) secretion caused by a GH secreting pituitary adenoma is considered, investigation should proceed as shown in Table 4.4.

Protocol for glucose tolerance test

Give 1.75 g carbohydrate orally (up to maximum of 75 g = two glasses of Lucozade). Serum GH at: −30, 0, 30, 60, 90, 120 and 150 minutes. Normal GH suppression is a value of <4 mU/L at some time during the test.

Causes of tall stature

Familial tall stature or constitutional advanced growth

This is the most common cause of referral of patients for tall stature. If the patient is a girl, it is frequently the mother who, having suffered herself from being tall as a child and adolescent, is concerned about her daughter. In groups of tall children, GH secretion has been shown to be statistically elevated when compared to normal or short stature children. However, in an individual child excess GH secretion is not usually apparent.

The tall stature is usually noticeable by primary school entry. Physical examination is normal. Assessment of bone age, which is likely to be advanced, and calculation

Table 4.1 Differential diagnosis of tall stature.

1 Familial tall stature

2 Syndromes associated with tall stature:
chromosomal defects
Klinefelter's syndrome
XXXY, XYY syndromes
overgrowth syndromes
Sotos' syndrome
Weaver's syndrome
Marshall–Smith syndrome
Beckwith–Wiedemann syndrome, hyperinsulinism
Marfan's syndrome
MEN 2B
ACTH resistance
Homocysteinuria

3 Tall stature of endocrine origin:
GH secreting pituitary tumour
precocious puberty
hyperthyroidism

4 Simple obesity

Abbreviations: ACTH, adrenocorticotrophic hormone; GH, growth hormone; MEN, multiple endocrine neoplasia.

Table 4.2 Procedures for the assessment of a patient with tall stature.

Height, weight, height velocity
Heights of parents, siblings
Birth weight, length, head circumference
History of previous growth, past medical history
Intellectual development
Systematic inquiry
Examination for dysmorphic features
Systematic examination
Pubertal development staging with measurement of testicular volume
Bone age and final height prediction

Table 4.3 Baseline investigations for tall stature.

Karyotype
T4, TSH
IGF-I
Bone age and final height prediction

Abbreviations: IGF-I, insulin-like growth factor; T4, thyroxine; TSH, thyroid-stimulating hormone.

Table 4.4 Investigations for suspected GH secreting pituitary adenoma.

Glucose tolerance test for GH secretion
MRI scan of pituitary
Visual fields
Cortisol (9.00 a.m.)
Prolactin
Testosterone, LH, FSH (depending on age)

Abbreviations: FSH, follicle-stimulating hormone; LH, luteinizing hormone; MRI, magnetic resonance imaging.

of final height prediction may be helpful. The likelihood of earlier than average puberty should be explained. Reassurance and growth monitoring are the principles of management.

Syndromes associated with tall stature

These disorders will not be described in detail. They are all rare; however, the principal phenotypic features of three important tall stature syndromes—Sotos', Marfan's and Beckwith–Wiedemann syndrome—are given in Table 4.5.

Endocrine causes of tall stature

The three endocrine causes of tall stature should be suspected after clinical examination. All will require hormone investigations to confirm the abnormality. Specialist referral at this stage is recommended.

GH secreting pituitary tumour

A GH-secreting tumour causes tall stature and gigantism in childhood and adolescence, and acromegaly in adult life. An association with McCune–Albright syndrome is recognized. Because of its extreme rarity in childhood, this disorder should be managed jointly with an adult endocrinologist, who will have far more experience. Suppression of GH secretion may require pituitary surgery, radiotherapy, somatostatin analogue or GH receptor antagonist therapy.

Treatment of familial (constitutional) tall stature

Occasionally, the degree of anxiety surrounding advanced growth, usually in girls, is so great that treatment is indicated to try to slow down growth and therefore reduce final height. Two forms of therapy are currently used:

Table 4.5 Principal clinical features of Sotos', Marfan's and Beckwith–Wiedemann syndromes.

Sotos' syndrome
Increased birth length
Increased birth head circumference
Recognizable facies
    downslanting eyes
    bossed forehead
    prominent jaw
Hypotonia, clumsiness
Early puberty
50% need special education
Rare, autosomal dominant inheritance

Marfan's syndrome
Autosomal dominant
Fibrillin gene defect
One in 10 000 births
Arm span 8 cm > height
Arachnodactyly
Skeletal features
    kyphoscoliosis
    joint laxity
    pectus excavatum
    pes planus
High arched palate
Aortic dilatation, aortic, mitral valve anomalies
Myopia, lens dislocation

Beckwith–Wiedemann syndrome
Increased birth weight and length
Growth velocity and bone age advanced during first 4–6 years
Macroglossia
Hemihypertrophy
Ear signs
    ear lobe creases (see Chapter 2)
    pits on pinna
Hypoglycaemia
Omphalocoele
Malignancies (e.g. Wilms' tumour)
Learning difficulties

high-dose sex-steroid therapy and GH-suppressive therapy using a somatostatin analogue. In future, GH receptor antagonist therapy may be appropriate.

Sex-steroid therapy

The indication for the use of sex steroids to reduce final height is based on evidence that abnormally high circulating levels will advance skeletal maturation and eventually cause early epiphyseal fusion. De Waal from the Netherlands has published the most extensive results. In girls, ethinylestradiol 100–300 µg/day orally combined with cyclical progesterone (i.e. norethisterone 5 mg/day for days 1–14 of each calendar month), if used relatively early, reduced final height by up to 7 cm. In boys, testosterone 250–1000 mg monthly caused a similar reduction. An early age of onset of treatment (bone age 10 years in girls, 12.5 years in boys) was associated with the best results. In an extensive inquiry, 10 years after final height, no significant adverse affects were identified.

Somatostatin analogue therapy

Suppression of GH levels should theoretically slow down growth and, if continued on a long-term basis, may reduce final adult height. Hindmarsh at the Middlesex Hospital, London, has reported that the use of the somatostatin analogue octreotide in a dosage of 37.5–50 µg once or twice daily caused significant decrease in height velocity, with reduction in height prediction of up to 5 cm.

Octreotide, which is given by subcutaneous injection, may cause gastrointestinal side-effects. It is likely that to reduce final height effectively, complete suppression of GH may be necessary. This treatment would be best organized jointly with an adult endocrinologist who has had experience of its use.

Future developments

• Molecular analysis of tall stature and overgrowth syndromes is likely to identify new genetic causes of these disorders.

When to involve a specialist centre

• Dysmorphic syndromes associated with tall stature.
• Tall stature associated with excess GH secretion.
• Difficult cases of tall stature associated with hyperthyroidism or precocious puberty.
• GH receptor antagonist treatment is likely to become established as the treatment of choice for constitutional tall stature.

Controversial points

• The treatment of tall stature in girls is controversial.

High-dose oestrogen therapy is rarely practised now. Treatment with a somatostatin analogue may be effective but is invasive and associated with side-effects. New therapy using a GH receptor antagonist is promising but not yet established to be beneficial.

• As tall stature is better tolerated by society, there seems to be less indication for therapy.

• Rare conditions, such as GH secreting pituitary tumours, are very infrequently seen in paediatric practice. These patients must be managed jointly with an adult endocrine unit.

Potential pitfalls

• Failure to consider the diagnosis of or examine the patient carefully enough for dysmorphic features suggestive of Marfan's syndrome. This diagnosis may have serious consequences as these patients need life-long cardiovascular surveillance.

• Failure to appreciate that tall stature and delayed puberty are an unusual combination. An important differential diagnosis is Klinefelter syndrome, which should be considered.

CASE HISTORY

A 9-year-old girl was referred because of tall stature. She was in good health. On examination there were no dysmorphic features. Her height was just above the 97th centile and her parents' heights were on the 90th and 97th centiles. Pubertal development was: breast, stage 2; axillary hair, stage 2; pubic hair, stage 3; and no menarche.

Baseline investigations (Table 4.3) were all normal. Consequently, an endocrine cause of her advanced growth was not identified. Bone age was 12.4 years and final height prediction was 188 cm. The parents, particularly the mother who had suffered as a result of her own tall stature, enquired about treatment. The child was not particularly concerned. Treatment was not advised.

Question
Are any further investigations indicated?

Answer
Probably not. She had occasional headaches so a magnetic resonance imaging (MRI) scan of the pituitary was performed which showed a pituitary gland with a convex upper border but no suprasellar extension.

She also had a height velocity of 9.2 cm/year. She therefore had an oral glucose tolerance test for GH suppression. Her GH levels during the glucose tolerance test suppressed to 0.5 mU/L, indicating that there was no evidence of increased GH secretion.

Diagnosis: constitutional (familial) advanced growth.

References and further reading

De Waal, W.J., Greyn-Fokker, M.H., Stijnen, T. *et al.* (1996) Accuracy of final height prediction and effect of growth reductive therapy in 362 constitutionally tall children. *Journal of Clinical Endocrinology and Metabolism* **81**, 1206–1216.

Drop, S.L.S. & Lamberts, S.W.J. (1998) Constitutional advanced growth and gigantism. In: *Growth Disorders: Pathogenesis and Treatment* (eds C.J.H. Kelnar, M.O. Savage, H.F. Stirling & P. Saenger), pp. 775–789. Chapman & Hall Medical, London.

Hindmarsh, P.C., Pringle, P.J., Di Silvio, L. & Brook, C.G.D. (1990) A preliminary report on the role of somatostatin analogue (SMS 201–995) in the management of children with tall stature. *Clinical Endocrinology* **32**, 83–91.

Patton, M.A. (1998) Genetic and dysmorphic syndromes with tall stature. In: *Growth Disorders: Pathogenesis and Treatment* (eds C.J.H. Kelnar, M.O. Savage, H.F. Stirling & P. Saenger), pp. 323–335. Chapman & Hall Medical, London.

5 Puberty

Physiology of normal puberty

Puberty occurs when the secretion of gonadotrophin-releasing hormone (GnRH) by the hypothalamus, which is largely but not entirely suppressed during childhood, increases so that pulsatile secretion of luteinizing hormone (LH) increases, resulting in sufficient sex steroid production to result in secondary sexual development (see Fig. 5.1).

In boys
- LH stimulates the Leydig cells to produce testosterone which induces the features of secondary sexual development. β human chorionic gonadotrophin (hCG) has similar structure and action to LH.
- Follicle-stimulating hormone (FSH) binds to receptors on the Sertoli cells, enhancing spermatogenesis.
- Spermatogenesis depends on the complex interaction of various paracrine factors; qualitatively normal spermatogenesis can occur without FSH and LH but quantitative production requires gonadotrophins.
- Testosterone modulates LH secretion.
- Inhibin B produced by the Sertoli cells exerts a negative feedback effect on FSH secretion.
- Sex hormone-binding globulin (SHBG) levels fall so that free androgen levels rise.

In girls
- LH stimulates proliferation of follicular and thecal cells, and during the follicular phase of the menstrual cycle induces androgen secretion by theca cells.
- FSH induces proliferation of granulosa cells; increases expression of LH receptors on granulosa cells; enhances aromatase activity so that androstenedione is converted to oestradiol (E2); and increases progesterone (P) production.
- E2 acts on FSH receptors on the granulosa cells to cause proliferation of the follicular cells in addition to inducing secondary sexual development.
- Inhibin B is produced by granulosa cells in small antral follicles, inhibin A by large antral follicles and by the corpus luteum. Inhibins may have a role in inhibiting FSH secretion and in dominant follicle selection.
- Ovulation results from interaction of LH, FSH and E2 on the developing primordial follicle (see below).
- SHBG levels decrease only slightly.

In both sexes
- GH and insulin-like growth factor (IGF-I) secretion are enhanced because of increased levels of sex steroids and insulin.
- Insulin secretion rises and is accompanied by an increase in insulin resistance.

Physiology of the menstrual cycle

During embryogenesis the primordial germ cells migrate

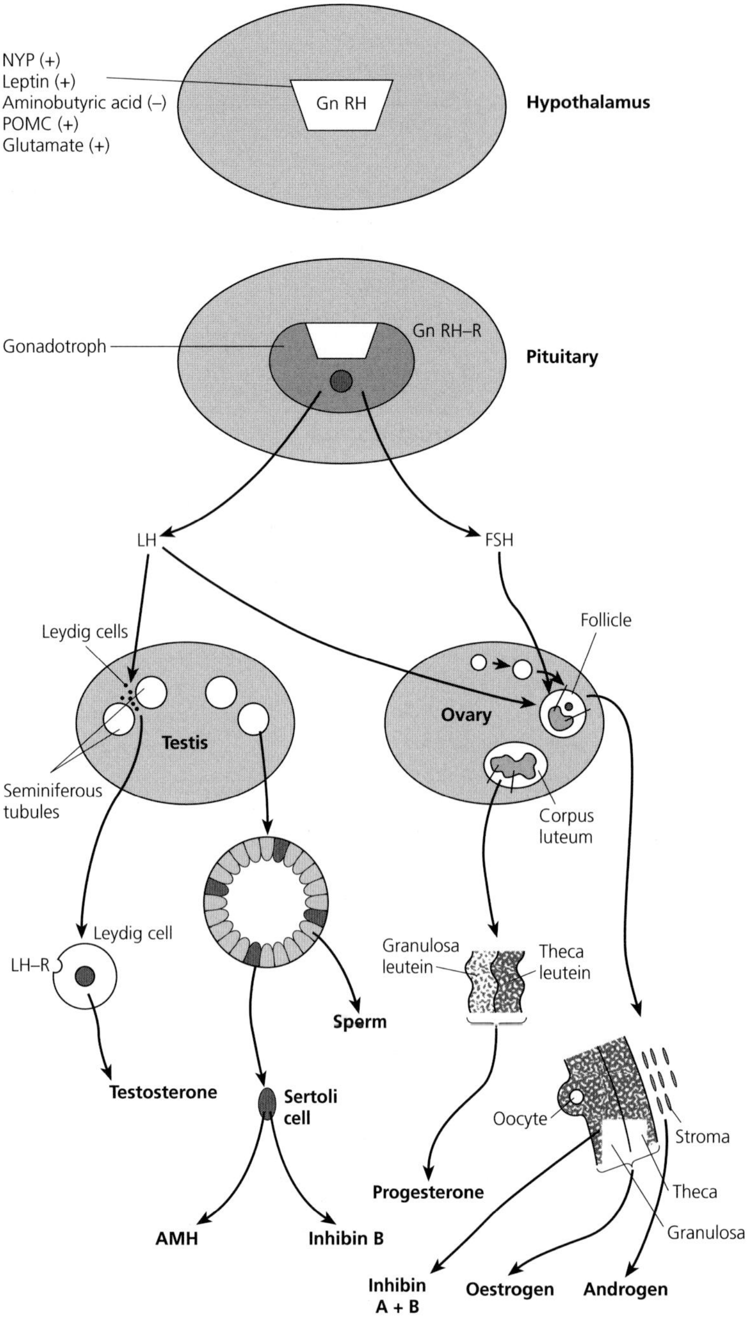

Fig. 5.1 Schematic representation of hypothalamic–pituitary–gonadal pathways.

to the ovary and develop into primordial follicles. In the fetus the pool of primordial follicles reaches a peak of about 7 million germ cells at 20 weeks gestation, falling to 1–2 million at birth, 500 000 at menarche, and about 100 at the menopause. FSH levels reflect the size of the primordial follicle pool at any given time. Each follicle contains an oocyte arrested in the prophase of the first meiotic division.

Follicular phase (approximately 14 days, but variable in duration)

- At the beginning of the menstrual cycle 15–20 primordial follicles develop of which only one ultimately develops into a Graafian follicle, the rest becoming atretic.
- On day 1 of the follicular phase FSH levels increase as a result of decreased inhibition from the falling levels of E2 and P at the end of the previous cycle.
- FSH stimulates the follicles to secrete E2 by increasing androstenedione secretion by the thecal cells and inducing aromatase expression in the granulosa cells. Increasing E2 levels cause a decrease in LH and FSH secretion.
- During this time one follicle emerges as dominant, with more FSH receptors than the others; it therefore recruits more of the diminishing supply of FSH, thus secreting more and more E2.
- At the crucial moment E2 feedback on the pituitary changes from negative to positive inducing the pre-ovulatory LH surge.

Luteal phase (always 14 days)

- LH stimulation results in the ovum entering the final phase of 1st meiotic division to become a secondary oocyte. The follicle swells and ruptures, releasing the ovum into the peritoneal cavity, and from there into the fallopian tube.
- LH induces luteinization of granulosa and thecal cells of the follicle to form the corpus luteum. This results in increased P synthesis which induces swelling and secretion of the endometrium.
- P levels peak 5–7 days post-ovulation, exerting a negative effect on GnRH and thus causing a decrease in pulse frequency.
- As GnRH pulse frequency falls, FSH and LH secretion decreases, causing the corpus luteum to lose its receptors.
- In the absence of pregnancy the corpus luteum becomes atretic (corpus albicans), levels of P and E2 fall, and FSH levels start to rise as a new cycle begins.

Onset of puberty

The GnRH secreting neurones are under the influence of controlling neurones of both excitatory (glutamate) and inhibitory (GABA) nature. In addition, they are under the control of glial cells (excitatory). At the time of puberty, changes in trans synaptic neurotransmission and glial inputs (such as that provided by prostaglandins released by astrocytes), result in the pulsatile secretion of GnRH and hence the pubertal cascade.

The following points should be noted.

- In girls the hypothalamus is more prone to 'break free' of suppression than in boys. Thus idiopathic precocious puberty is more common in girls, and girls exposed to cranial irradiation and CNS disorders, such as hydrocephalus, are prone to enter puberty earlier than boys.
- Exposure of the hypothalamus to high levels of sex steroids (e.g. poorly controlled salt-wasting 21 hydroxylase deficiency) may activate puberty; this phenomenon is known as priming.

Clinical aspects of normal puberty

Pubertal staging

This involves an assessment of breast (B) development in girls, genital (G) development and testicular volume in boys, and pubic (P) and axillary (A) hair development in both sexes. Whenever possible it is preferable for males to stage boys and for females to stage girls. Male doctors should ensure that a female member of staff is present during the examination of a girl.

Breast staging

B1 Prepubertal
B2 Breast budding
B3 Development of actual breast mound (in obese girls it is difficult to distinguish between B1 and B3)
B4 Areola projects at an angle to breast mound
B5 Adult configuration

Genital staging

G1 Prepubertal penis (unstretched length 2.5–6 cm), scrotum and testes (volume ≤3 mL)
G2 Testes ≥4 mL ± scrotal laxity, but no penile enlargement
G3 Penile lengthening with further development of testes and scrotum
G4 Penile lengthening and broadening, further development of the testes (volume usually 10–12 mL)
G5 Adult genitalia, testes usually 15–25 mL

N.B. Testicular volume should be gauged using the Prader orchidometer. Penile size (useful for serial staging and important if hypogonadism is suspected) is measured from the base of the penis to tip of the glans (not the foreskin). Obese individuals are sometimes referred because of small penis size. However, firm compression of the suprapubic fat pad reveals normal penile size in almost all cases.

Pubic hair staging

P1 No pubic hair
P2 Fine hair over mons pubis and/or scrotum/labia
P3 Adult type hair (coarse, curly) but distribution confined to pubis
P4 Extension to near adult distribution
P5 Adult

Axillary hair staging

A1 No axillary hair
A2 Hair present but not adult amount
A3 Adult

Milestones and growth patterns of puberty in girls and boys

In girls (Table 5.1), breast budding is accompanied by acceleration in growth rate with PHV at B2–3 and usually marked deceleration in height velocity after menarche. Boys (Table 5.2) enter puberty about 6 months later than girls. In boys, at G2 growth rate is either the same as or slower than at G1. The increase in growth rate coincides with testicular volumes of 6–10 mL.

In both sexes, the age of onset and duration of pubertal development is subject to marked individual variation. Early puberty is associated with a higher PHV, and delayed puberty with a lower PHV.

The 12.5–14 cm difference in height between adult males and females relates to three factors:

1 The difference in age of PHV—12 years in girls and 14 years in boys—means that boys have two extra years of 'childhood' growth.

2 The intensity of the growth spurt is greater in boys than girls.

3 Boys are slightly taller than girls during the childhood years.

Pubertal assessment

Clinical

- Height of adolescent.
- Mid-parental height and target range.
- Height velocity.
- Pubertal stage.
- Bone age.

Pelvic ultrasound

- Assessment of uterine size, shape and endometrial echo reflect the effect of oestrogen.
- Ovarian volumes and the size/number of follicles identified reflect gonadotrophin effect.

Table 5.1 Mean ages of breast (B) stages in girls with corresponding height velocities including peak height velocity (PHV). Data from Tanner *et al.* 1966.

	Age (years)	Height velocity (cm/year)
B1	Prepuberty	approx 4–7 from 7 years
B2	11.2	7
PHV	12.1	8.3 (6.2–10.4)
B3	12.2	8.2
B4	13.1	5
Menarche	13.5	3.6
B5	15.3	=1

Breast budding is accompanied by acceleration in growth rate with PHV at B2–3 and usually marked deceleration in height velocity after menarche.

Table 5.2 Mean ages of genital (B) stages in boys with corresponding height velocities including peak height velocity (PHV). Data from Tanner *et al.* 1966.

	Age (years)	Height velocity (cm/year)
G1	Prepuberty	approx 4–7 from 7 years
G2	11.6	5
G3	12.9	6.3
G4	13.8	9.3
PHV	14.0	9.5 (7.2–11.7)
G5	14.9	6.2

At G2 growth rate is either the same as or slower than at G1. Increase in growth rate coincides with testicular volumes of 6–10 mL.

Biochemical

This is required where there is diagnostic uncertainty and/or when treatment is contemplated. The biochemical investigation of puberty is given below. Normative data are shown in Table 5.3.

- Karyotype.
- Basal LH and FSH.
- LHRH 2.5 µg/kg (max 100 µg) IV with LH and FSH sampling at 0, 15, 30 and 60 minutes.
- Serum testosterone/oestradiol and SHBG.
- In boys serum testosterone measurement 4 days after single s.c. injection of hCG 100 units/kg (max 1500 units).
- Measurement of serum androstenedione, 17 OHP and DHEAS together with testosterone and oestradiol before

Table 5.3 Normative data for LH and FSH before (basal) and after (peak) stimulation with 100 μg intravenous LHRH, derived for 85 subjects aged 3–17 years with no evidence of endocrine disease (Tawfik, Galloway and Donaldson). Reference range for testosterone and estradiol is from the Institute of Biochemistry, Glasgow Royal Infirmary.

Tanner stage	LH (units/L)		FSH (units/L)		Testosterone (nmol/L)	Estradiol (pmol/L)
	Basal	Peak	Basal	Peak		
Girls						
B1	0.5	2.4	2.0	12.0		<50
	(0.5–2.4)	(0.5–4.9)	(0.2–5.0)	(2.2–26.4)		
B2	0.55	9.7	3.3	9.9		
	(0.5–2.6)	(1.6–16.4)	(0.5–8.9)	(6.8–22.2)		
B3–4	1.6	23.6	5.8	14.3		
	(0.5–4.8)	(6.1–50.6)	(2.5–7.0)	(12.0–26.7)		
Boys						
G1	0.5	2.0	1.0	4.4	<0.3	
	(0.2–0.5)	(0.5–5.11)	(0.2–4.7)	(1.0–11.6)		
G2	1.1	8.3	1.7	2.5		
	(0.5–2.0)	(4.4–13.8)	(0.3–4.2)	(0.9–11.2)		
G3–5	1.9	16.6	3.2	6.3		
	(1.9–4.0)	(10.4–21.1)	(1.8–10.6)	(2.8–17.0)		
Adult					8.7–35.0	180–1500

and after simulation with synacthen, and 24-hour urine for steroid profile are of value in the work-up of selected cases.
• Basal gonadotrophins are of limited value in diagnosing puberty, but elevation of FSH (>10 units/L) indicates primary gonadal failure.
• Prepubertal luteinizing hormone-releasing hormone (LHRH) test shows LH peak <5 units/L, with LH response less marked than FSH response. A pubertal LHRH test shows LH peak >5 units/L, LH response usually greater than FSH response.
• A prepubertal LHRH test is indistinguishable from central hypogonadism with GnRH or LH and FSH deficiency.

Sexual precocity

Definitions
Sexual precocity: a general term meaning early sexual development.
True central precocious puberty (TCPP): normal puberty, resulting from activation of the hypothalamus, and following a normal sequence, but occurring abnormally early. In the UK, this is defined as before 8 years in girls and 9 years in boys.
Precocious pseudopuberty: sexual precocity caused by the abnormal secretion of sex steroids independent of hypothalamo–pituitary control.
Thelarche: isolated breast development, commonly in infants and preschool children, in the absence of other symptoms and signs of sexual precocity.
Thelarche variant: a descriptive term for girls in which thelarche is persistent or slowly progressive, often associated with a moderate increase in height velocity and bone age, and sometimes vaginal bleeding, but a prepubertal LHRH test.
Exaggerated adrenarche: in some individuals adrenarche (adrenal puberty occurring between 6 and 8 years) is associated with sufficient androgen secretion to cause symptoms and signs of sexual precocity. This phenomenon is often mistakenly referred to as '**premature adrenarche**', a term which should be confined to adrenarche occurring before 6 years of age.
Premature menarche: cyclical uterine bleeding (confirmed by identifying an endometrial echo on pelvic ultrasound at the time of vaginal bleeding) in the absence of other symptoms and signs of sexual precocity.

Clinical assessment and diagnosis of boys and girls with sexual precocity

Tables 5.4 and 5.5 show the types and causes of sexual precocity in boys and girls. The data illustrate that:
- idiopathic TCPP is very rare in boys;
- precocious pseudopuberty is rare;
- in secondary precocious puberty, the underlying cause is usually self evident (e.g. known CNS disorder); and
- exaggerated adrenarche is more common in girls than boys.

History

Two key aspects must be addressed:
1 Symptoms relating to sex steroid production.
2 Features suggesting aetiology of sexual precocity.

Symptoms related to sex steroid production

Androgen-related
- Greasy skin
- Acne
- Greasy hair
- Body odour
- Pubic and/or axillary hair
- Enlargement of penis or clitoris
- Deepening of voice
- Increase in growth rate
- Mood swings/behaviour problems ± aggression

Table 5.4 Types of sexual precocity encountered at Royal Hospital for Sick Children, Glasgow 1989–2004.

	Girls	Boys
True central precocious puberty		
Idiopathic	106	2
Secondary	29	13
Precocious pseudopuberty	9*	6†
Adrenarche	190	29
Thelarche	89	
Thelarche variant	39	
Premature menarche	24	
Unclassified	5	

*Feminizing adrenal adenoma (1); feminizing ovarian tumour (1); virilizing ovarian tumour (1); McCune–Albright syndrome (2); 11-hydroxylase deficiency (1); cause unknown (2). †Simple virilizing 21-hydroxylase deficiency (2); testotoxicosis (1); virilizing adrenal adenoma (1); oxymethalone (2).

Oestrogen-related
- Breast tenderness and development (often asymmetrical initially)
- Mood swings/behaviour problems
- Vaginal discharge
- Cyclical vaginal bleeding

Mood swings and behaviour changes, important in deciding whether or not to treat precocious puberty, must be gauged carefully, and where possible separated from 'normal' difficult behaviour!

Features suggesting cause of sexual precocity
- Family history of early puberty.

Table 5.5 Aetiology of true central precocious puberty (onset <8 years in girls and <9 years in boys) seen at RHSC, Glasgow 1989–2004.

	Girls	Boys
Idiopathic	106	2
Cranial irradiation		
ALL	2*	0*
Medulloblastoma	1	0
Other tumour	1	0
NHL	0	0
Tumour		
Optic nerve glioma (NF)	6 (4)	5 (3)
Craniopharyngioma	1	1
Hypothalamic hamartoma	0	1
Germinoma	0	1
3rd ventricle cyst	1	1
Neurological disorder		
Learning disability +/epilepsy	8†	3†
Hydrocephalus/spina bifida	7	1
Tuberculous meningitis	1	0
Cerebral palsy	2	0
Priming		
11-OHD	1	0
SV 21-OHD	0	2
Oxymethalone	0	1
Testotoxicosis	0	1

ALL, acute lymphoblastic leukaemia; NF, neurofibromatosis; NHL, non-Hodgkin's lymphoma; SV21-OHD, simple virilizing 21 hydroxylase deficiency. *Between 1989–2004 an additional 28 girls and 3 boys were seen with early (cf precocious) puberty related to cranial irradiation for ALL. †Between 1989–2004 an additional 34 girls and 9 boys were seen with early puberty associated with CNS disorder/learning disability.

- History of headache, vomiting or visual disturbance, suggestive of intracranial tumour.
- Perinatal problems resulting in periventricular haemorrhage with hydrocephalus.
- Neurological deficit (e.g. cerebral palsy).
- Cranial irradiation (e.g. for CNS prophylaxis in leukaemia).
- Drug therapy, e.g. oxymethalone.

Physical assessment
- Height.
- Weight.
- Bone age.
- Pubertal status, including examination of the genitalia in girls with history suggestive of androgen excess.
- Blood pressure.
- Examination of fundi.
- Systemic examination including nervous system.
- Examination for *café au lait* patches (seen in neurofibromatosis (Fig. 5.2) and McCune–Albright syndrome) and axillary freckling (seen in neurofibromatosis).

Diagnosis and management of sexual precocity in girls

Oestrogen-mediated sexual precocity

True central precocious puberty (Table 5.5)

Clinical features
In a straightforward case there will be a history of breast development followed by other features of normal puberty including increase in growth rate, development of pubic and axillary hair, vaginal discharge, mood swings and sometimes vaginal bleeding. Examination will show a girl who looks older than her chronological age, with a height centile above the parental target range, features of normal puberty and bone age advanced by usually more than 2 years. Pelvic ultrasound will confirm oestrogen effect—enlarged uterus showing fundal swelling ('heart-shaped' configuration) often with several millimetres of endometrial echo; and gonadotrophin effect—ovaries usually above 3 mL in volume with several 6 mm follicles.

Investigations (in addition to bone age and pelvic ultrasound assessment)
- LHRH test to confirm pubertal response.
- Serum oestradiol.

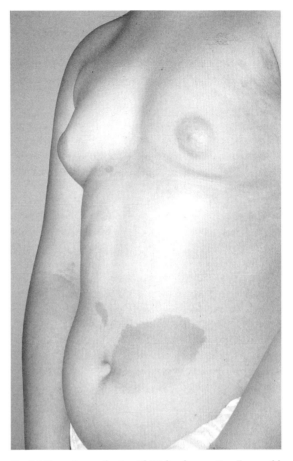

Fig. 5.2 Precocious puberty with B4 development in a 7-year-old girl with neurofibromatosis and optic nerve glioma.

- In selected cases thyroid function tests, serum and urine steroid measurement to exclude precocious pseudo-puberty.
- Pituitary imaging if TCPP confirmed.

Magnetic resonance imaging (MRI) is the investigation of choice, since resolution is better than with CT scanning. Imaging is now regarded as good practice in all children with TCPP, including girls, although parents can be reassured that an abnormality requiring intervention with surgery or radiotherapy is very unlikely to be found in an otherwise well girl with no clinical features to suggest an underlying lesion.

Management
The object of treatment is to prevent early epiphyseal closure with compromise in final height, and to alleviate psychological distress to the girl and her family. In some cases

the progress of puberty is so indolent that treatment is not indicated. If treatment is to be undertaken, the drug of choice is a GnRH analogue which, when given in pharmacological doses, downregulates GnRH receptors, thus inhibiting LH and FSH secretion. Available preparations are:

- buserelin spray 400 µg four times daily;
- goserelin 3.6 mg s.c. monthly or long acting preparation giving 10.8 mg s.c. 3-monthly;
- leuprorelin 3.75 mg s.c. monthly; and
- triptorelin 3.75 s.c. or 4.2 mg i.m. 3–4 weekly or long-acting preparation giving 11.25 mg i.m.

Note that:

1 Nasal spray preparations require frequent administration and have been largely superseded by depot injections.

2 Long-acting Goserelin (Zoladex LA) given as a subcutaneous dose of 10.8 mg 9–12 weekly has been the preparation of choice in Glasgow since 1996. It has proved to be efficacious and well tolerated with no adverse effects recorded.

3 The Triptorelin preparation Gonapeptyl 3.75 mg (Ferring) has recently been licensed for use in precocious puberty and at the time of writing is the only GnRH analogue to be licensed for use in children in the UK.

Follow-up
Three- to four-monthly clinical and auxological assessment is indicated initially, then six-monthly once the symptoms have largely settled. Pelvic ultrasound is a useful adjunct to clinical assessment. Bone age should be performed annually. Total suppression of symptoms is rarely achieved, but reasonable control with cessation of menses will occur. Occasionally, the addition of cyproterone acetate 25–50 mg/day is required for girls who are particularly difficult to suppress. However, this drug can cause malaise, weight gain and tiredness, and we are reluctant to use it.

The question as to when to stop LHRH-suppressive therapy should be discussed in advance with the family. We have found, using 3-monthly Goserelin, that menses occur 12–18 months after discontinuing the injections. This has led us to recommend stopping therapy at the end of the penultimate year of primary school, so that menses will tend to start during the first year of secondary school. Families whose girls have learning disability may wish to continue treatment for longer but suppressive therapy beyond 11–12 years of age carries the theoretical risk of preventing normal calcium accretion by the skeleton, and so we advise against continuing beyond this age.

Precocious pseudopuberty — feminizing (Table 5.4)
The diagnosis is suspected when there is progressive feminizing precocity associated with a prepubertal LHRH test. Causes include adrenal adenoma, granulosa cell tumour of the ovary and the McCune–Albright syndrome. The last disorder may present with breast development and vaginal bleeding in a girl with *café au lait* patches and bony symptoms or signs on X-ray.

Investigations
Imaging of the ovaries by pelvic ultrasound, adrenal CT/MRI, urine steroid analysis, LHRH test, measurement of the tumour markers α fetoprotein and β hCG, and a skeletal survey may be required.

Treatment
Surgery is the treatment of choice for adrenal and ovarian tumours. Medical treatment for precocious pseudopuberty is directed at restricting or antagonizing sex steroid production. Useful agents include:

- Androgen receptor blockers — cyproterone acetate, flutamide and spironolactone
- 5α-reductase inhibitors — finasteride
- Testosterone biosynthesis inhibitors — ketoconazole
- Aromatase inhibitors — testolactone, anastrozole.

Secondary true puberty resulting from priming of the hypothalamus will require additional GnRH therapy.

Thelarche

Clinical features
Premature thelarche is usually seen in girls of pre-school age (Fig. 5.3). Sometimes the breast development has been present from birth. More commonly, the mother notices breast development, often asymmetrical and with a tendency to wax and wane, from the age of 6–12 months. There are no other features of sexual precocity and height velocity is normal. The bone age and pelvic ultrasound are consistent with chronological age.

Investigations
Bone age and pelvic ultrasound may be waived in mild cases of premature thelarche. In more florid cases these, together with an LHRH test should be performed. The FSH response is often pronounced, with 30- or 60-minute values of up to 25 units/L while LH values are below 4 units/L. Plasma oestradiol is usually unrecordable using standard assays.

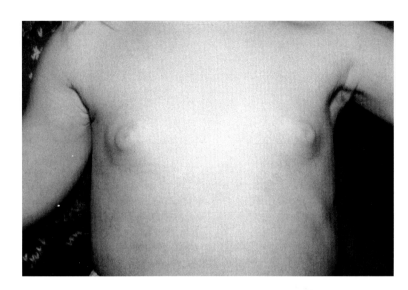

Fig. 5.3 Premature thelarche with stage 2–3 breast development.

Treatment
None is required.

Follow-up
Three- or four-monthly clinic visits over a 1-year period to confirm that breast development is static or regressing.

Thelarche variant
Girls with thelarche variant are usually between 5 and 8 years of age and present with breast development which persists and may progress slightly in association with slight increase in height velocity and modest advance in bone age. Vaginal bleeding sometimes occurs. Pelvic ultrasound may show an oestrogen effect on the uterus, but is less marked than for TCPP. Ovaries may show some enlargement with an increase in follicular activity.

Diagnosis
Thelarche variant is diagnosed in the context of the clinical and pelvic ultrasound pattern in conjunction with a prepubertal LHRH test, normal imaging of the adrenal glands and an indolent clinical course. Thelarche variant probably includes a variety of conditions including TCPP that is too mild to be detected on the LHRH test, and subtle alterations in responsiveness of the ovaries to normal prepubertal LH and FSH levels.

Management
Usually no treatment is required but the girls must remain under surveillance and undergo serial auxology, pubertal staging and pelvic ultrasound examination. Rarely, girls may show unacceptable progression of symptoms and signs so that treatment is requested. Under these circumstances specialist referral is recommended. Peripheral antagonists such as cyproterone may be tried.

Premature menarche
This condition occurs in girls usually between 4 and 8 years of age in whom cyclical vaginal bleeding occurs in the absence of other features of sexual precocity. The diagnosis is made by identifying an endometrial echo on pelvic ultrasound when the child is experiencing vaginal bleeding.

Diagnosis
It is essential not to diagnose premature menarche unless the above criteria are satisfied and other causes of vaginal bleeding have been excluded. These include recurrent vulvovaginitis, foreign body, child sexual abuse, other causes of trauma and vaginal tumours (e.g. rhabdomyosarcoma).

Investigations
Pelvic ultrasound examination is usually sufficient but an LHRH test may be required if there is any suspicion of symptoms other than vaginal bleeding.

Treatment
None is required.

Follow-up
Three- to four-monthly review to confirm normal auxology and no development of other features of sexual precocity.

Androgen-mediated sexual precocity

Exaggerated adrenarche

Clinical features
This is by far the most common cause of androgenicity in girls, and presents from 6 years of age with a history of body odour, greasy skin and hair, weight gain and sometimes mood disturbance, usually in association with some pubic and/or axillary hair development.

Diagnosis
Adrenarche must be distinguished from simple virilizing and non-classical 21-hydroxylase deficiency, and androgen-secreting tumours of the adrenal glands or ovaries. This is usually easy on clinical grounds as the symptoms and signs of adrenarche are relatively mild and in particular there is no clitoromegaly. Bone age may be advanced by 1 year, sometimes more if obesity is an accompanying feature.

Investigations
In all but the mildest cases blood should be taken for serum testosterone, androstenedione, 17-hydroxy progesterone (17-OHP) and dehydroepiandrosterone sulphate (DHEAS) (see Chapter 8 for normal values). Measurement before and after synacthen stimulation is advised if the clinical features are particularly marked.

Treatment and follow-up
No treatment is required. Three- to four-monthly clinical review over a 1-year period is advisable to confirm normal growth rate and lack of progressive virilization. Although a link between low birth weight and smallness for gestational age, exaggerated adrenarche, and subsequent hyperandrogenism (e.g. polycystic ovary syndrome) has been described, the majority of girls are of normal birth weight and clinical features of androgen excess are mild. We do not therefore recommend long term treatment in these patients.

Precocious pseudopuberty—virilizing (Table 5.4)
The simple virilizing variety 21-hydroxylase deficiency is suggested by the combination of advanced growth, clitoromegaly, pubic/axillary hair development and bone age advance, especially if the girl is younger than 6 years. Virilizing tumours of the adrenal or ovary are suggested by a shorter history, so that features such as tall stature may not have had time to become manifest (Fig. 5.4).

Investigations
Measurement of serum testosterone, 17-OHP, androstenedione and DHEAS under basal conditions and after stimulation with Synacthen will confirm abnormal elevation of plasma androgens. Urine steroid analysis will help identify adrenal enzyme defects. Adrenal CT or MRI must be performed as well as careful evaluation of the ovaries on ultrasound. If, despite imaging, a tumour cannot be identified, then measurement of serum androgens by selective venous sampling from the adrenal veins should be carried out in a specialist centre.

Treatment and monitoring
Simple virilizing 21-hydroxylase deficiency is discussed in Chapter 8. Virilizing tumours of the adrenal glands and ovaries are treated surgically.

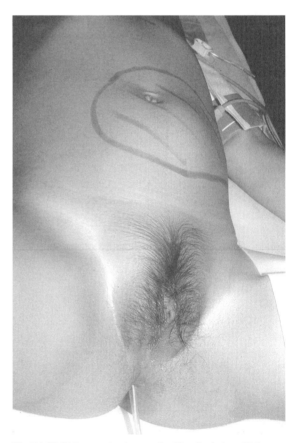

Fig. 5.4 Virilizing ovarian tumour (outline shaded on skin) causing pubic hair and clitoromegaly in a 3-year-old girl. Height status was normal.

Follow-up

This involves 3- to 4-monthly assessment to oversee regression of the features of sexual precocity and a normal growth rate. Depending on availability, MRI or CT scanning of the adrenals or ovaries should be performed annually. Long-term follow-up is needed to pre-empt the development of TCPP because of priming.

Diagnosis and management of sexual precocity in boys

Androgen-mediated sexual precocity

True central precocious puberty (Table 5.5)

This condition is rare in boys, and its occurrence must prompt a search for an underlying cause (Fig. 5.5). Clinical symptoms include rapid growth rate, behaviour disturbances, a deepening of the voice and enlargement of the genitalia. Examination will demonstrate symmetrical enlargement of the testes to volumes >4 mL.

Diagnosis

The combination of sexual precocity with bilateral testicular enlargement makes the diagnosis of TCPP in boys easy. If the testes are prepubertal in volume and/or asymmetrical the causes of precocious pseudopuberty must be sought (see below).

Investigations

LHRH test to confirm true puberty, with measurement

of serum testosterone; imaging of the hypothalamo–pituitary area by MRI (or CT if MRI unavailable). The tumour markers β-hCG and α-fetoprotein should be measured to detect germinomas.

Treatment

Treatment is with an LHRH analogue as described for girls with TCPP. Any underlying cause should be treated.

Monitoring

As for TCPP in girls. In cases where no tumour is found on initial imaging, serial brain imaging at 6- to 12-monthly intervals for a 2- to 3-year period is required to detect an evolving lesion.

Precocious pseudopuberty (Table 5.4)

Simple virilizing 21-hydroxylase deficiency will result in excessive androgen secretion from the adrenal glands. Adrenal tumours may be androgen secreting. In the testes an activating LH receptor mutation affecting all the Leydig cells (germline) causes the condition known as testotoxicosis. An activating LH receptor mutation affecting only a group of cells (somatic) results in a Leydig cell tumour (Fig. 5.6). Precocious pseudopuberty may be seen in boys receiving the anabolic steroid oxymethalone which exerts a direct androgenic effect, as well as priming the hypothalamus and causing true precocious puberty.

Common to all these rare conditions are testes that are either prepubertal in volume (in the case of adrenal disorders or an exogenous cause), modestly and symmetrically enlarged (i.e. 3–4 mL in testotoxicosis and hCG secreting

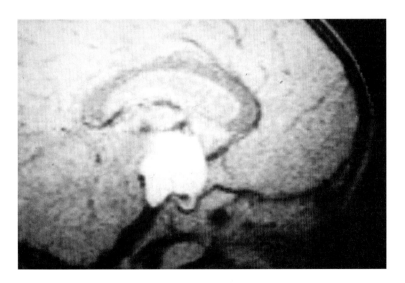

Fig. 5.5 Hypothalamic hamartoma in a 6-year-old boy, causing gelastic seizures and true central precocious puberty.

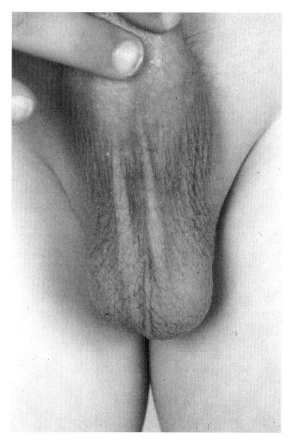

Fig. 5.6 Leydig cell tumour causing slight enlargement of left testis with contralateral atrophy, and precocious pseudopuberty in a 5-year-old boy.

tumours) or unilaterally enlarged with contralateral atrophy (in Leydig cell tumours). By contrast in TCPP both testes are >4 mL in volume.

Investigations
The LHRH test will show suppressed LH and FSH values in precocious pseudopuberty unless the primary disorder has activated the hypothalamus. Investigations of the underlying cause may include β-hCG and α-fetoprotein measurement; serum testosterone, 17-OHP, androstenedione and DHEAS before and after Synacthen stimulation; urine steroid analysis; testicular ultrasound and adrenal CT.

Treatment
Surgery is the treatment of choice for tumours. Medical treatments include ketoconazole, cyproterone, testolactone and flutamide.

Adrenarche
Adrenarche is less common in boys than girls, but is still the most common cause of androgenicity. The clinical diagnosis, investigations and management are as for girls.

Oestrogen-mediated sexual precocity
Feminizing tumours of the adrenal glands and testes are extremely rare. Gynaecomastia, caused either by enhanced oestrogen production from aromatization of testosterone at puberty, or by increased tissue sensitivity to normal circulating oestrogen levels, is a relatively common problem in boys and is discussed below.

Delayed puberty and pubertal failure

Definitions
Delayed puberty: this is arbitrarily defined as absence of signs of secondary sexual development in a girl aged 13 years or a boy aged 14 years. A more practical definition is delay in the onset, progression or completion of puberty sufficient to cause concern to the adolescent, parents or physician.
Pubertal failure: puberty that either fails to begin, or having begun, fails to complete (in which case the term mid-pubertal arrest is often used).
Delayed menarche: first period after 15 years.
Primary amenorrhoea: failure to start periods.
Secondary amenorrhoea: cessation of established menses.
Oligomenorrhoea: infrequent periods (<6/year).

Classification
Delayed puberty is described as **central** or **peripheral**, depending on whether the site of the problem lies in the hypothalamo–pituitary axis or in the gonads. Central delayed puberty can be further subdivided into delay with intact hypothalamo–pituitary axis, and delay caused by impairment of the axis. Table 5.6 gives a working classification of delayed puberty and its causes.

Clinical assessment of boys and girls with delayed puberty

Almost all boys, and most girls, with delayed puberty have simple constitutional delay in growth and adolescence (CDGA). In pathological delayed puberty, the cause may be obvious from the past medical history. The challenge is to diagnose the occasional case of pathological

Table 5.6 Classification of delayed and abnormal puberty (including delayed/absent menarche).

Central (both sexes)		
Intact H–P axis	CDGA	
	Chronic systemic disease	
	Poor nutrition (including anorexia nervosa)	
	Psychosocial deprivation	
	Steroid therapy	
	Hypothyroidism	
Impaired H–P axis	Tumours adjacent to H–P axis	
	Craniopharyngioma	
	Optic glioma	
	Germinomas, astrocytomas	
	Congenital anomalies	
	Septo-optic dysplasia	
	Congenital panhypopituitarism	
	Irradiation	
	Pituitary tumour/optic glioma	
	Craniospinal axis for medulloblastoma	
	Trauma	
	Surgery, e.g. for craniopharyngioma	
	Head injury	
	GnRH/LH/FSH deficiency	
	Congenital idiopathic	
	Kallmann's syndrome	
	Prader–Willi syndrome	
	Laurence–Moon–Bardet–Biedl syndrome	
Peripheral	*Boys*	*Girls*
	Bilateral testicular damage	Gonadal dysgenesis
	Cryptorchidism	Turner's syndrome
	Failed orchidopexy	Pure gonadal dysgenesis
	Atresia	
	Torsion	
	Syndromes associated with cryptorchidism	Irradiation/chemotherapy
	Noonan's	Abdominal irradiation
	Prader–Willi	(for Wilms' tumour)
	Laurence–Moon–Bardet–Biedl	Total body irradiation
		Cyclophosphamide, busulphan
	Gonadal dysgenesis	Intersex disorders
	Klinefelter's	Including CAIS
	Other XY aneuploidy syndromes	
	XO/XY	Polycystic ovary syndrome
	Irradiation/chemotherapy	Toxic damage
	Testicular irradiation	Galactosaemia
	Total body irradiation	Iron overload (thalassaemia)
	Cyclophosphamide	

Abbreviations: CAIS, complete androgen insensitivity syndrome; CDGA, constitutional delay in growth and adolescence; FSH, follicle-stimulating hormone; GnRH, gonadotrophin-releasing hormone; H–P, hypothalamo–pituitary; LH, luteinizing hormone.

delay in puberty in which the cause is not evident and also the more complicated cases with a multifactorial aetiology (e.g. constitutional, nutritional, social).

History
• *Growth pattern*. The history of long-standing short stature followed by a widening gap in height status between the patient and peer group from secondary school entry onwards is suggestive of CDGA.
• *General health*. An enquiry should be made for any symptoms of chronic ill health. Asthma may be associated with delayed puberty, especially when inhaled steroids have been used.
• *Features/associations with gonadal impairment*. These include a previous history of cryptorchidism, orchidopexy, and gonadal irradiation. An idea of sense of smell can be determined by asking whether the adolescent can smell toast burning or unpleasant odours such as rotten eggs.
• *Family patterns*. An enquiry should be made concerning age at menarche in the mother and delayed growth spurt/voice breaking in the father. Where applicable the pubertal milestones of siblings should be sought.
• *Social and educational aspects*. A tactful enquiry as to the occupation and lifestyle of the family may indicate whether or not there is social disadvantage. The presence of learning disability is established by asking about the need for learning support in mainstream or special education. Learning disability may be a component of dysmorphic syndromes associated with delayed puberty (e.g. Noonan's syndrome).

Examination
• Height, weight.
• Measured or (much less reliable!) reported parental heights.
• Measured or reported sibling heights.
• Pubertal staging.
• Nutrition.
• Dysmorphic features.
• General examination with particular attention to clubbing, blood pressure, and fundi.

Investigations
(If indicated)
• Bone age.
• Chromosomes.
• Basal FSH and LH and serum oestradiol/testosterone.
• Pelvic ultrasound in girls.
• LHRH test.
• Serum testosterone 4 days after hCG 100 units/kg (max 1500 units).

• Urinalysis for blood and protein.
• Test of sense of smell.

Causes of delayed puberty and pubertal failure

Central delay with intact axis

Constitutional delay in growth and adolescence in boys
By far the most common cause of delayed puberty, CDGA is usually easily diagnosed by the history of long-standing short/borderline short stature during childhood. Following secondary school entry at 11 years there is a decline in height status so that the boy becomes progressively shorter for age. Commonly there is a family history of delayed puberty.

Frequently, the boy expresses distress to his parents, sometimes related to teasing, but more often because of discomfort at being small and young-looking for age. There is frequently embarrassment about taking showers at school. In boys of 13 years and over the testes usually show some enlargement (4 mL), but no penile enlargement (Tanner stage G2).

Diagnosis
CDGA should usually be a positive diagnosis and not one of exclusion. However, the presence of possible contributory factors such as poor nutrition, socioeconomic and psychological difficulties, and chronic ill health (e.g. severe asthma) can render assessment difficult. Endocrine disturbance is suggested when the short stature and delayed puberty are out of context with the family pattern, when the testes are undescended or abnormal, when there are symptoms and signs such as headache or optic atrophy suggestive of craniopharyngioma, or when penis and testes are hypoplastic, especially in association with an impaired sense of smell (Kallmann's syndrome).

Investigation
None is necessary in CDGA except for bone age estimation, which usually shows delay.

Management
The boy should be reassured that he is normal, simply a late developer. Prediction of adult height is helpful providing that a single experienced observer performs the bone age assessment. In the UK the RUS (TW2) method of Tanner and Whitehouse is preferred. The following medical treatments can be offered in order to enhance growth

rate and expedite the features of puberty without affecting final height outcome.

• In boys aged 11.5–13.5 years, oxandrolone 1.25–2.5 mg at night for 3–6 months may be helpful in maintaining a reasonable prepubertal height velocity (4–6 cm/year). Occasionally, such treatment may increase the height velocity to 6–7 cm/year.

• In boys over 13.5 years of age, testosterone therapy may be offered. This can be given as Sustanon 100 mg intramuscularly once a month for 3 months, or as testosterone undecanoate 40 mg orally daily for 3 months. Such treatment should be given only if the clinician is confident that the delay in puberty is physiological, and not a manifestation of underlying disease (e.g. Crohn's disease).

Follow up

Six-monthly visits to the clinic may be helpful in reassuring untreated boys. Boys treated with oxandrolone or testosterone should be seen 6-monthly for two visits following treatment to ensure satisfactory progress. Occasionally, a repeat course of testosterone is indicated. If there is any doubt about the diagnosis of CDGA it is prudent to keep the boy under observation until testicular volumes are >10 mL.

Constitutional delay in growth and adolescence in girls (Fig. 5.7)

CDGA in girls is less common than in boys but remains the most common cause of delayed puberty. Characteristically, the tempo of puberty, when it starts, is slower and a gradual increase in height rather than a discernible adolescent growth spurt is observed (Fig. 5.7).

Diagnosis

CDGA in girls must be distinguished from Turner's syndrome as well as other pathological causes of delayed puberty. In doubtful cases, the chromosomes and basal gonadotrophins should be checked and a pelvic ultrasound performed. It should be noted that failure to identify one, and occasionally both, ovaries may occur in normal girls.

Treatment

In contrast to boys, who can be given a sizeable dose of testosterone with no ill effect on final height, oestrogen therapy in girls is both less effective and more likely to cause premature epiphyseal closure. Occasionally, pubertal delay is so marked and growth rate so slow that there is a need for treatment. In these circumstances growth hormone levels should be measured. Daily ethinyloestradiol 2 µg for a 1- to 2-year period can be given, with concurrent

growth hormone administration if stimulation testing shows growth hormone insufficiency.

Delayed puberty caused by chronic disease

Sometimes the chronic disease is obvious, and the child is referred simply to confirm that no other pathology is responsible and to advise as to possible treatment. The clinician must assess the severity of the chronic disease and confirm that the severity of the delay in growth and adolescence matches the severity of the chronic condition. If this is not the case, then further investigation is indicated.

A small proportion of girls and boys presenting with delayed puberty will be found to have chronic disease as the underlying cause. Gastrointestinal conditions such as coeliac disease and Crohn's disease can be notoriously silent. The following screening investigations are of value in selected cases.

• Chromosomes.

• TFT, LH and FSH, cortisol, prolactin (screening for endocrine disease).

• Full blood count, ferritin, red cell folate, erythrocyte sedimentation rate (screening for gastrointestinal disease).

• IgA anti-transglutaminase antibodies (screening for coeliac disease).

• Creatinine, urea and electrolytes, calcium, phosphate, alkaline phosphatase, urine analysis and culture, renal ultrasound (screening for renal disease).

Impairment of the hypothalamo–pituitary–gonadal axis in boys

Central (Table 5.6)

Some adolescents have clear evidence of damage to the hypothalamo–pituitary axis (e.g. craniopharyngioma) and will clearly not enter or complete puberty without treatment. Adolescents with delayed puberty who do not fulfil the criteria of CDGA pose some difficulty, for the LHRH test cannot distinguish between physiological central delay and true GnRH or gonadotrophin deficiency.

A history of impaired sense of smell, testicular maldescent and/or surgery and assessment of academic performance must be sought. Examination includes a search for dysmorphic features, systemic examination and detailed examination of the external genitalia. Investigations are detailed above.

Management

In doubtful cases it is best to induce puberty with testosterone from the age of 13–14 years onwards until either full secondary sexual development has been achieved or

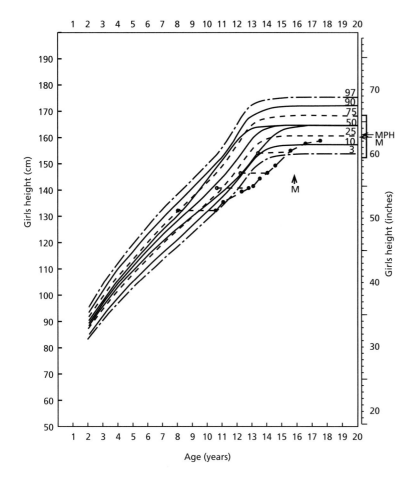

Fig. 5.7 Growth chart of girl with delay in growth and adolescence showing attenuated and late growth spurt with menarche at 15 years old. Final height is equal to the mid parental height (MPH). M, menarche.

spontaneous testicular development to >10 mL has taken place (indicating intact endogenous gonadotrophin secretion). If spontaneous testicular enlargement has not occurred by the age of 16–18 years, replacement therapy should be discontinued and the gonadal axis fully re-evaluated.

Peripheral (Table 5.6)

Primary hypogonadism is suggested by the combination of:
• history compatible with testicular injury (bilateral cryptorchidism, testicular surgery, testicular irradiation, total body irradiation, bilateral torsion);
• behaviour and learning difficulties (evocative of a chromosomal disorder, such as Klinefelter's syndrome);
• abnormal genital examination with one or both testis cryptorchid or abnormally small; and

• testicular volumes may which are inappropriate for genital and pubic hair stage (e.g. 4 mL testes in the context of G4, P4).

Investigations
These will show elevated FSH (above 10 units/L) with exaggerated LH and FSH responses to LHRH (FSH often above 50 units/L). Human chorionic gonadotrophin test may show impaired testosterone rise, or no rise in severe cases.

Management
Anorchic subjects will clearly require therapy, as will individuals with poor progression of secondary sexual development, particularly if testosterone levels are low with poor response to hCG. By contrast, boys with low testicular volumes but normal genital and pubic hair develop-

ment and acceleration of linear growth will not require treatment. As with central hypogonadism, it is best to treat doubtful cases pre-emptively rather than waiting, which carries the risk that development may not progress satisfactorily, resulting in distress to the patient.

Treatment of hypogonadism

We recommend giving intramuscular testosterone as follows:

- Sustanon 100 mg every 6 weeks for the first year.
- Sustanon 100 mg every 4 weeks for the second year.
- Sustanon 250 mg every 4 weeks for the third year, then 250–500 mg every 3–4 weeks depending on clinical factors and serum testosterone levels.

Alternatives include oral testosterone undecanoate 40 mg/day for the first year, 80 mg/day for the second year and 120 mg/day thereafter. Testosterone pellets implanted every 3–6 months can be used once secondary sexual development is established but are not currently used to induce puberty. Testosterone patches are available for adults, but experience of inducing puberty with this method is still limited.

Impairment of the hypothalamo–pituitary–gonadal axis in girls

Central

The causes of hypothalamic and pituitary gonadotrophin deficiency in girls are similar to those in boys, although isolated GnRH and gonadotrophin deficiency is rarer. Investigations will show low LH and FSH levels. As for boys, management involves inducing puberty in doubtful cases (see below).

Peripheral

Gonadal dysgenesis as a result of Turner's syndrome or iatrogenic damage from total body irradiation are the main causes of primary gonadal failure in girls.

Investigation
Basal FSH and LH will be elevated in frank ovarian impairment. An LHRH test may be required to demonstrate milder germ cell damage. Pelvic ultrasound may show a less developed uterus than would be expected from the pubertal stage, while ovaries may be small or unidentifiable.

Management
In doubtful cases pubertal induction should be offered from 13 years.

Treatment
It is important for oestrogen replacement to be gradual, not only to avoid premature fusion of the epiphyses, but also to prevent unsightly overdevelopment of the areolae of the breast. We recommend the following regimens.

- Ethinyloestradiol 2 µg/day for 1 year followed by 4 µg/day for a further year.
- Ethinyloestradiol 6, 8 and 10 µg/day during the third year, in 4-monthly steps.
- Norethisterone 5 mg/day for the first 5 days of each calendar month once the ethinylestradiol dosage reaches 10 µg/day, or sooner if breakthrough bleeding occurs.
- Low-dose combined contraceptive pill, e.g. Loestrin 20 (21 days on and 7 days off) during fourth year.
- Involvement of a gynaecologist once pubertal induction is complete so that further modes of oestrogen replacement (such as transdermal patches) can be discussed.

Other pubertal disorders

Menstrual problems

The most common complaint is that of irregular, prolonged and heavy uterine bleeding, sometimes associated with considerable discomfort. This is related to immaturity of the hypothalamic–pituitary–ovarian axis during the first few years after onset of menses, and should be considered a normal phenomenon. Usually no treatment is required other than simple analgesia. However, the symptoms are sometimes so intrusive that the family demand treatment. Under such circumstances the following strategies may help:

- Norethisterone 5 mg/day for the first 5–10 days of menstrual bleeding. This is to help shed the endometrial lining following anovulatory cycles (when no corpus luteum is produced).
- Low-dose contraceptive pill for a 1-year period.
- In cases where the contraceptive pill alone does not settle irregular uterine bleeding, norethisterone 5 mg/day can be added to days 10–20 of the cycle.

Amenorrhoea and oligomenorrhoea are commonly seen as part of normal delayed puberty, and are particularly likely to occur in the context of low body mass caused by extreme physical training, poor nutrition and eating disorders such as anorexia nervosa.

Primary amenorrhoea is seen in girls with pubertal failure, anatomical disorders of the reproductive tract and in the syndrome of complete androgen insensitivity (see Chapter on Intersex).

Investigation

None is required where the history and examination indicate the diagnosis. Pelvic ultrasound assessment and blood samples for chromosomes, gonadotrophins and sex steroids are helpful in selected cases.

Hirsutism and hypertrichosis

There is an overlap between hirsutism (inappropriate/excessive hair growth in androgen-dependent sites such as moustache and beard area, chest, etc.) and hypertrichosis (generalized increase in body hair).

Hirsutism may be seen in the following instances:
- certain ethnic groups, e.g. Mediterranean, Indian subcontinent;
- caused by androgen secretion by ovarian or adrenal tumours and adrenal enzyme disorders;
- as part of the polycystic ovary syndrome (PCOS); and
- idiopathic, presumably caused by increase in end organ sensitivity.

Hypertrichosis may be seen in:
- certain ethnic groups as for hirsutism;
- primary hypothyroidism;
- Cushing's syndrome, especially iatrogenic;
- certain dysmorphic syndromes;
- secondary to drugs such as diazoxide and cyclosporin A; and
- idiopathic.

Diagnosis and management

Androgen excess can be gauged by accompanying features such as tall stature, bone age advance, clitoromegaly, etc. PCOS is suggested by accompanying oligomenorrhoea and/or obesity.

Investigations

These are unnecessary if the hirsutism is mild and the cause obvious (e.g. racial). In selected cases investigations should be performed as for PCOS.

Treatment

Treatment is directed at the underlying cause, and where this is not possible, cosmetic strategies include bleaching of facial hair, removal of hair by electrolysis and referral to a dermatologist for consideration of laser treatment.

Polycystic ovary syndrome

Polycystic ovary syndrome (PCOS) is defined as hyperandrogenism with ovulatory dysfunction, is not usually seen before the third decade of life, but may occur in postmenarchal teenagers and, very occasionally, in premenarcheal girls. The clinical features of PCOS include obesity, hirsutism, greasy skin and hair, acne, oligo/amenorrhoea and subfertility. Polycystic ovaries are diagnosed if there are 10 or more follicular cysts measuring 2–8 mm in diameter and arranged either peripherally around a dense core of stroma or scattered throughout an increased amount of stroma. Polycystic ovaries have been reported in over 20% of volunteer women and are not therefore diagnostic of PCOS. Moreover, polycystic ovaries are not always present in women with PCOS. Laboratory features of PCOS include elevated serum androgens (particularly testosterone and androstenedione), LH hypersecretion, hyperinsulinism and low SHBG. Frequently, only some of the clinical and laboratory features are present.

The cause of PCOS is controversial. Insulin resistance appears to be an inherent feature, even in non-obese patients. One hypothesis for the pathophysiology of PCOS concerns the type of phosphorylation of the insulin receptor. Under normal circumstances the insulin receptor is activated by *tyrosine* autophosphorylation leading to increased tyrosine kinase activity. There is evidence that in some patients with PCOS *serine* phosphorylation of the insulin receptor occurs, resulting in an inhibition of insulin signaling with consequent hyperinsulinaemia and insulin resistance. However, as the insulin receptor on steroidogenic cells is normally phosphorylated, the increase in insulin levels results in hyperandrogenism by increasing 17-hydroxylase and 17,20-desmolase enzyme activity. The resultant ovarian hyperandrogenism leads in turn to LH hypersecretion and enlarged polycystic ovaries.

Diagnosis and management

In a girl with a history suggestive of PCOS and enlarged ovaries on ultrasound, investigations are directed at confirming the diagnosis and excluding conditions such as non-classical 21 hydroxylase deficiency and other causes of hyperandrogenism. The full investigation of PCOS with exclusion of 21 hydroxylase deficiency is as follows:
- pelvic ultrasound;
- basal LH and oestradiol;
- fasting plasma insulin and SHBG measurement;
- basal serum androstenedione, testosterone, DHEAS, and 17-OHP
- if basal 17-OHP is elevated a standard Synacthen test (250 μg) and 24 hr urine for steroid analysis are indicated to exclude non-classical CAH.

Treatment

Mild cases do not require treatment. The cornerstone of non-medical management is weight reduction which reduces the hyperinsulinism. Medical treatment is directed at the hyperinsulinaemia and hyperandrogenism. Metformin 500 mg once, twice or three times daily is used in hyperinsulinaemic girls especially in the context of obesity. The dose may need to be adjusted according to side effects such as diarrhea. Dianette (containing cyproterone and ethinyloestradiol) is useful in combating signs of androgen excess. It is important to manage PCOS in collaboration with an adult endocrine physician or gynaecologist experienced in the field.

Breast problems

Breast problems can be divided into gynaecomastia in boys and either asymmetrical or symmetrical smallness or largeness of breast size in girls.

Boys with gynaecomastia

An unfortunate emphasis in fat distribution towards the breast area in simple obesity causes apparent gynaecomastia. Exaggerated breast development at puberty is the most common cause of true gynaecomastia in boys. Normal genital and testicular development should be verified. In severe or doubtful cases, chromosomes for Klinefelter's syndrome, basal gonadotrophins and serum oestradiol should be checked. Occasionally, drugs such as spironolactone will cause gynaecomastia.

Treatment

If gynaecomastia is severe and causing distressing problems (Fig. 5.8), e.g. the boy will not participate in physical activities or have showers in front of his peers, then plastic surgery referral is indicated with a view to mammary reduction by either liposuction or subareolar incision and removal of excess tissue.

Girls with asymmetrical or symmetrical smallness or largeness of breasts

Symmetrical enlargement

Occasionally, breast size is unacceptably large to the girl and family, in which case referral to a plastic surgeon for consideration of reduction mammoplasty is indicated.

Symmetrical smallness

Girls with delayed puberty will have smaller breasts than their peers and can be reassured accordingly. Poor breast growth may occur in girls who have received chest irradiation for cancer (e.g. lung metastases). Once optimal breast size has been achieved by waiting for endogenous puberty to complete, or by oestrogen administration in girls with gonadal failure, referral for augmentation mammoplasty should be discussed with the family. If there is reluctance

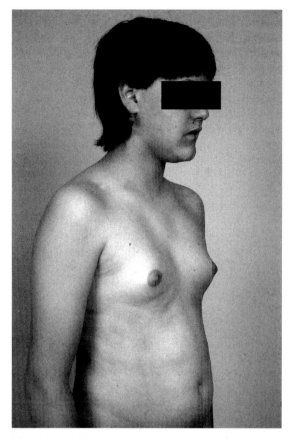

Fig. 5.8 Idiopathic gynaecomastia in an adolescent boy.

to inject foreign material, such as silicone, into the breasts of teenage girls on the part of the plastic surgeon, then reconstructive surgery should be considered.

Asymmetrical largeness or smallness

Asymmetrical breast development is very common in the early stages of puberty, particularly in girls with sexual precocity. Occasionally, postpubertal girls present with an unacceptable discrepancy in breast size. Investigation is unhelpful and referral to a plastic surgeon is indicated for either reduction mammoplasty on one side or augmentation mammoplasty on the other.

Future developments

• A more physiological approach to delivering sex steroid replacement is needed. The most common form of maintenance replacement in adolescent and young adult girls is still the oral contraceptive pill, which delivers no oestrogen for 3 months of the year.

• Measures of the adequacy of sex steroid replacement in adolescents and young adults will include bone mineral density, cardiovascular risk factors and, in females, uterine morphology.

• There is interest in offering males with central hypogonadism, who have completed pubertal induction with testosterone, therapy with LH and FSH to increase testicular volume.

• The psychological assessment and counselling of adolescents and young adults with hypogonadism and infertility is an important area for further development.

Potential pitfalls

• Girls with apparent breast development in association with weight gain, tall stature, and pubic hair may be considered to have precocious or early puberty when the actual diagnosis is exaggerated adrenarche in association with simple obesity (causing increased growth rate) and giving the impression of true breast development. Pelvic ultrasound is useful in showing a prepubertal uterus, but a GnRH test may be required to clarify the diagnosis in some cases.

• The diagnosis of true puberty cannot be made by measurement of basal gonadotrophins. A stimulation test with GnRH is needed. In the early stages of true puberty the GnRH test may show a pre-pubertal response.

Controversial points

• What is the preferred option for the hormonal treatment of CDGA in boys?

• What hCG regimen (dose, number of injections, and time scale) should be used in the gonadal assessment of boys?

• What is the optimal treatment in girls with CDGA?

• There is no consensus as to the most physiological and acceptable methods of long-term sex-steroid replacement in boys and girls with hypogonadism.

When to involve a specialist centre

• Girls with sexual precocity when: (a) diagnosis unclear; or (b) treatment contemplated.

• All boys with sexual precocity.

• Hypogonadism.

• Polycystic ovary syndrome should be managed jointly with an adult/reproductive endocrinologist, or gynaecologist.

CASE HISTORIES

Case 1

A 7-year-old girl presents with breast enlargement and slight vaginal discharge, together with moodiness and body odour. There is no relevant past history and she is well with no headaches, visual disturbance or polydipsia. Mother and two elder sisters had early menarche at 10–11 years. At the age of 7.8 years the girl looks more like an 11-year-old and bone age is advanced at 10.8 years. Height is on the 90th centile and mid-parental height 50th centile. Examination shows Tanner stage B3, P2, A1. Pelvic ultrasound shows heart-shaped uterus with 4-mm endometrial echo, uterine length 5 cm. Ovaries are 3.5 mL in volume with five or six 6-mm follicles in each. GnRH test shows basal/stimulated values of 2.6/20 units/L for LH, and 3.2/15 units/L for FSH.

Question
What is the diagnosis, what further investigations should be carried out, and what treatment should be offered?

Answer
This girl has true precocious puberty—onset of pubertal development before the age of 8 years in a girl with a pubertal LHRH test. Idiopathic TCPP is the likeliest cause but it is now regarded as good practice to carry out pituitary imaging with MRI in girls as well as boys with TCPP. Given the age of the girl, the intensity of pubertal tempo and the behaviour disturbances, most clinicians would recommend suppressive therapy with an LHRH analogue but this must be carefully discussed with the family.

Case 2

A boy of 14 is referred with short stature and concern over pubertal development. He is a somewhat reticent historian but systematic inquiry reveals a fall-off in school attendance and performance over the past year. Further questioning indicates that he has been experiencing some diarrhoea and abdominal pain. On examination the boy does not look unwell, but weight has dropped from 42 kg at clinic 3 months ago to 39.2 kg now. Height at 138 cm is below the 3rd centile (mid-parental height 25th centile). There is mild finger clubbing. The testes are enlarged (4 mL) with scrotal laxity but prepubertal penis and no pubic or axillary hair. Examination is otherwise unremarkable, blood pressure 110/70. Bone age is delayed at 11.2 years.

Question

What is the pubertal stage in this boy? What is the clinical diagnosis? What (if any) investigations should be carried out. What treatment should be offered?

Answer

The pubertal stage is G2, P1, A1. While physiological delay in puberty is by far the most common cause of short stature and delayed puberty in boys, the vague abdominal symptoms, poor school performance, and finger clubbing suggest that the boy should be investigated for chronic disease. Barium meal and follow-through showed extensive abnormality in the small bowel, particularly the terminal ileum and the diagnosis of Crohn's disease was subsequently confirmed.

This case illustrates the importance of history taking and general examination in endocrine practice It would be inappropriate to carry out a height prediction on this boy, whose delayed puberty was caused by illness. Successful treatment of the underlying disease, rather than testosterone therapy, is indicated here.

Case 3

A girl of 14 years is seen in the joint oncology/endocrine clinic with concern over delayed menarche. She developed acute lymphoblastic leukaemia aged 10 years, relapsed 18 months after treatment and was successfully managed with autologous bone marrow transplantation. Total body irradiation in the dose of 1400 centigray and cyclophosphamide were given as part of her conditioning pretransplant. On examination she is on the 25th centile for height (mid-parental height 75th centile), Tanner stage B3, P3, A2. Pelvic ultrasound shows a cylindrical uterus measuring 3.2 cm with no endometrial echo, ovaries 1.2 and 1.8 mL in volume with no follicles seen. Basal FSH is 58 units/L, LH 20 units/L, oestradiol <50 pmol/L.

Question

What is the diagnosis, what further data are required, and how should this girl be managed?

Answer

This girl has primary ovarian failure caused by total body irradiation, resulting in mid-pubertal arrest. Pelvic ultrasound shows reduced uterine size and immature configuration attributable to oestrogen insufficiency. She will require oestrogen replacement, but before instituting this her bone age and stimulated growth hormone level should be tested. Bone age was 11.6 years and peak GH level 14 mU/L following insulin hypoglycaemia. Treatment with growth hormone therapy was declined by the girl and her family but she agreed to starting low-dose ethinyloestradiol aiming for a full replacement dose within 18 months.

Further reading

Carr, B.R. (1998) Disorders of the ovaries and female reproductive tract. In: *Williams Textbook of Endocrinology* (eds J.D. Wilson, D.W. Foster, H.M. Kronenberg & P.R. Larsen), 9th edn, pp. 751–818. W.B. Saunders.

Griffen, J.E. & Wilson, J.D. (1998) Disorders of the testes and male reproductive tract. In: *Williams Textbook of Endocrinology* (eds J.D. Wilson, D.W. Foster, H.M. Kronenberg & P.R. Larsen), 9th edn, pp. 819–876. W.B. Saunders.

Griffin, I.J., Cole, T.J., Duncan, K.A., Hollman, A.S. & Donaldson, M.D.C. (1995) Pelvic ultrasound measurements in normal girls. *Acta Paediatrica* **84**, 536–543.

Kelly, B.P., Paterson, W.F., Donaldson, M.D.C. (2003). Final height outcome and value of height prediction in boys with constitutional delay in growth and adolescence treated with intramuscular testosterone 125 mg per month for 3 months. *Clinical Endocrinology* **58**: 267–272.

Marshall, W.A. & Tanner, J.M. (1969) Variations in pattern of pubertal changes in girls. *Archives of Disease in Childhood* **44**, 291–303.

Marshall, W.A. & Tanner, J.M. (1970) Variations in the pattern of pubertal changes in boys. *Archives of Disease in Childhood* **45**, 13–23.

Paterson, W.F., Hollman, A.S., McNeill, E. & Donaldson, M.D.C. (1998) Use of long acting goserelin in the treatment of girls with precocious and early puberty. *Archives of Disease in Childhood* **79**, 323–327.

Tanner, J.M. (1962) *Growth at Adolescence*, 2nd edn, Blackwell, Oxford.

Tsilchorozidou, T., Overton, C. & Conway, G.S. (2004) The pathophysiology of polycystic ovarian disease. *Clinical Endocrinology* **60** (1):1–17.

6 Thyroid disorders

Embryology, anatomy and physiology of the thyroid gland

Embryology and anatomy

The thyroid gland develops from the floor of the pharynx at 4 weeks gestation in the form of a diverticulum which travels inferiorly leaving the thyroglossal tract in the neck. The latter normally disappears but cystic remnants may remain and form a thyroglossal cyst. The diverticulum becomes bi-lobed and fuses with the ventral aspect of the fourth pharyngeal pouch. Organogenesis is under genetic control and the transcription factors TTF1, TTF2 and Pax8 are known to have a crucial role.

Physiology

The main function of the thyroid gland is to synthesize thyroxine (T_4) and triiodothyronine (T_3).

Control of thyroid metabolism

The hypothalamus secretes thyrotrophin-releasing hormone (TRH) which stimulates the anterior pituitary to secrete thyroid-stimulating hormone (TSH). TSH acts on the thyroid cell by binding to a specific receptor (TSH-R) as shown in Fig. 6.1. The occupied receptor activates the G stimulatory protein which then stimulates thyroid metabolism via the adenylate cyclase, calcium and phospholipase C pathways.

Thyroxine synthesis

Figure 6.2 shows the main steps in T_4 synthesis. Dietary iodine is actively taken up by the thyroid follicular cells and oxidized to iodide. Tyrosyl residues on the thyroglobulin molecule are then iodinated to form monoiodotyrosine (MIT) and diiodotyrosine (DIT). These iodinated tyrosine molecules are coupled to form the iodothyronines, followed by cleavage of the residues from the thyroglobulin molecule to release MIT, DIT, T_3 and T_4. The tyrosine molecules then undergo deiodination to salvage the iodide. The thyroid gland is the sole producer of T_4 and produces 20% of T_3. Most T_3 is produced by deiodination in the peripheral tissues. T_3 is 3–4 times more potent than T_4 and is responsible for most thyroid activity. Gene mutations encoding various thyroid enzymes, eg thyroid peroxidase, may occur resulting in dyshormonogenesis. These mutations are inherited in an autosomal recessive manner.

Thyroxine metabolism

After T_4 is secreted by the thyroid gland, it is metabolized by the tissue enzymes deiodinase type I, II and III. Type II deiodinase catalyses T_4 to T_3 conversion by outer ring deiodination (ORD) (Fig. 6.3). Type III deiodinase converts T_4 to the inactive reverse T_3 (rT_3) by inner ring deiodination (IRD) while type I deiodinase catalyses both ORD and IRD. Seventy per cent of circulating T_4 and 50% of circulating T_3 is bound to thyroxine-binding globulin (TBG), the remainder to other proteins, primarily albumin. Only

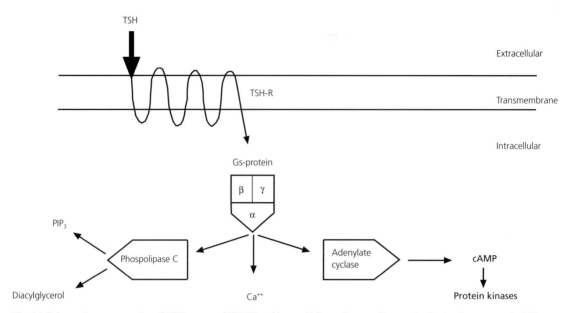

Fig. 6.1 Schematic representation of TSH receptor (TSH-R) and intracellular pathways. Gs-protein, G stimulatory protein; PIP_3, phosphatidyl inositol triphosphate.

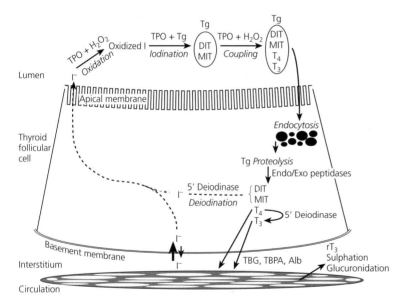

Fig. 6.2 Schematic representation of thyroxine (T_4) and triiodo-thyronine (T_3) synthesis. TPO, thyroid peroxidase; H_2O_2, hydrogen peroxide; Tg, thyroglobulin; MIT, monoiodo-tyrosine, DIT, diiodo-tyrosine; TBG, thyroxine-binding globulin; TBPA, thyroid binding pre-albumin; Alb, albumin; rT_3, reverse T_3.

0.03% of circulating T_4 and 0.3% of T_3 is unbound. Thus, total T_4 and T_3 concentrations reflect the TBG concentration, while free hormone measurements represent the active hormones and are therefore a more accurate assay of thyroid function.

Action of the thyroid hormones

The thyroid hormones have profound effects on growth, neurological development, metabolism, and cardiovascular function. T_4 and T_3 bind to α, β1 and β2 receptors in the target tissues, e.g. pituitary and hypothalamus (β2), liver (β1 and β2), heart (α), and brain (α and β1). This results in an increase in oxygen consumption, altered protein carbohydrate and lipid metabolism and potentiation of the action of catecholamines.

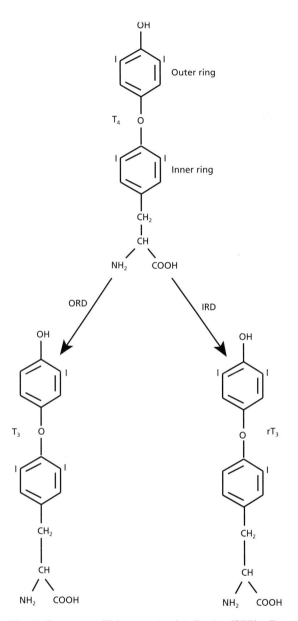

Fig. 6.3 Conversion of T_4 by outer ring deiodination (ORD) to T_3 and inner ring deiodination (IRD) to reverse T_3 (rT_3).

Fetal and neonatal thyroid metabolism

Fetal thyroid metabolism

During the first trimester the fetus is largely dependent on small amounts of maternal T_4 and T_3 that cross the placenta. Levels of TSH start to rise from the second trimester onwards. Total T_4 rises in response to this and also to increasing TBG levels. However, plasma T_3 and T_4 levels are low in fetal life compared with high inactive rT_3 levels because of the fetal predisposition to inactivation of the thyroid hormones. Although plasma T_4 and T_3 are low, these hormones are present in relatively high concentrations in target tissues, such as the brain. Furthermore, while only small amounts of maternal T_4 and T_3 cross the placenta, the quantities are significant so that thyroxine is measurable in babies with thyroid agenesis shortly after birth. Maternal iodine deficiency and maternal hypothyroidism are both associated with intellectual impairment in the child, proof of the vital importance of the maternal contribution to fetal thyroid function.

Thyroid function in term neonates

At birth there is an acute release of TSH. This TSH surge results in high T_4 and T_3 levels (Fig. 6.4). The ratio of T_4 and T_3 to rT_3 rises corresponding to preferential ORD of T_4 and decreased thyroid hormone inactivation. Levels of T_4 and T_3 are high by 7 days, falling thereafter so that by 14 days of age concentrations are similar to those found in infancy and childhood.

Thyroid function in preterm neonates

The preterm infant, especially below 34 weeks gestation, shows the fetal pattern of low plasma T_3 and T_4 with high rT_3. Factors contributing to this pattern include immaturity of the hypothalamic–pituitary axis, premature cessation of the small but significant maternal contribution to circulating thyroid hormone levels, and persistence of the fetal tendency towards inactivation of T_4 and T_3. It is uncertain whether or not the preterm thyroid state should be regarded as physiological, or pathological and requiring intervention. The situation is complicated by the knowledge that concentrations of thyroid hormones in the tissues may be substantially different to those found in the plasma. The issue of low T_4 levels in preterm infants is discussed further below.

Thyroid function tests

Table 6.1 shows the normal values for the commonly measured thyroid function tests. Free T_4 (FT_4) or T_4 and TSH measurement are the mainstay of assessment in hypothyroidism, with TSH the most sensitive indicator of primary disease. In primary hyperthyroidism, TSH is suppressed and there is preferential conversion of T_4 to T_3, so that the latter should be measured in suspected cases. TBG measurement is helpful in distinguishing between spurious

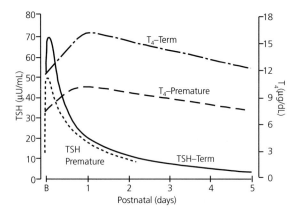

Fig. 6.4 Changes in serum TSH and T_4 concentrations in full-term and premature infants during the first 5 days of life. (From Fisher & Klein 1981,).

and true hypothyroxinaemia but is redundant if FT_4 is measured. Measurement of thyroid peroxidase antibodies (previously antimicrosomal and antithyroglobulin antibodies were measured) is used in the diagnosis of autoimmune thyroiditis. Stimulatory TSH receptor antibodies are positive in Graves' disease. In pituitary and hypothalamic disease, TSH levels will be inappropriately low for the low FT_4 (or T_4) level. The TRH test has traditionally been used to help differentiate secondary and tertiary hypothyroidism. Recent improvements in the quality of hypothalamic and pituitary MRI have provided a further means of assessment.

TRH test

Preparation: non-fasting.

Precautions: may cause mild flushing and desire to micturate.

Protocol: T = 0: 7 µg/kg TRH (protirelin), 200 µg max., intravenously over 1 minute. T = 0, 20, 60 minutes: serum TSH.

Interpretation: normally TSH peaks at 10–30 mU/L at 20 minutes with a fall by 60 minutes. In pituitary disease, TSH levels fail to rise normally in response to TRH. In contrast, in hypothalamic disease there may be a delayed TSH response, with TSH higher at 60 minutes than at 20 minutes.

Table 6.1 Normal values for the common thyroid function tests.

Free T_4	10–26 pmol/L	0.8–2.4 mg/dL
Free T_3	2.5–5.3 pmol/L	2.0–4.0 pg/mL
Total T_4	58–140 nmol/L	4.6–10.5 microgm/dL
Total T_3	1.1–2.2 nmol/L	80–185 ng/dL
TSH	0.5–6.0 mU/L	

Abbreviations: T_3, triiodothyronine; T_4, thyroxine; TSH, thyroid-stimulating hormone.

Definition and classification of thyroid disorders

The term **hypothyroxinaemia** describes the phenomenon of low levels of thyroxine in the context of normal plasma TSH levels. It is encountered in the preterm infant, in acute non-thyroidal illness (e.g. during malnutrition, trauma and diabetic ketoacidosis) and in association with certain drugs. During recovery, thyroid hormone levels spontaneously return to normal.

Hyperthyrotropinaemia refers to mild elevation of TSH (e.g. 7–15 mU/L) in the context of normal FT_4 (or T_4) concentrations.

Hypothyroidism is a state in which the hypothalamic–pituitary–thyroid axis is failing, or is in danger of failing, to produce sufficient T_4. Hypothyroidism can be classified according to:
- site of abnormality: thyroid (primary), pituitary (secondary), hypothalamus (tertiary);
- timing of abnormality: prenatal (congenital) or postnatal (acquired); and
- severity: thyroid axis jeopardized but able to produce normal T_4 levels (compensated hypothyroidism); thyroid axis unable to maintain normal T_4 levels (decompensated hypothyroidism).

Hyperthyroidism refers to overproduction of T_4 and is almost invariably primary.

The term **goitre** refers to thyroid gland enlargement. A goitre is best inspected with the child's neck slightly extended. Asking the child to swallow will make a goitre more obvious. The gland is best palpated with the examiner standing behind the child and can be described in terms of size, texture (e.g. smooth or nodular), consistency and symmetry. A goitre may be subclassified according to thyroid function—hypothyroid, hyperthyroid or euthyroid goitre.

Neonatal hypothyroxinaemia, hyperthyrotropinaemia and transient neonatal hypothyroidism

Neonatal hypothyroxinaemia

Preterm infants have relative hypothyroxinaemia which may become more marked during acute illness (e.g. respiratory distress syndrome). There is some evidence that mortality and neurodevelopmental outcome is worse in preterm infants who have been hypothyroxinaemic, prompting interest in giving thyroid replacement. However, T_4 administration is ineffective, FT_4 and T_4 levels rise but T_3 remains low and it is likely that the administered T_4 is converted to rT_3. Preliminary data suggest that T_3 administration is also ineffective. Moreover, the safety of exposing preterm infants to thyroid hormones is unknown. A recent Cochrane review concluded that there is insufficient evidence at present to support the use of thyroid hormones in preterm infants.

Hyperthyrotropinaemia

Neonatal hyperthyrotropinaemia may reflect the physiological TSH surge or be caused by delayed maturation of the hypothalamic–pituitary–thyroid axis. No treatment is required but the infant should be kept under surveillance.

Transient neonatal hypothyroidism (Table 6.2)

Transient TSH elevation, with or without a low FT_4 (or T_4), accounts for roughly 25% of cases referred by the screening laboratory if TSH is measured on day 5. If TSH elevation is mild (<20 mU/L) and FT_4 (or T_4) is normal then surveillance may be justified. However, if there is any doubt about the thyroid status then thyroxine replacement should be started and the child re-evaluated at a later date.

Table 6.2 Causes of transient neonatal hypothyroidism.

Iodine deficiency
Iodine excess (e.g. following antiseptic administration for sterile procedures)
Perinatal stress (e.g. birth asphyxia, respiratory distress, sepsis)
Down's syndrome
Transplacental transfer of maternal antibodies
Maternal drugs (e.g. carbimazole, amiodarone)

Congenital hypothyroidism

Permanent congenital hypothyroidism is one of the most common disorders in paediatric endocrinology with an incidence of approximately 1 in 4000 births.

Aetiology (Table 6.3)

Thyroid dysgenesis accounts for approximately 85% of congenital hypothyroidism. Inherited or de novo gene mutations affecting the transcription factors TTF1, TTF2 and PAX8 may be responsible for a small number (probably <2%) of cases. In thyroid ectopia, initial thyroid dysfunction may be mild but can deteriorate in later childhood. Autosomal recessive defects in thyroid hormone synthesis account for approximately 10% of congenital hypothyroidism in the UK. A number of gene mutations responsible for these defects have been discovered. Pendred's syndrome-sensorineural deafness with a dyshormonogenetic goitre- is due to a mutation in the pendrin gene. In contrast to infants with thyroid dysgenesis, in-

Table 6.3 Causes of congenital hypothyroidism.

Thyroid dysgenesis
Thyroid agenesis
Hypoplastic gland
Ectopic (usually sublingual) gland

Synthetic defects
TRH and TSH deficiency
TSH receptor defect
G-protein defect (as part of Albright's hereditary osteodystrophy)
Defects in T_4 synthesis (dyshormonogenesis)
    iodide transport defect
    organification defect
    peroxidase deficiency
    thyroglobulin defect
    deiodinase deficiency
Pendred's syndrome

Maternal disease
Thyroid disease with transplacental transfer of thyroid peroxidase antibody or thyrotropin receptor blocking antibody
Maternal drugs, e.g. carbimazole

Miscellaneous
Down's syndrome

Abbreviations: T4, thyroxine; TRH, thyrotrophin-releasing hormone; TSH, thyroid-stimulating hormone.

fants with synthetic defects will have goitrous hypothyroidism provided that the defect is distal to the TSH receptor.

Other causes of congenital hypothyroidism are rare. TSH or TRH deficiency account for hypothyroidism in approximately 1 in 100 000 births and usually occur in the context of disorders causing multiple anterior pituitary deficiencies, e.g. septo-optic dysplasia. TSH receptor mutations are rare and may be clinically indistinguishable from thyroid dysgenesis as the gland will be severely hypoplastic or apparently absent. Rarely, autoimmune thyroiditis from transplacental passage of thyroid antibodies can result in permanent hypothyroidism.

Screening

The combination of difficulty in achieving an early clinical diagnosis and the severe neurodevelopmental consequences of late diagnosis, especially beyond 3 months of age, led to the establishment of screening programmes in the late 1970s and early 1980s in most developed countries. In the UK, screening is usually performed between days 5 and 7 of life. Capillary blood is collected from the baby's heel. Screening options include TSH measurement only (which will miss secondary and tertiary hypothyroidism), T_4 measurement only (which will miss compensated hypothyroidism) and measurement of both T_4 and TSH. In the UK, TSH measurement is used. Practices vary in different centres, but the following is fairly standard.

• If TSH >30 mU/L the laboratory notifies the paediatric endocrinologist.

Notification should be by day 14 of life.

The infant should then be seen and treatment started within 24 hours of notification.

• If TSH is 6–29 mU/L a repeat capillary sample is requested by the laboratory and the paediatrician notified if the repeat value is >6 mU/L. Formal TFTs will then be performed.

A recent study has suggested that preterm babies <1500 g and acutely ill babies >1500 g should have their thyroid function re-checked as they may have undergone an intervention, e.g. iodine exposure, a blood transfusion or a dopamine infusion, which may have effected the results of the initial screening. Re-testing may be particularly important in term infants with cardiac disease due to the association of congenital heart disease and congenital hypothyroidism. It could be performed at 2 and 4 weeks with babies <1500 g also being tested at discharge. Several cases of delayed thyrotropin elevation were detected in this study with some infants also having low thyroxine levels. Though most were due to transient thyroid dys-

function detection was considered important due to the critical role of thyroid hormones on neuro-development. Some centres routinely retest all newborns or selected groups of patients (e.g. patients in NICU). However, this practice is not widespread and further data is required before rescreening guidelines become universal.

It is important to note that no screening programme is perfect and occasional errors will occur, e.g. mislabelling and loss of samples.

Clinical features

Awareness of clinical symptoms and signs is required for the detection of infants missed on the screening programme and for the assessment of infants with high TSH values.

History
• Sleepiness.
• Poor feeding.
• Prolonged jaundice.
• Constipation.
• Hoarse cry.
• Family history of congenital hypothyroidism.
• Maternal history of thyroid disease.

Signs
• Lethargy.
• Jaundice.
• Large tongue.
• Goitre.
• Coarse facies.
• Umbilical hernia.
• Dry skin.
• Wide posterior fontanelle.
• Hypothermia.
• Peripheral cyanosis.
• Oedema.

There is a slightly increased prevalence (5%) of nonthyroidal malformations—particularly cardiac—and a thorough examination is therefore indicated.

Investigations

If hypothyroidism has been diagnosed on neonatal screening then an urgent venous sample for FT_4 (or T_4) and TSH measurement should be performed to confirm the diagnosis. In most laboratories the result can be obtained on the same day. In a well term baby with unequivocal TSH elevation (>30 mU/L) the likelihood of true congenital hypothyroidism is such that treatment should be started immediately. If the TSH <30 mU/L and there are no clinical features of hypothyroidism then treatment can be deferred until the results of the venous sample are known (see transient neonatal hypothyroidism).

The role of isotope scanning in the assessment of babies with congenital hypothyroidism is controversial. ^{99m}Tc-pertechnetate or ^{123}I-labelled sodium iodide scans will, if performed within a few days of starting thyroxine treatment, provide information about the anatomy and site of the thyroid gland and help to distinguish between thyroid dysgenesis and dyshormonogenesis with goitre. However, caution is needed in interpreting the data as decreased or absent uptake of isotope may occur in babies with anatomically normal thyroid glands following exposure to iodine, in the presence of maternal blocking antibodies or if the scan is performed after thyroxine treatment has led to TSH suppression.

In cases where the scan has shown normal or high uptake of isotope, and normal thyroid position and anatomy, the likely diagnosis is dyshormonogenesis or occasionally transient hypothyroidism. In some centres more detailed investigations are carried out in order to reach a more specific diagnosis. Occasionally, a perchlorate discharge test is performed. This test can help diagnose the most common dyshormonogenetic defect, peroxidase deficiency. In this condition there is a 60–70% discharge of radioactive iodide within 1 hour of administering perchlorate (normally less than 10% is discharged within 1 hour). Increasingly in cases of suspected dyshormonogenesis specific gene mutations are being identified and the perchlorate discharge test is being performed less often.

Thyroid ultrasound scanning is a promising but relatively untried technique. Failure to identify thyroid tissue in the neck strongly suggests thyroid dysgenesis with either absent or ectopic gland, while identification of a small, normal or enlarged thyroid gland *in situ* indicates the need for further investigation. In some centres both isotope and ultrasound scanning are performed.

X-ray of knee in newborns with congenital hypothyroidism gives an index of the severity of intrauterine hypothyroidism but is of no diagnostic value and is rarely performed now in the UK.

All infants with congenital hypothyroidism should have their hearing tested. In countries with universal neonatal hearing screening this will be routinely done. Where there is no such programme a hearing assessment should be arranged.

Treatment

Initial treatment regimens are controversial. FT_4 (or T_4)

should be maintained in the upper half of the normal range but there is no consensus as to whether the high TSH should be suppressed quickly or allowed to normalize over a period of weeks or months. Most paediatricians advocate a high dose regimen of 10–15 µg/kg/day. One such regimen consists of administering thyroxine 50 µg/day for 1 week followed by 37.5 µg/day thereafter. This regimen results in rapid normalization of thyroid function tests with FT_4 (or T_4) in the high/normal range. Untoward symptoms such as tachycardia, irritability and diarrhoea are rare. Thyroid function should be measured after 2 weeks of treatment. If there are clinical or biochemical signs of overtreatment on 37.5 µg/day the dosage can be reduced to 25 µg/day. An alternative regimen consists of giving 6–9 µg/kg/day which often equates to a starting dosage of 25 µg/day.

Advocates of the high-dose regimen believe that it optimizes the child's IQ and neuro-development. Advocates of the low-dose regimen cite the absence of the side-effects of overtreatment, the rare possibility with overtreatment of premature craniosynostosis and evidence that a higher starting dose may lead to later behavioural difficulties.

The normal range of TFTs is higher in neonates than in older children and many laboratories will have slightly different normal ranges for the different age groups.

The dosage of thyroxine is increased as the infant grows and in line with the TFTs. Often a dose of 50 µg/day is required at approximately 1 year of age and 75 µg/day at about 2 years of age. The dosage of thyroxine is approximately $100 \mu g/m^2/day$ and doses of up to 200 µg once daily may be required in adulthood. Thyroxine in infants can be administered as crushed tablets (smallest tablet 25 µg, but this can be halved and dose changes of 12.5 µg can be made) or as a suspension. However, the latter has a shelf-life of only 1 week, will require frequent repeat prescriptions and is best avoided.

Soy milk formulas and iron medication administered in close time proximity to thyroxine can interfere with thyroxine absorption. These infants may require more frequent follow-up and higher doses of thyroxine.

Follow-up

Developmental progress, growth and thyroid function should be checked monthly from 1 to 3 months of age, every 2–3 months from 3 months to the end of the first year, every 3–4 months between 1 and 3 years of age and every 4–12 months thereafter until growth is completed. Follow-up should be more frequent if there are concerns about compliance or if abnormal values are obtained.

At all stages the aim is to keep the FT_4 (or T_4) in the upper half of the normal range. In the case of low treatment regimens it may take several months for the TSH levels to fall to normal. Failure to comply with treatment, especially during the first 3 years of life, may impair normal brain development. Conversely, overtreatment may cause features of thyroxine excess. If the TSH is >5 mU/L then the dose may need to be raised by 12.5–25 μg/day and the TFTs should be repeated in 4–6 weeks. Conversely, the dose should be reduced by similar amounts if the TSH level is <0.5 mU/L. Information leaflets are very useful, as is contact with a similarly affected child and family or a support group.

A period off treatment for 3 weeks with measurement of FT_4 (or T_4) and TSH before and after stopping treatment is indicated in selected cases at about 3 years of age to exclude transient hypothyroidism. This is unnecessary in infants shown to have an aplastic, hypoplastic or ectopic thyroid gland on a thyroid scan and in cases with a TSH >10 mU/L on treatment after 12 months of age.

Outcome

Neonatal screening programmes have revolutionized the outlook for babies with congenital hypothyroidism and the prognosis is now excellent. However, there is still controversy as to whether very early treatment can completely reverse the effects of hypothyroidism. A large American retrospective controlled trial of pregnant mothers with thyroid disease demonstrated a deficit of 4 IQ points in infants of mothers with a high TSH and a normal FT_4 and a deficit of 7 IQ points in infants of mothers with a low FT_4 level (a small number of whom were treated in pregnancy) compared to the control group of infants (none of the babies had congenital hypothyroidism). This suggests that some of the prenatal effects of hypothyroidism may be irreversible.

The infants at greatest risk of neuro-developmental impairment are those with thyroid agenesis and low initial FT_4 levels. Delay in starting treatment and poor compliance with treatment are further exacerbating factors. Neuro-developmental impairment is subtle and selective and can effect a wide range of areas, including sensorineural hearing and speech delay, visuospatial abilities, motor skills, memory, arithmetic abilities, attention and behaviour. A 1996 meta-analysis performed on seven major follow-up studies demonstrated that children with congenital hypothyroidism had IQ levels that were, on average, 6 points lower than those of the control group. As a result of the above, children with congenital hypothyroidism tend to mildly underachieve at school. It is possible that the more recently used high-dose initial thyroxine regimens may improve developmental outcome but further studies are needed to substantiate this.

Acquired hypothyroidism

This condition can be difficult to recognize as onset may be very insidious and it has often been present for a number of years prior to diagnosis.

Aetiology

Causes of acquired hypothyroidism

Primary
- Iodine deficiency.
- Autoimmune (Hashimoto's) thyroiditis.
- Thyroid surgery.
- Following irradiation to neck (e.g. craniospinal irradiation, total body irradiation).
- Radioiodine therapy.
- Antithyroid drugs (e.g. carbimazole).
- Goitrogens.

Secondary and tertiary
- Craniopharyngioma and other tumours impinging on the hypothalamic–pituitary axis.
- Neurosurgery.
- Cranial irradiation.

Iodine deficiency

Although this is the most common worldwide cause of hypothyroidism, it more commonly results in a euthyroid goitre. Clinical iodine deficiency is extremely rare in the UK but is more common in other European countries, such as Germany and Poland. The condition is suspected in cases of goitre, a family history of iodine deficiency and from a knowledge of the regional iodine status. It is diagnosed by urinary iodine measurements and treated with trace amounts of iodine. The iodination of salt is reducing the prevalence of this problem.

Autoimmune (Hashimoto's) thyroiditis

This is the most common cause of acquired hypothyroidism in the Western world. It is more common in girls—particularly in adolescence—and there may be a family history. Presentation may be with a goitre with compensated hypothyroidism or with decompensated hypothyroidism with a goitre or an atrophic gland. Autoantibodies are present in 95% of cases. Autoimmune thyroiditis may be associated with other autoimmune diseases, such as diabetes mellitus and Addison's disease, as well as with skin disorders, such as alopecia areata and vitiligo. It is particularly common in Down's syndrome in whom annual capillary TSH screening is recommended from 1 year of age onwards. Girls with Turner's syndrome are also at increased risk.

Miscellaneous causes
These include the hypothalamic–pituitary disorders in which other anterior pituitary hormone deficiencies will almost invariably be present. Dietary goitrogens, such as iodide, cabbage and soya beans, have been reported to cause hypothyroidism.

Clinical features (Fig. 6.5)

History
- Weight gain.
- Tiredness.
- Constipation.
- Cold intolerance.
- Slowing of linear growth ± short stature.
- Poor school performance.
- Delayed puberty (occasionally precocious puberty).
- Menstrual irregularity.
- Presence of other autoimmune disorders.
- History of slipped femoral epiphysis.
- Family history of thyroid or other autoimmune disorders.

Signs
- Myxoedematous facies.
- Short stature.
- Goitre.
- Obesity.
- Dry skin.
- Increase in body hair.
- Pallor.
- Vitiligo.

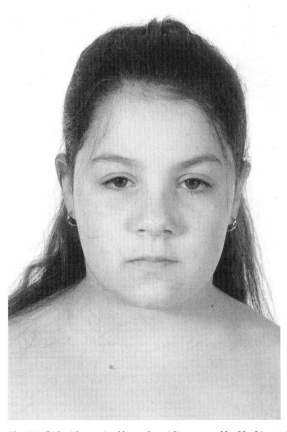 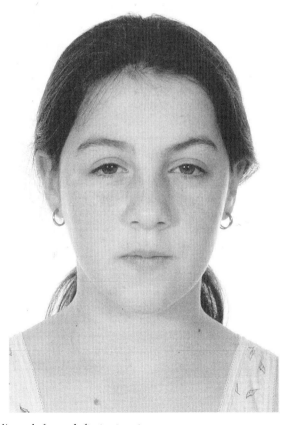

Fig. 6.5 Girl with acquired hypothyroidism caused by Hashimoto's disease before and after treatment.

- Proximal muscle weakness.
- Delayed relaxation of ankle reflexes.
- Delayed puberty (occasionally precocious puberty).

This condition can be very insidious and in retrospect it may become apparent that it has been present for several months or even 2 to 3 years. The principal symptoms of hypothyroidism are tiredness and weight gain, while the key signs are pallor, myxoedematous facies and short stature relative to the mid-parental height. If previous heights are available it may be possible to pinpoint the start of the hypothyroidism. The goitre is usually diffuse and non-tender but may be nodular and is occasionally tender. Usually puberty is delayed, but occasionally cross-stimulation of FSH and LH by TRH may lead to incomplete sexual precocity with enlarged ovaries on ultrasound scan in girls and testicular enlargement in boys. Paradoxically, in all but the most severe cases of acquired hypothyroidism, children do well at school, methodically doing their homework until it is completed.

Investigations

These will depend on the cause of the hypothyroidism. FT_4 (or T_4) and TSH measurement are required to confirm the diagnosis. In acquired hypothyroidism, thyroid peroxidase (TPO) antibodies should always be measured. A bone age is often performed and will show delay. If there is no goitre and the autoantibody screen is negative then an isotope scan should be performed to exclude a late presentation of thyroid dysgenesis. Inappropriately low or normal TSH values in the face of a low FT_4 (or T_4) suggests pituitary or hypothalamic disease which can be further investigated with the TRH test (page 94). Proven secondary and tertiary hypothyroidism should be investigated by further anterior pituitary testing and by magnetic resonance imaging (MRI).

Treatment

Treatment is with thyroxine $100\,\mu g/m^2/day$ given as a single dose. Children with clinical hypothyroidism should start with a quarter of the target dosage during the first month, building up gradually to the full dosage over a period of 2–3 months. Catch-up growth with increased height velocity and weight loss will occur. Treatment for severe hypothyroidism, however gradual, is often associated with marked adverse symptoms including fatigue, irritability, poor concentration and emotional lability, particularly in children with learning difficulties. School performance may also deteriorate.

There is controversy as to whether euthyroid patients with compensated autoimmune thyroiditis should be treated. A pragmatic approach is to give thyroxine replacement if the TSH value is >15 mU/L, or if the TSH is above 6 mU/L in the presence of a goitre. Occasionally, treatment may be associated with the development of a slipped femoral epiphysis or Perthes' disease, both of which cause leg pain and a limp. However, the former is more likely to be seen as a presenting feature of hypothyroidism.

Follow-up

Considerable surveillance and reassurance may be required by some families during the first few months following diagnosis. Thereafter, clinic visits and thyroid function tests should take place every 6–12 months. The TSH level is a sensitive marker of under- or over-replacement. In the case of non-compliance, FT_4 (or T_4) will be normal if thyroxine was taken on the day of the clinic visit but TSH levels will be raised.

Outcome

The prognosis for autoimmune thyroiditis is very good and the outlook partly depends on whether the child will develop other autoimmune diseases. Most patients need treatment for life, but very occasionally spontaneous remission occurs. Complete catch-up growth following treatment can be expected in mild to moderate cases. However, complete catch-up may not occur in severely affected children with prolonged hypothyroidism. Parents of children with severe hypothyroidism should be warned that it may take up to 2 years before their child is completely back to normal.

Hyperthyroidism

The causes of hyperthyroidism are the following.
- Graves' disease.
- Neonatal thyrotoxicosis.
- Autoimmune (Hashimoto's) thyroiditis.
- Syndrome of selective T4 resistance.
- Autonomous nodules.
- TSH-dependent hyperthyroidism.
- Activating mutations of the TSH receptor.

Graves' disease (Fig. 6.6)

Graves' disease is rare, with an incidence of 0.8 per 100 000 children per year. It usually occurs in the second decade, is six times more common in girls and in up to 60% of cases there is a family history of thyroid disease. It occurs more commonly in children with other autoimmune disorders and there may also be a family history of non-thyroidal autoimmune disease. It is caused by stimulation of the TSH receptor by immunoglobulins. The associated exophthalmos is because of infiltration of the orbit and surrounding structures with lymphocytes, mucopolysaccharides and oedema.

Clinical features
The onset of Graves' disease is usually insidious, over several months, but may be acute.

History
- Anxiety.
- Irritability and hyperactivity.
- Tiredness.
- Deteriorating school performance and handwriting.

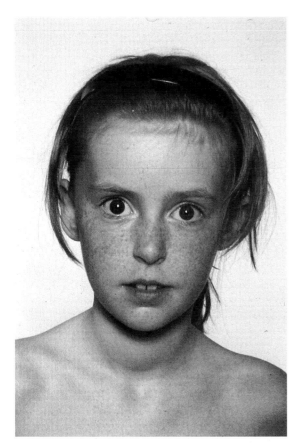

Fig. 6.6 Girl with Graves' disease.

- Weight loss in spite of increased appetite.
- Rapid height increase.
- Palpitations.
- Heat intolerance.
- Sleep disturbance.
- Diarrhoea.
- Menstrual irregularities or amenorrhoea.
- Family history.

Examination
- Goitre (usually diffuse).
- Exophthalmos, rarely associated with ophthalmoplegia.
- Tachycardia.
- Hypertension.
- Facial flushing.
- Tremor.
- Sweatiness.
- Relative tall stature (height centile usually above parental target range centiles).
- Thyroid bruit.
- Heart murmur.
- Choreiform movements.

   Thyroid crisis or storm is a form of thyrotoxicosis characterized by an acute onset which may be precipitated by surgery, infections, drug withdrawal/non-compliance and radioiodine treatment. The patient develops hyperthermia, severe tachycardia and restlessness and may become delirious, comatose or die. It is rare in childhood.

Diagnosis
The diagnosis is usually obvious and is confirmed by finding elevated FT_4 (or T_4) and T_3 concentrations, with TSH suppression. Rarely, FT_4 (or T_4) levels are normal but T_3 levels are elevated, so called 'T_3 toxicosis'. TSH receptor antibodies (TRAb) are elevated and in most cases thyroid peroxidase (TPO) antibodies are also positive. Bone age is usually advanced.

Treatment
The majority of patients do not require admission. If symptoms are severe, e.g. marked tachycardia and hypertension, then admission may be necessary till the propranolol has taken effect and the patient can then be reviewed in clinic the following week.

   The three modalities of treatment in Graves' disease are medical, radioactive iodine and surgery.

Medical treatment
Treatment is with one of the following antithyroid drugs:

1 Carbimazole or methimazole initial dose 0.25 mg/kg three times a day in children up to 12 years of age and 10 mg three times a day in children aged 12 to 18 years. The maximum total daily dose is 40 mg a day.
2 Propylthiouracil 5–10 mg/kg/24 hours given in three divided doses. Treatment should be started at the lower dose. It may take 2 weeks to become euthyroid.

There is some evidence that carbimazole and methimazole have fewer side effects than propylthiouracil. The most serious side-effect of these drugs is agranulocytosis and neutropenia. It is idiosyncratic and not predictable from regular blood tests but may be commoner with higher drug doses. Routine monitoring of the full blood count is not indicated. Neutropenia occurs in approximately 0.3% of patients usually within the first 3 months. A slightly greater percentage may develop mild to moderate leucopenia. Patients should be asked to report symptoms of infection—especially sore throat, mouth ulcers and bruising. In such instances treatment should be stopped and an urgent full blood count performed. Ideally, written information should be provided to back up the verbal advice. Stopping the medication nearly always leads to resolution of the problem after 1–2 weeks. In severe cases granulocyte colony-stimulating factor may be used. The alternative drug can often be successfully substituted but in such cases closer monitoring of the full blood count is required to avoid a recurrence. Anti-thyroid drugs can also cause itchy rashes in 2–5% of patients. These are usually transient, can be treated with antihistamines and rarely necessitate a change in therapy. Hepatotoxicity, nausea, headaches and arthralgia may also occur.

Propranolol (dose 250–750 µg/kg/dose three times a day, dose adjusted according to response) is also required during the first few weeks in most cases to help control the signs of sympathetic overactivity, such as tachycardia and tremor. Propranolol can be reduced and stopped once thyroid function returns to normal and should not be used in patients with asthma or heart failure.

After 4–8 weeks of starting antithyroid drugs FT_4 (or T_4) and FT_3 will fall to normal although TSH may remain suppressed for several more weeks. The rapidity of the response is usually proportional to the size of the gland. When the FT_4 (or T_4) and FT_3 fall to within the lower half of the reference range (usually after 6–12 weeks of treatment) there are two possible approaches:
1 Approximately half the previous total dose of antithyroid is administered. In the case of carbimazole or methimazole this can be given as a single daily dose but in the case of propylthiouracil it is given in two divided doses.

The dosage is titrated to maintain normal thyroid hormone concentrations; or
2 the initial antithyroid dosage—sufficient to cause hypothyroidism—is continued, and a small replacement dose of thyroxine, initially 25 µg, is commenced. The dose of thyroxine may need to be increased subsequently depending on the TFTs (block and replace regimen).

Both methods have their advocates. The advantages of the more popular dose titration regimen are that there are fewer side effects on the lower drug doses and that compliance is better on one rather than two drugs. The advantages of the block-and-replace regimen are improved stability with fewer episodes of hyperthyroidism and hypothyroidism, a reduced number of blood tests and clinic appointments and possibly an improved remission rate following a larger antithyroid drug dose.

Eye disease is milder in children than in adults. If the patient develops symptoms such as dry or painful eyes hypromellose eye drops, one drop to each eye up to four times a day may be indicated. In the case of significant symptoms or impaired eye movements early referral to an ophthalmologist is required.

Attempts to stop antithyroid medication after 24 months are usually unsuccessful, particularly in prepubertal children and in those with a moderate or large goitre at presentation. Therefore, a cautious reduction in treatment rather than a sudden discontinuation of antithyroid drugs is recommended. In the majority of cases, ≥75%, the patient relapses. In such cases the options are further medical treatment, radioactive iodine or surgery. Poor compliance with drug treatment and drug side-effects may also lead to consideration of radioiodine treatment or surgery.

Radioactive iodine
Radioiodine therapy should be conducted in collaboration with an adult endocrinologist with a special interest in thyroid disorders.

Radioiodine is administered orally and is given with the aim of ablating the thyroid gland and inducing hypothyroidism. Antithyroid medication should be stopped 5 days prior to treatment and can be re-started if necessary, 1 week later. Following treatment, patients should be reviewed after a few days because of the small risk of a thyroid crisis and subsequently every 6 weeks so that thyroxine treatment can pre-empt the onset of severe hypothyroidism. A small number of patients require a second dose of radioiodine, especially if a low initial dose was used. In a recent study of children and adolescents an average radioiodine dose of 14.7 mCi (approximately 540 MBq), led to the development of hypothyroidism between 40 and 90 days in 75% of patients. Treatment leads to a marked diminution in thyroid volume.

Traditionally there has been a reluctance to give radioiodine treatment to children because of concerns about cancer. There have been cases of thyroid cancer in children who received radioiodine treatment. However, this is rare and thyroid cancer is also commoner in patients with Graves' disease who have not had radioiodine treatment. Long-term follow-up studies of both thyroid and extrathyroid cancer risk in patients who received radioiodine have been reassuring. In any case if a relatively high dose of radioiodine is used this should lead to thyroid gland ablation and the risk of a subsequent malignancy should be extremely low. Nevertheless, further long-term follow-up data of patients treated with the currently used doses of radioiodine is required and in the UK radioiodine treatment is generally considered only in children over 10 years of age. In a minority of patients radioiodine treatment can lead to a marked deterioration in eye disease. Some endocrinologists therefore avoid radioiodine in patients with severe ophthalmopathy.

Thyroid surgery
Euthyroid status must be induced prior to surgery. Some surgeons perform a subtotal thyroidectomy with the aim of rendering the patient euthyroid on no treatment. Such surgery is particularly suitable in non-compliant patients. However, if an insufficient volume of the gland is removed a relapse will occur; if too much is removed hypothyroidism will follow. Furthermore, close follow-up is required to monitor these two eventualities which can occur many years after surgery.

An alternative approach, now considered to be the treatment of choice in many centres, consists of performing a total thyroidectomy. Hypothyroidism results and standard thyroxine treatment is administered. Surgery should be carried out by an experienced thyroid surgeon to minimize the risk of complications. These include recurrent laryngeal nerve palsy with a resultant hoarse voice, hypoparathyroidism causing hypocalcaemia and unsightly keloid scar formation.

Neonatal thyrotoxicosis
This rare condition is caused by the transplacental transfer of maternal TSH receptor antibodies which stimulate the fetal and neonatal thyroid. The higher the thyroid-stimulating immunoglobulin level in pregnancy the greater the risk that the infant will develop thyrotoxicosis. This disease may occur in infants of mothers with active hyperthyroidism who are on treatment and in those with inactive hyperthyroidism. Only a minority of infants of mothers with Graves' disease, <10%, are affected.

The degree of thyroid dysfunction will depend on the net effect of maternal thyroid-stimulating and blocking TSH receptor antibodies, maternal hyperthyroxinaemia and maternal antithyroid drugs. A scheme for the investigation of babies of mothers with Graves' disease and hypothyrodism is outlined in Figure 6.7. TSH and T_4 levels rise in the first few days of life and the assessment of the infant's thyroid status should be made with reference to the normal TSH and T_4 levels at that postnatal age. Babies at high risk of thyrotoxicosis (e.g. thyroid-stimulating immunoglobulin level raised or not measured in pregnancy, clinical thyrotoxicosis or drug therapy in third trimester, evidence of fetal thyrotoxicosis) may need to be observed in hospital for a few days following delivery. Infants at low risk, for instance those whose mothers had normal thyroid-stimulating immunoglobulin levels, may be discharged immediately but parents should be aware of the possible symptoms. These usually develop at 24–48 hours of age, but may be delayed for up to 10 days in babies whose mothers are on antithyroid drugs which can cross the placenta. Most infants have biochemical thyrotoxicosis with no or few symptoms but a minority will be severely affected with goitre, tachycardia, arrhythmias, hypertension, cardiac failure, increased appetite, weight loss, diarrhoea, irritability and exophthalmos. Cord bloods may be normal, especially in infants of mothers on antithyroid drugs, but subsequently T_3 and T_4 levels will rise, while TSH concentrations will fall below the lower limit of normal. The half-life of thyroid stimulating immunoglobulins is approximately 12 days and resolution of the disease corresponds to their degradation so that the disorder is self-limiting over 3–12 week.

Treatment is as shown in Table 6.4. Usually treatment with propylthiouracil, carbimazole or methimazole together with propranolol is sufficient but iodine may also be required and occasionally a sedative such as chloral hydrate is also helpful. In severe cases prednisolone (2 mg/kg/day) may also be needed. The clinical features should significantly improve within 48 hours. After 1 week of treatment the iodine can be stopped and the propranolol reduced. Babies should be reviewed weekly until stable. Subsequently visits can be extended to 2 weekly. The antithyroid drugs may be needed for 6 weeks to 3 months with the dose being gradually reduced to

1. Maternal Graves disease

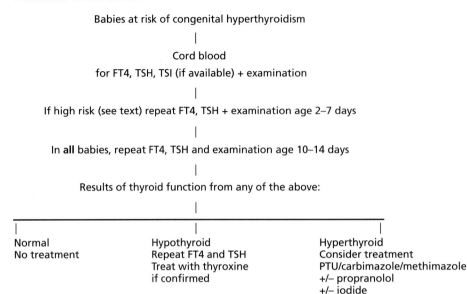

Babies at risk of congenital hyperthyroidism

|

Cord blood

for FT4, TSH, TSI (if available) + examination

|

If high risk (see text) repeat FT4, TSH + examination age 2–7 days

|

In **all** babies, repeat FT4, TSH and examination age 10–14 days

|

Results of thyroid function from any of the above:

|

Normal	Hypothyroid	Hyperthyroid
No treatment	Repeat FT4 and TSH	Consider treatment
	Treat with thyroxine	PTU/carbimazole/methimazole
	if confirmed	+/– propranolol
		+/– iodide

Fig. 6.7 Investigation of babies of mothers with thyroid disease. TSI, thyroid-stimulating immuno-globulin; PTU, propylthiouracil. Amended and reproduced from A. L. Ogilvy-Stuart *Archives of Disease in Childhood* (2002) **87**, 165–171 with permission from the BMJ Publishing Group.

2. Maternal hypothyroidism
This is usually secondary to autoimmune thyroiditis and the mother may be producing thyroid inhibiting or rarely thyroid stimulating antibodies so the baby may develop transient hypothyroidism or, very rarely, hyperthyroidism. These babies should be reviewed at 10 days to 2 weeks and thyroid function (TSH and FT4) measured.

If the maternal hypothyroidism is secondary to congenital aplasia or hypoplasia of the thyroid gland, there is only a slightly increased risk to the baby of hypothyroidism and the Guthrie test should suffice.
If the hypothyroidism is secondary to treatment (surgery or radioiodine) for Graves' disease, the baby is at risk of neonatal thyrotoxicosis and will need to be managed as above.

Table 6.4 Treatment for neonatal thyrotoxicosis.

1 Propylthiouracil 5–10 mg/kg/day orally in three divided doses; or carbimazole (or methimazole) 0.5–1.5 mg/kg/day orally in three divided doses
2 Lugol's solution (5% iodine, 10% potassium iodide = 126 mg iodine/mL) 1 drop (about 8 mg) orally, 8-hourly
3 Propranolol 0.25–0.75 mg/kg orally 8-hourly
4 Chloral hydrate 30 mg/kg/dose orally, 8-hourly as required

keep the baby euthyroid. Mortality rates of up to 20% have been reported, usually from arrhythmias and/or heart failure but occasionally from tracheal compression or infection. There are few data on the long-term sequelae of neonatal thyrotoxicosis. Documented long-term side-effects include an increased risk of intellectual impairment and of craniosynostosis and these babies should therefore be followed up in clinic.

Other causes of hyperthyroidism

Hashimoto's thyroiditis
Hashimoto's thyroiditis may cause thyrotoxicosis in 5–10% of patients. TPO (thyroid peroxidase) antibodies are present and TRAb antibodies (TSH receptor antibodies) are usually absent. Treatment is as for Graves' disease but as the condition is milder and remits more readily; neither radioactive iodine nor surgery are indicated. The patient may subsequently become hypothyroid.

Selective T4 resistance syndrome
The syndrome of selective T_4 resistance results from an inactivating mutation of the gene encoding the β2 thyroid hormone receptor which is present in the hypothalamus and pituitary. This causes hypothalamic–pituitary axis insensitivity to T_4, whereas other tissues (e.g. heart) remain sensitive. Presentation is with a goitre and features of hy-

perthyroidism, and investigations show raised T_3 and T_4 concentrations with inappropriately normal or elevated TSH levels. Treatment is with T_3 (to try and suppress TSH) and propranolol, reserving carbimazole therapy for refractory cases.

Autonomous nodules

Very rarely an autonomous nodule or nodules may cause hyperthyroidism. McCune–Albright syndrome is associated with autonomous thyroid adenomas. The nodule(s), which are follicular adenomas, can be diagnosed clinically and by isotope scanning and are very rarely malignant. Treatment is generally surgical.

TSH-dependent hyperthyroidism

TSH-dependent hyperthyroidism is a very rare condition which is caused by a pituitary TSH-secreting tumour. Neurological signs, e.g. visual changes, are often present. Neuroradiological evaluation is required.

Activating mutations of the TSH receptor

Rarely activating mutations of the TSH receptor can be responsible for familial and sporadic cases of non-immune hyperthyroidism. These patients may present in the neonatal period or in childhood with goitres and suppressed TSH levels. Hyperthyroidism with a multinodular goitre occasionally occurs in patients with the McCune–Allbright syndrome as a result of an activating mutation of the α subunit of the G protein.

Thyroid neoplasia

Solitary or multiple thyroid nodules are very rare in childhood. Over 50% of isolated thyroid nodules are cysts or benign adenomas, 30–40% are malignant while hyperfunctioning adenomas are very rare. Of the malignant nodules over 90% are papillary or follicular carcinomas. The classification of neoplastic thyroid nodules is shown in Table 6.5.

Children with thyroid neoplasia may have a history of head and neck irradiation, a painless rapidly enlarging nodule, hoarseness or dysphagia. Examination may reveal a hard nodule, lymphadenopathy or evidence of metastases (e.g. lung). Of patients with autoimmune thyroiditis 10–15% will have nodules and these are nearly always benign. Patients are usually euthyroid and autoantibody-negative. An ultrasound may identify a cystic lesion which is nearly always benign. Patients with non-cystic lesions may require a radioisotope scan. Nodules which concentrate iodide are usually benign. If there is *any* doubt following the above investigations then a fine-needle biopsy, if feasible, should be performed.

If the clinical picture is suggestive of malignancy, or if the needle biopsy is positive or suspicious, then surgery is indicated. Surgery consists of removal of the affected lobe followed by total thyroidectomy if frozen sections confirm malignancy. Postoperative thyroxine therapy should lead to complete suppression of TSH so as not to stimulate tumour regrowth. Radioactive iodine treatment is also given if there is evidence of metastatic disease or distant lymph node involvement. Follow-up consists of regular clinical assessment and measurement of thyroid function tests to ensure TSH suppression. Thyroglobulin is also measured as it indicates the presence or absence of functioning thyroid tissue. Ultrasound is also useful in detecting neck recurrences. The prognosis in the papillary and follicular carcinomas is very good, even in those with metastases, and life expectancy is normal. The prognosis in the much rarer cancers, e.g. anaplastic carcinoma, is much poorer and more aggressive treatment is necessary.

Medullary thyroid carcinoma arises from the parafollicular C cells and usually secretes calcitonin and occasionally other hormones, such as adrenocorticotrophic hormone (ACTH). It may be isolated or associated with other tumours in one of the multiple endocrine neoplasia (MEN) syndromes which are autosomal dominant. MEN type 2 consists of:
- MEN 2A: medullary thyroid carcinoma, pheochromocytoma and hyperparathyroidism; and
- MEN 2B: medullary thyroid carcinoma, pheochromocytoma and multiple mucosal neuromata.

In children with a family history of MEN 2A or 2B in whom genetic studies have shown that the child is affected, complete thyroidectomy is now recommended before the age of 5 years to pre-empt the inevitable development

Table 6.5 Classification of neoplastic thyroid nodules.

Follicular tumours
Follicular adenoma
Follicular carcinoma
Papillary carcinoma
Anaplastic carcinoma

Non-follicular tumours
Medullary carcinoma
Lymphoma
Teratoma
Metastatic
Miscellaneous

of medullary thyroid cancer, which has a poor prognosis once it has become clinically evident. Follow-up includes calcitonin monitoring.

Miscellaneous disorders

Colloid (simple) goitre

During adolescence the thyroid gland may become diffusely enlarged. Thyroid function tests and an autoantibody screen should be performed and, if both of these are normal, the diagnosis—by elimination—is that of a colloid goitre. The goitre usually resolves spontaneously.

Subacute thyroiditis

In this condition the thyroid gland is acutely inflamed because of a viral infection. There is often evidence of a recent or intercurrent upper respiratory tract infection. The patient may be febrile and the gland may be tender and painful. Usually there is an increase in T_4 and T_3 with symptoms and signs of hyperthyroidism. Treatment is with analgesics and non-steroidal anti-inflammatory drugs and, in severe cases, steroids may be needed. Propranolol may also be necessary. Hyperthyroidism usually lasts for 1–4 weeks and may be followed by a period of hypothyroidism as the gland recovers. The total course of the illness is 2–9 months with most patients making a complete recovery, but occasionally permanent hypothyroidism may occur.

> ### When to involve a specialist centre
>
> - Neonatal thyrotoxicosis.
> - Investigation of familial and / or goitrous congenital hypothyroidism.
> - Graves' disease that is difficult to control or relapsing.
> - A thyrotoxic crisis
> - Suspected thyroid neoplasia.
> - Hypothyroidism secondary to pituitary disease.

Future developments

- Advances in molecular genetics are likely to lead to: a better understanding of the aetiology of congenital hypothyroidism; clearer guidelines on the investigation, treatment and prognosis of congenital hypothyroidism.
- It is likely that there will be an increase in the use of radioactive iodine in thyrotoxosis.
- Further insight into the affect of maternal thyroid dysfunction on fetal development may lead to thyroid screening in pregnancy.

Controversial points

- Should preterm infants with hypothyroxinaemia be treated with thyroid hormones?
- Should preterm neonates <1500 g or acutely ill neonates >1500 g have repeat TFTs and, if so, when?
- Should imaging be performed on all infants with congenital hypothyroidism? If so, should an isotope scan, an ultrasound, or both be performed?
- Should first-degree relatives of children with autoimmune thyroiditis or Graves' disease have their thyroid function checked?
- What initial dosage regimen should be administered to infants with congenital hypothyroidism?
- Should patients with Graves' disease who have relapsed after 2 years of medical treatment be offered further medical treatment, radioactive iodine or a thyroidectomy?
- Should all pregnant women have their TFTs measured to avoid possible adverse effects on their infants?
- In thyrotoxicosis which medical regimen should be adopted: a dose titration regimen or a block replace regimen?

> ### Potential pitfalls
>
> - A normal thyroxine with a high TSH level may indicate that thyroxine has been taken on the day of the clinic visit but irregularly prior to that. Diplomatic questioning should help determine if the problem is non compliance or if a higher thyroxine dose is needed.
> - Children with congenital hypothyroidism who at the age of 3 years are on a small dose of thyroxine and in whom investigation has shown a normally located thyroid gland may require re-evaluation. They may have had transient hypothyroidism and not require life-long treatment.
> - In children with autoimmune thyroiditis thyroxine treatment should be started in a stepwise fashion to diminish the risk of behavioural problems (especially in children with learning difficulties).
> - Children with thyrotoxicosis with a normal FT_4 (or T_4) and a suppressed TSH level who still have symptoms should have their FT_3 measured. The FT_3 may be elevated and the cause of their symptoms and the suppressed TSH.
> - A low FT_4 (or T_4) level with a normal or only slightly elevated TSH level (TSH <10 mU/L) should prompt consideration of the possibility of secondary or tertiary hypothyroidism.

CASE HISTORIES

Case 1

A 13-year-old girl presented at clinic having been diagnosed as having hypothyroidism by her family doctor who had confirmed the diagnosis with thyroid function tests. She also had a 2-year history of a limp in her left leg. On examination she was short and obese with a goitre and other signs of hypothyroidism. She had limitation of movement of her left hip and a limp.

Questions
1 What is the most likely diagnosis?
2 What investigations should be done?
3 What is the treatment?

Answers
1 Slipped femoral epiphysis and Hashimoto's disease.
2 Anterioposterior and 'frog-leg' view X-rays (an A–P X-ray alone may not demonstrate the slipped epiphysis) and thyroid autoantibodies.
3 In spite of the long history, urgent referral to an orthopaedic surgeon and urgent surgery are necessary. An acute on chronic slippage of the epiphysis may cause avascular necrosis of the femoral head. Prophylactic pinning of the other femoral head is advocated by some surgeons. Thyroxine treatment should also be started.

Case 2

An endocrinological opinion was sought about the following series of thyroid function tests. They were taken from a boy with congenital hypothyroidism caused by an ectopic gland who had been treated with thyroxine from day 15 of life. At 5 years of age he was in a mainstream school but had speech delay and behavioural problems (Table 6.6).

Questions
1 What is your interpretation of these results?
2 Are there any measures that could have been taken or that could be taken now to alter the situation?

Answers
1 These results indicate poor compliance. The FT_4 values are normal as a result of the tablets having been taken in the few days prior to the

Table 6.6 Thyroid function tests.

Age	FT_4 (normal 12–26 pmol/L or 0.8–2.4 mg/dL)		TSH (normal 0.5–6.0 mU/L)
10 months	20.9	1.6	2.5
1.5 years	22.9	1.8	3.7
2.1 years	9.0	0.7	53.8
2.2 years	10.6	0.8	79.6
2.3 years	32.7	2.4	0.91
2.6 years	9.3	0.7	44.2
3.1 years	22.8	1.8	32.5
4.7 years	23.9	1.9	34.5
5.1 years	18.5	1.5	29.3

Abbreviations: FT_4, free thyroxine; TSH, thyroid-stimulating hormone.

blood test. However, the half-life of TSH is longer and the elevated TSH values point to the lack of compliance.
2 Earlier recognition and action may well have reduced this boy's poor compliance, developmental delay and behavioural problems. If, despite full explanations and maximum support, the situation did not improve then there would be grounds for considering child-protection proceedings.

Case 3

A 13-year-old boy was referred to the regional endocrine clinic for consideration of growth hormone treatment. He also had delayed puberty and intermittent headaches. On examination his height was >–4.0 SD with evidence of growth failure for at least 4 years. His weight was –1.0 SD and he was entirely prepubertal. A recent growth hormone stimulation test at the referring hospital showed a maximum response to a diethylstilbestrol primed clonidine test of 5 mU/L. He was said to have had normal thyroid function tests 2 years previously with a FT_4 = 9.2 pmol/L (9–24) and a TSH of 1.2 mU/L (0.4–4.0)

Questions
1 Are these thyroid function tests normal?
2 What is the likely overall diagnosis?
3 Is there a problem in interpreting his clonidine test?

Answers

1 Highly suggestive of secondary or tertiary hypothyroidism.

2 Panhypopituitarism secondary to a pituitary tumour.

3 Yes, one can get a low growth-hormone level in any form of untreated hypothyroidism. However, he is likely to be growth-hormone deficient and in fact had a large cystic craniopharyngioma.

Case 4

An 11-year-old girl with Down's syndrome is referred with tiredness, mild diarrhoea and a TSH of 9.2 mU/L (0.4–4.0) and an FT_4 of 14.1 pmol/L (9–24) [1.13 mg/dL (0.8–2.4)]. She also had a raised thyroid peroxidase (TPO) antibody titre.

Questions

1 Would you treat this child with thyroxine?

2 What two other investigations would you consider doing?

3 What is the likely diagnosis?

Answers

1 The thyroid function is only mildly deranged with a normal FT_4 and a slightly raised TSH. This slight abnormality is unlikely to cause any symptoms. Children with Down's syndrome may have an atrophic thyroiditis with no goitre. TSH levels sometimes rise transiently and can fluctuate. If the TSH rises to above 10 mU/L the child should have TFTs 6 monthly. If the TSH rises above 15 mU/L the child should have TFTs every 3–6 months and is likely to eventually require thyroxine. In the above situations the family should be told of the symptoms to look out for. If the TSH >20 mU/L with a normal FT_4 the patient should be treated with thyroxine.

2 A general paediatric approach should be taken looking for the large number of causes of tiredness and diarrhoea in a child with Down's syndrome. The two most important investigations are a full blood count looking for anaemia and a coeliac screen.

3 The likeliest diagnosis is coeliac disease. The anti-transglutaminase antibodies were positive and a jejunal biopsy confirmed coeliac disease. Coeliac disease is an immunological disorder and is commoner in Down's syndrome. The tiredness and diarrhoea resolved on a gluten-free diet.

References and further reading

Birrell, G. & Cheetham, T. (2004) Juvenile thyrotoxicosis; can we do better? *Archives of Disease in Childhood* **89**, 745–750.

Brown, R.S. (2001) The thyroid gland. In: *Clinical Paediatric Endocrinology* (ed. C.G.D. Brook & P.C. Hindmarsh), 4th edn, pp 288–320. Blackwell Science, Oxford.

Haddow, J.E., Palomaki, G.E., Allan, W.C. *et al.* (1999) Maternal thyroid deficiency during pregnancy and subsequent neuropsychological development in the child. *New England Journal of Medicine* **341**, 549–555.

LaFranchi, S (2004) Disorders of the thyroid gland. In: *Nelson's Textbook of Pediatrics* (ed. R.E. Behrman, R.M. Kliegman & H.B. Jenson) 17th edn, pp 1870–1889. Saunders, Philadelphia.

Larson, C., Hermos, R., Delaney, A. *et al.* (2003) Risk factors associated with delayed thyrotropin elevations in congenital hypothyroidism. *Journal of Pediatrics* **143**, 587–591.

Kelnar, C.J.H. & Butler, G.E. (2003) Endocrine gland disorders. In: Forfar and Arneil's *Textbook of Paediatrics* (ed. N. McIntosh, P. Helms & R. Smyth) 6th edn, pp 443–559. Churchill Livingstone, London.

Ogilvy-Stuart, A.L. (2002) Neonatal thyroid disorders-a review. *Archives of Disease in Childhood* **87**, F165–F171.

Osborn, D.A. (2001) Thyroid hormones for preventing neurodevelopmental impairment in preterm infants. Cochrane Database *Systematic Review* (4): CD001070.

Rovet, J. (2003) Long term follow up of children born with sporadic congenital hypothyroidism. Annals of Endocrinology **64**, 1:58–61.

7 Intersex and other disorders of sexual differentiation

Introduction

Intersex is when the genotype (usually but not always 46,XX or 46,XY) is at partial or complete variance with the sexual phenotype. **Ambiguous genitalia** describes a type intersex where the external phenotype is sufficiently abnormal to cause uncertainty as to which gender should be assigned. The term **complex genital anomaly**, which is more descriptive than ambiguous genitalia and does not have the same unfortunate connotation, should now be used.

Understanding the physiology of sexual differentiation is a prerequisite for developing diagnostic and management models in the field of intersex.

Physiology of sexual differentiation

Embryology

Sex *determination* concerns the determination of gonadal type and occurs in this sequence:

• Development of indifferent gonad from urogenital ridge.

• Migration of primordial germ cells during the 4th and 5th weeks of gestation from the dorsal endoderm of the yolk sac, reaching the urogenital ridge by 6–8 weeks.

• Testicular differentiation and testosterone production by 9 weeks' gestation.

• Ovarian differentiation with germ cell meiosis at 11–12 weeks' gestation.

Sex *differentiation* involves the development of internal genitalia, urogenital sinus and external genitalia.

Internal genital development (Fig. 7.1)

• At 7 weeks' gestation the fetus possesses a double system—the Wolffian ducts with potential for male development and the Mullerian ducts with potential for female development.

• In the presence of a testis, the Mullerian system involutes while the Wolffian system develops into the epididymis, vas deferens, seminal vesicles and ejaculatory ducts.

• In the absence of a testis, the Wolffian system involutes and the Mullerian system develops into the fallopian tubes, uterus and upper third of the vagina.

Development of urogenital sinus (Fig. 7.1)

• Under the influence of androgen the sinus narrows to form the posterior urethra. Outgrowths of the urogenital sinus form the prostate gland and bulbourethral glands of Cowper.

• In the absence of androgen the urogenital sinus differentiates into the lower two-thirds of the vagina and the urethra. Outgrowths form the paraurethral glands of Skene and the vestibular glands of Bartholin.

External genitalia (Fig. 7.2)

In contrast to the internal genitalia, the external genitalia arise from a *common anlage*; a mid-line genital tubercle formed at 8 weeks' gestation with lateral urethral folds flanked by labioscrotal swellings.

• The genital tubercle develops into the glans penis in the male and the clitoris in the female.

• The urethral folds develop into the corpus spongiosum

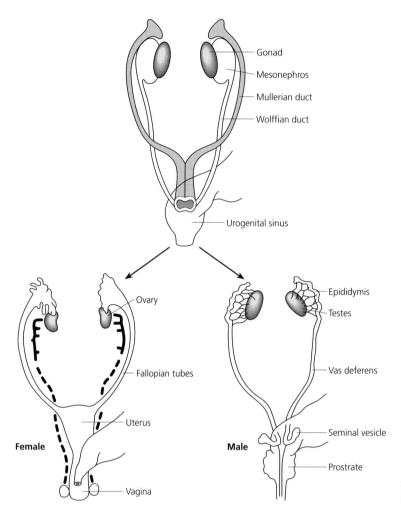

Gonad
Mesonephros
Mullerian duct
Wolffian duct

Urogenital sinus

Ovary
Fallopian tubes
Uterus
Female
Vagina

Epididymis
Testes
Vas deferens
Seminal vesicle
Male
Prostrate

Fig. 7.1 Differentiation of the internal genitalia.

enclosing the urethra in the male, and into the labia minora in the female.

• The labioscrotal folds fuse in the mid-line to form the scrotum and ventral part of the penis in the male, and remain separate to form the labia majora in the female.

Hormonal control of primary sexual differentiation (Fig. 7.3)

The fetus has an inherent tendency towards female differentiation so that, in the absence of a gonad, normal female internal and external genitalia will develop. By contrast, normal male differentiation requires:

1 an intact testis with functioning Leydig and Sertoli cells; and

2 the presence of the enzyme 5α-reductase.

Male differentiation will then proceed as follows.

• Development of the Wolffian system under the influence of testosterone, secreted by the Leydig cells.

• Regression of the Mullerian system under the influence of anti-Mullerian hormone (AMH), a peptide produced by the Sertoli cells.

• Development of the common anlage and the urogenital sinus under the control of dihydrotestosterone (DHT), synthesized from testosterone in tissues which contain 5α-reductase.

The following points should be noted:

• The testes exert a paracrine effect on adjacent tissues so that a testis on one side will result in Wolffian development and Mullerian regression, while a streak gonad on

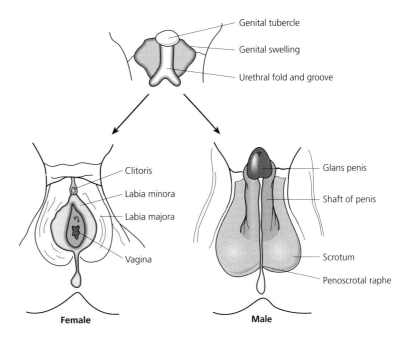

Fig. 7.2 Differentiation of the external genitalia from the common anlage.

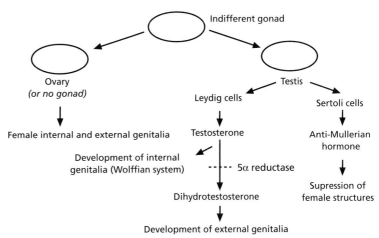

Fig. 7.3 Hormone control of primary sexual differentiation.

the other side may be associated with Wolffian regression and Mullerian development. This situation may be encountered with 45,X/46,XY mosaicism (often called mixed gonadal dysgenesis).

• The presence of a uterus in a newborn with ambiguous genitalia indicates that either an ovary is present or there is no gonad or, if testicular tissue is present, it must be dysgenetic with poor Sertoli cell function.

• 46,XY individuals with complete or partial androgen resistance will secrete and respond normally to AMH so

that development of fallopian tubes, uterus and upper third of the vagina will not occur.

Genetic control of gonadal sex determination

Table 7.1 gives a glossary of some of the genes and proteins currently known to be involved with sex determination and differentiation. Gonadal sex determination results from an interplay between SRY protein and other proteins. AMH secretion by the Sertoli cells is under the control of the AMH gene, situated on chromosome 19p.

Table 7.1 Glossary of genes and proteins involved in primary sex determination.

Gene abbreviated name	Full name	Protein	Function
SRY	Sex determining region of the Y chromosome	SRY protein	Male-specific factor; mutations in SRY → XY female
HMG Box	High Mobility Group Box		The DNA-binding domain of a number of transcription factors, including SRY and SOX proteins
SOX	SRY-like HMG Box	SOX proteins	A family of genes with homology to SRY which are involved in sex determination. Mutation in SOX-9 → XY female; associated with camptomelic dysplasia
DAX-1	Dosage sensitive sex reversal, adrenal hypoplasia congenita on the X chromosome, gene 1	470 amino acid protein	Located at Xp21. Involved in gonadotrophin, adrenal and gonadal development Mutations → adrenal hypoplasia and gonadotrophin deficiency. Duplication → XY sex reversal.
WT-1	Wilms' tumour-1	WT-1 protein	? Involved early in sex determination. Mutations in 46,XY individuals associated with gonadal dysgenesis, urogenital malformations, and malignancy (e.g. Denys Drash, Frasier, and WAGR syndromes)
SF-1	Steroidogenic Factor-1	461 amino acid protein	Regulates genes involved in sex determination and differentation, and steroidogenesis.

Table 7.2 Classification of intersex.

	Karyotype	Gonad	Phenotype
Male undermasculinization	46,XY or abnormal karyotype with major Y-bearing cell line (including 45,X/46,XY)	Testis (may be dysgenetic)	Partial or complete failure of masculinization
Female masculinization	46,XX	Ovary	Partial or complete masculinization
True hermaphroditism	46,XX or 46,XX/46,XY chimerism or 46,XY (rare)	Ovarian and testicular tissue as: bilateral ovotestis or unilateral ovotestis with contralateral testis or ovary	Ambiguous genitalia with persistence of both Wolffian and Mullerian systems

Classification of disorders of sexual differentiation

Classification of intersex

Intersex is classified into male undermasculinization (previously called male pseudohermaphroditism), female masculinization (previously known as female pseudohermaphroditism) and the very rare true hermaphroditism (Table 7.2).

The wider area of disordered sexual differentiation (which includes intersex) can be classified according to the genotype.

Karyotype includes both X and Y chromosomes

• Male undermasculinization caused by androgen deficiency or resistance, gonadal dysgenesis, or moderate to severe idiopathic developmental anomaly.

• Less severe disorders of penile and testicular dif-

Table 7.3 Causes of male undermasculinization due to androgen and AMH deficiency/resistance.

Karyotype	Gonad	Diagnosis	Defect	Phenotype
46,XY	Testis	*Defects in androgen synthesis with normal AMH secretion*		
		Gonadotrophin deficiency	Congenital hypopituitarism	Micropenis ± hypospadias
		Leydig cell hypoplasia	LH receptor gene mutation → inactivating defect	Female or ambiguous. Elevated LH and FSH levels
		Enzyme defects resulting in failure of cortisol synthesis	StAR mutation → deficiency of steroidogenic protein	Female external genitalia with cortisol and aldosterone deficiency
			HSD 3B2 mutation → 3β HSD deficiency	Severe hypospadias/ambiguous genitalia ± salt loss
			CYP 17 gene mutation → 17α-hydroxylase deficiency	Female with hypertension and hypokalaemia
		Biosynthetic defect with intact cortisol synthesis but failure of androgen production	CYP 17 gene mutation → 17, 20 desmolase deficiency	Female/ambiguous/hypoplastic male, depending on severity of enzyme defect
			17β-HSD3 gene mutation → 17β HSD deficiency	Predominantly female external genitalia but virilization at puberty because of increased androstenedione levels
		Failure of tissue conversion of testosterone to dihydrotestosterone	SRD 5A2 gene mutation → 5α-reductase type II deficiency	Female phenotype/ambiguous genitalia at birth because of DHT deficiency. Masculinization at puberty, largely testosterone-mediated
		Androgen resistance with normal AMH secretion		
		CAIS	Androgen receptor mutations → inactivating defect	Female external genitalia, blind vagina, testes intra-abdominal/in inguinal canals, absent internal genitalia
		PAIS	→ incomplete activation	Ambiguous genitalia; small phallus and urogenital sinus, impaired response to exogenous androgens
		AMH failure with normal androgen function		
			AMH and AMH receptor mutations	Phenotypic male with uterus and fallopian tubes

Abbreviations: AMH, anti-Mullerian hormone; CAIS, complete androgen insensitivity syndrome; DHT, dihydrotestosterone; FSH, follicle-stimulating hormone; LH, luteinizing hormone; PAIS, partial androgen insensitivity syndrome; StAR, steroidogenic acute regulatory.

ferentiation, and breast anomalies, in the absence of an identifiable hormonal cause.

- Aneuploidy syndromes.

Karyotype includes the X but not the Y chromosome

- Female masculinization.
- Female phenotype with little or no virilization.
- Aneuploidy syndromes.

Disorders of sexual differentiation with normal/abnormal karyotype involving both X and Y chromosomes

Male undermasculinization

Biosynthetic defects (Table 7.3)

Synthetic defects in the pathways leading to ineffective androgen function may occur at any point between gonadotrophin-releasing hormone (GnRH) production in the hypothalamus and 5α-reductase production in the target tissues. Gonadotrophin deficiency leads to micro-penis with small testes. Leydig cell hypoplasia is suggested by severe undermasculinisation with sex reversal in a genetic male with identifiable gonads and raised gonadotrophins. Three of the five enzyme defects causing congenital adrenal hyperplasia, and deficiency of the enzymes 17,20 desmolase and 17β hydroxysteroid dehydrogenase, will result in androgen deficiency (see Fig. 7.4 and Chapter 8). The phenotype and clinical features will depend on the site, severity and selectivity of the enzyme defect (Fig. 7.5). 5α-reductase deficiency is an autosomal recessive disorder, most often seen in consanguinous

families (Fig. 7.6), resulting in moderate to severe micro-penis with hypospadias, labioscrotal folds and palpable gonads. Diagnosis is suggested by normal or high testosterone (T) levels with low plasma DHT levels, reduced DHT metabolites in the urine, and decreased DHT:T ratio following human chorionic gonadotrophin (hCG) administration.

Androgen resistance

Complete androgen insensitivity syndrome (CAIS) is an X-linked disorder caused by a variety of inactivating androgen receptor (AR) mutations. The mother is a healthy

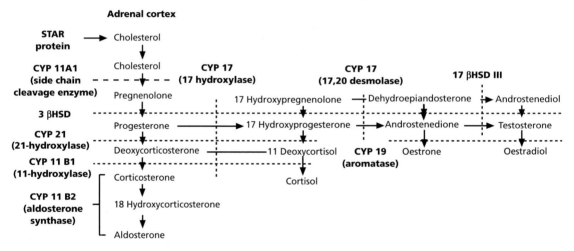

Fig. 7.4 Pathways of steroid synthesis in adrenal gland and gonads.

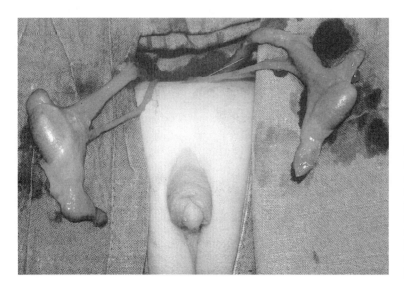

Fig. 7.5 3β-hydroxysteroid dehydrogenase deficiency in a 46,XY individual causing severe undermasculinization but no cortisol or aldosterone deficiency. Five years old at presentation, the child was established in the female gender and underwent gonadectomy (note morphologically normal testis, epididymis and vas deferens on each side) together with phallic reduction and vaginoplasty.

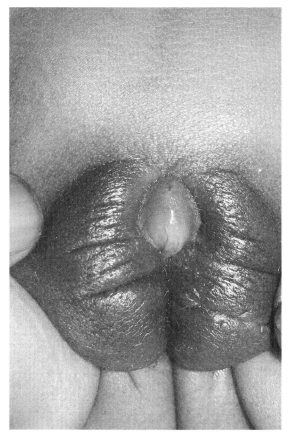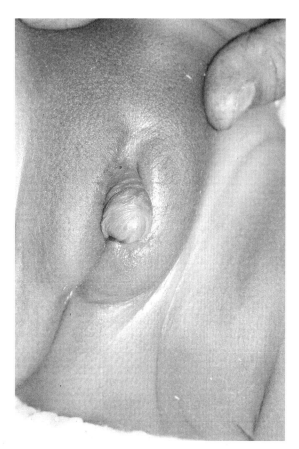

Fig. 7.6 5α-reductase deficiency causing severe micropenis with hypospadias and labio-scrotal folds containing gonads (left). Application of dihydrotestosterone cream (right) resulted in sufficient penile development for reconstructive surgery to be carried out.

carrier, while half of her genetically male offspring will be phenotypic females with absent female structures, intraabdominal testes and blind vagina. The diagnosis is usually made in the index case by the presence of hernia ± gonad during infancy, or by primary amenorrhoea in the adolescent. Although completely insensitive to androgen, individuals are exquisitely sensitive to oestradiol which is aromatized from the high/normal testosterone levels. This results in ample breast development and female habitus, but there is little or no body hair because of the androgen resistance (Fig. 7.7). Management of CAIS includes gonadectomy, examination under anaesthetic to ensure vaginal adequacy, and life-long oestrogen replacement together with screening of phenotypically female family members. This is discussed in more detail below.

Partial androgen insensitivity syndrome (PAIS) is the term applied to a number of AR mutations which are par-tially inactivating so that individuals are variably undermasculinized in conjunction with complete suppression of female structures other than the distal vagina (Fig. 7.8). The management of these cases is difficult and controversial unless the degree of undermasculinization is relatively mild.

Dysgenetic testes ± abnormal karyotype (Table 7.4)
Mixed gonadal dysgenesis is the term applied to 45,X/46,XY mosaicism causing complex external genital anomaly with a streak gonad on one side and a dysgenetic testis on the other. The external and internal phenotype will depend on the degree of testicular dysgenesis. With severe androgen and AMH deficiency the external genialia will be undermasculinised and both vagina and uter-us will be present. If testicular dysgenesis is relatively mild, undermasculinization will also be mild and female internal structures suppressed. Depending on the pre-

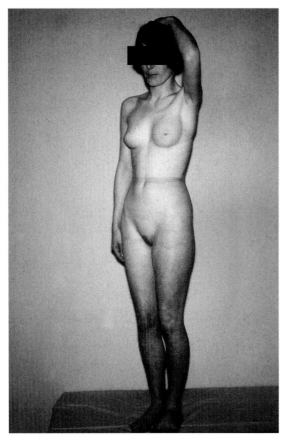

Fig. 7.7 46,XY individual with complete androgen insensitivity. Note ample breast development but absent/sparse auxillary and public hair.

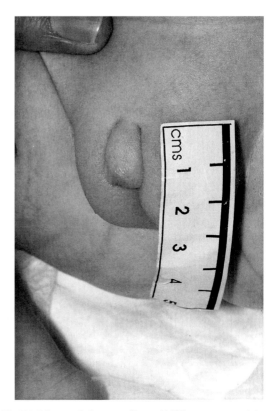

Fig. 7.8 Micropenis, hypospadias and bifid scrotum containing gonads in a 46,XY infant with partial androgen insensitivity. Assignment of female gender would be difficult technically in view of infact AMH secretion and suppression of female structures. However, the adequacy of the phallus in adult life is of concern.

dominance of the 45,X cell line there may be features of Turner's syndrome.

Vanishing testes syndrome is a descriptive term applied to genetically normal males with anorchia and variable undermasculinization in whom the testes have undergone regression *in utero*. Some 46,XY individuals have streak gonads and complete or near complete sex reversal. This phenomenon is known as pure gonadal dysgenesis.

Developmental anomalies

Some genetic males with hypospadias and other genital anomalies have evidence of intact AMH secretion with suppression of female structures and normal androgen production.

Disorders of penile, testicular and breast differentiation in XY individuals

While severe micropenis and hypospadias with bifid scrotum will come under the category of male undermasculinization, most penile disorders are less severe, idiopathic, and will present to the surgeon. Testicular disorders include micro- and macro-orchidism, unilateral and bilateral cryptorchidism, and absence (anorchia). Gynaecomastia, almost always idiopathic, is the most common breast anomaly. Management of these conditions is discussed below.

Aneuploidy syndromes

Klinefelter's syndrome (47,XXY) is the commonest male chromosomal disorder and usually results from paternal

Table 7.4 Causes of gonadal dysgenesis associated with 46,XY or other Y bearing karyotype.

Diagnosis	Karyotype	Defect	Clinical features
Mixed gonadal dysgenesis	45,X/46,XY	Non-disjunction early in mitosis	Dysgenetic gonads with variable phenotype (including normal female, ambiguous, and complete/near complete male). Variable Turner phenotype
Vanishing testes syndrome	46,XY	Unknown	Variable undermasculinization related to timing of prenatal testicular failure
Pure gonadal dysgenesis	46,XY	SRY gene mutations X-linked recessive defect Autosomal recessive defect Duplication of DSS locus (Xp21 region) → suppression of testicular differentiation	Phenotypic female ± clitoromegaly with streak gonads Gonadectomy required to prevent development of gonadoblastoma
ATR-X syndrome	46,XY	XH2 mutation (at Xq 13.3)	Associated with α-thalassaemia and mental retardation
10q deletion	46,XY ± unbalanced translocation deletion involving 10q	Deletion of 10q	Sex reversal ± dysmorphism and other congenital anomalies
9p deletion	46,XY ± unbalanced translocation deletion involving 9p	9p deletion	Sex reversal ± dysmorphism and other congenital anomalies
Denys Drash syndrome	46,XY	Mutation of WT-1 gene (Xp 13 region)	Ambiguous genitalia with streak/dysgenetic gonads associated with Wilms' tumour, mesangial sclerosis and renal failure
WAGR	46,XY	WT-1 mutations	Wilms' tumour, aniridia, genitourinary abnormalities, mental retardation (WAGR) with hypospadias and cryptorchidism
Camptomelic dwarfism	46,XY	SOX9 gene mutation (17q24–25 region)	Camptomelic dwarfism with normal ovaries and female phenotype in 46,XX subjects, sex reversal in most 46,XY individuals.

or maternal non-disjunction during the first meiotic division. The condition is often not diagnosed until adult life but may be diagnosed in childhood as a chance finding (e.g. in the course of amniocentesis) or in the assessment of boys with learning and behaviour problems. Examination may show relatively long legs (eunuchoid habitus). Adolescents have small testes due to seminiferous tubule dysgenesis, with high gonadotrophins, low normal androgens, azoospermia, gynaecomastia and exacerbation of eunuchoid proportions. Adolescents can be offered testosterone therapy during puberty to augment Leydig cell production and limit disproportion. Individuals with a Y chromosome and more than two X chromosomes (e.g. 48,XXXY or 49,XXXXY) have features similar to

Table 7.5 Causes of moderate to severe female masculinization.

Karyotype	Gonad	Diagnosis	Defect	Phenotype
46,XX	Ovary	Congenital adrenal hyperplasia	CYP 21 mutation → 21 hydroxylase deficiency	Mutation and degree of enzyme deficiency influences phenotype including salt wasting variety with moderate to severe virilization, and simple virilizing variety without manifest salt loss
			CYP 11 B1 mutation → 11β-hydroxylase deficiency	Rare. Degree of virilization depends on severity of enzyme defect. Hypertension occurs because of high deoxycorticosterone levels
			HSD 3B2 mutation → 3β-HSD deficiency	Rare. High levels of the weak androgen DHEAS result in mild virilization
		Aromatase deficiency	Aromatase gene mutation	Tall stature with non-fused epiphyses; mild virilization caused by elevated testosterone
		Maternal ovarian/adrenal tumour	Androgen production → fetal virilization	Very rare
		Drugs with androgenic effects (e.g. danazol)	Androgen production fetal virilization	Very rare
		Developmental anomaly with no identifiable endocrine cause	Various, aetiology unknown	May occur with urological and other congenital anomalies
46,XX	Testis	XX male with normal phenotype/mild undermasculinization, e.g. hypospadias	Y → X translocation involving SRY gene in 80%; 20% SRY-negative? caused by mutation(s) elsewhere on X chromosome or autosomes	Complete or near complete male phenotype relative short stature, germ cell impairment similar to Klinefelter's syndrome

Abbreviation: DHEAS, dehydroepiandrosterone.

Klinefelter's syndrome but with greater gonadal and mental impairment and may require testosterone supplementation beyond puberty. Individuals with the 47,XYY syndrome are usually normal except for tall stature but may have important behaviour problems during childhood and adolescence. Endocrine treatment is not required.

Disorders of sexual differentiation with normal/abnormal karyotype involving X but not Y chromosome

Female masculinization (Table 7.5)
Three of the enzyme defects causing congenital adrenal hyperplasia will cause virilization in affected 46,XX individuals (see Fig. 7.4 and Chapter 8). Aromatase deficiency is extremely rare as are maternal drugs and androgen secreting tumours. In some cases congenital anomalies occur in association with ano-rectal malformations in the absence of any identifiable endocrine cause.

Normal female genitalia with little or no virilization (Table 7.6)
17α-hydroxylase and 17,20-lyase deficiency may cause failure of oestrogen secretion resulting in pubertal failure, while the StAR protein defect is (surprisingly) associated with normal puberty in 46,XX individuals but premature ovarian failure.

Pure gonadal dysgenesis is the term applied to 46,XX (and 46,XY) individuals with streak gonads and essentially normal phenotype. This condition presents with failure to enter puberty in the context of normal rather

Table 7.6 Disorders of sex differentiation with 46,XX or 48,X karyotype and little or no virilization.

Karyotype	Gonad	Diagnosis	Defect	Phenotype
46,XX	Ovary	Steroidogenic enzyme disorders	StAR protein mutation → deficiency in steroidogenic protein responsible for cholesterol transport	Premature ovarian failure in affected females
			CYP 17 mutation → 17α-hydroxylase deficiency	Hypertension, hypokalaemia and failure of oestrogen secretion at puberty
			→ 17,20-lyase deficiency	Failure of oestrogen secretion by ovaries at puberty but no hypertension or hypokalaemia
46,XX	Streak	Gonadal dysgenesis	Usually unknown. In some cases: 2p mutation → FSH receptor defect (autosomal recessive) trisomy 13 and 18	Occasional clitoromegaly; eunuchoid body proportions
45,X or 46,XX with abnormal second X ± mosaicism	Dysgenetic/Streak	Turner's syndrome	Nondisjunction at or shortly after conception	Characteristic dysmorphic features with short stature, primary ovarian failure, cardiac and renal anomalies, specific learning difficulties and middle ear problems
47,XXX	Ovary	Triple X syndrome	Maternal nondisjunction	Tall stature with behaviour and learning difficulties in some cases
				Delayed menarche/premature ovarian failure may occur

Abbreviation: StAR, steroidogenic acute regulatory.

than short stature, elevated gonadotrophin levels and hypoplastic uterus on pelvic ultrasound.

Turner's syndrome, the commonest disorder of sexual differentiation in phenotypic females, is discussed in Chapter 3.

Aneuploidy syndromes

These include the Triple X syndrome (47,XXX), associated with learning disability, tall stature and premature ovarian failure. The 48,XXXX and 49,XXXXX syndromes are associated with learning disability and tall/short stature respectively, but normal ovarian function.

Clinical diagnosis and investigation of intersex and related disorders

Complex genital anomaly

This distressing problem is usually identified at birth and poses the dilemma of gender assignment.

Complex genital anomaly in the newborn

Both parents should be seen as soon as possible. The key points in counselling are the following:
• Initial counselling by attending staff, backed up as swiftly as possible by senior paediatrician.
• Key phrase 'there is something the matter with the way that the baby's genitals have been formed, so that we cannot at present say whether the child should be brought up as a boy or a girl'.
• Infant should be referred to as 'the baby' or 'the child' not as he, she or it!
• Mother and baby should be in a single room.
• Registration of name should be postponed.
• Urgent investigations should lead to definite gender assignment within 2 weeks.

History
• Consanguinity.
• Maternal medications.
• Maternal health including androgenic symptoms, such as increase in body hair.

Examination
• General examination to rule out dysmorphic syndrome ± congenital anomalies.
• Palpation of the abdomen and inguinal regions for gonads.
• Meticulous description ± diagram of abnormal genitalia, including:

labioscrotal folds;
clitorophallus;
nature and size of opening below clitorophallus;
identification where possible of urethral meatus and vaginal opening; and presence and site of gonad(s).
• Examination of anus.
• Medical photography.

The degree of masculinization can be expressed as a Prader stage (see Chapter 8) or by using the external masculinization score devised by Ahmed *et al*. This score comprises the degree of labioscrotal fusion, phallic size, site of urethral meatus and position of each gonad.

Further investigation and management

The following professionals should be informed as soon as possible.
• Paediatric endocrinologist.
• Paediatric surgeon or other surgeon with expertise in intersex management (i.e. urologist, plastic surgeon).
• Radiologist.
• Biochemistry department.
• Medical genetics department.

If access to the professionals listed above is difficult then transfer to a specialist centre for specific tests or for general management may be necessary.

The following investigations should be carried out as quickly as possible:
• Genotype. Conventional karyotyping using peripheral lymphocytes takes a minimum of 3 days. A much quicker method is to determine the presence of a Y chromosome using the technique of fluorescent *in situ* hybridization (FISH) on heparinized blood. Using FISH analysis a provisional karyotype can be obtained within hours.
• 17α-hydroxyprogesterone (17-OHP).
• Urine collection for steroid analysis to exclude enzyme defect.
• Pelvic ultrasound to define the following structures:
uterus; and
intra-abdominal, inguinal or labioscrotal gonad(s).
• In selected cases, genitography to define:
vagina;
urethra; and
bladder.

N.B. Transplacental transfer of maternal 17-OHP can lead to spuriously elevated levels in the baby's blood for the first 48–72 hours. However, these will be less than the grossly raised values seen in babies affected by 21-hydroxylase deficiency. There is therefore a case for taking an initial 17-OHP sample without delay in newborns with complex genital anomalies, sending a further sample at 48 hours if necessary. Because attempts at a 24-hour urine collection often result in repeated applications of urine bags and perineal excoriation a timed (e.g. 4–6 hours) urine collection is more practical.

Diagnosis and gender assignment

Figure 7.9 shows a flow diagram giving the main diagnostic possibilities. Gender assignment may be straightforward, for example in a 46,XX baby with 21-hydroxylase deficiency and mild to moderate virilization. However,

some cases are very difficult, for example an infant with partial androgen insensitivity with doubtful adequacy of the phallus for adult life. Criteria for gender assignment include:

- diagnosis;
- presence of female structures (i.e. vagina, uterus);
- adequacy of phallic tissue;
- parental wishes; and
- cultural aspects.

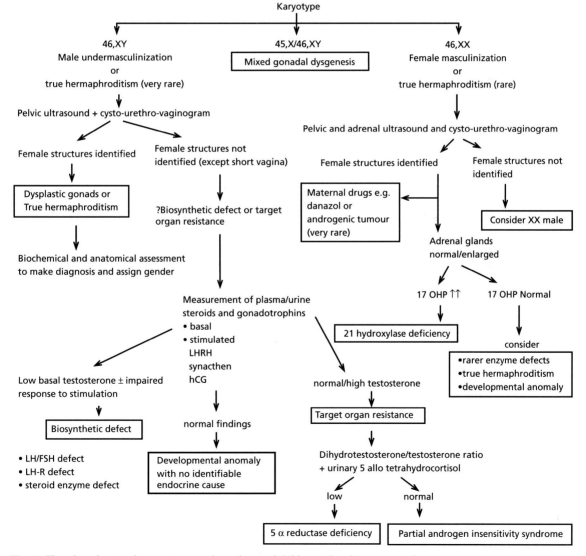

Fig. 7.9 Flow chart showing diagnostic approach to infants and children with ambiguous genitalia.

Disorders with no ambiguity: male phenotype

Penile problems

Micropenis

True micropenis is when the phallus measures less than 2.5 cm from the base of the penis to the tip of the glans penis (not the tip of the foreskin). We recommend measurement with the penis unstretched and the clinician firmly pressing back the suprapubic fat.

Most boys referred with micropenis have simple obesity with the penis 'buried' in surrounding suprapubic fat, and penile length within the normal prepubertal range of between 2.5 and 6 cm. Simple explanation and reassurance should suffice in this situation.

True micropenis with no other penile anomaly may be caused by the following:
• Gonadotrophin deficiency (e.g. as a result of panhypopituitarism or Kallmann's syndrome).
• Prader–Willi syndrome.
• Severe growth hormone deficiency or insensitivity.
• Androgen deficiency or resistance.
• Idiopathic.

Investigations should comprise the following.
• Assessment of growth status in comparison with the parental heights.
• Karyotype.
• Luteinizing hormone-releasing hormone (LHRH) test followed by hCG 100 U/kg (max 1500 U) subcutaneously and testosterone measurement 4 days later.
• Testing sense of smell.

Treatment, if required, is of the underlying cause and either application of DHT cream twice daily for 6 weeks, or a single injection of Sustanon 75 mg intramuscularly.

Hypospadias

Hypospadias is defined as incomplete fusion of the urethra with the meatus on the ventral aspect of the penis — the glans, corona, shaft of penis, and (most severe) the perineum. This abnormality is commonly accompanied by chordee – curvature of the penis – caused by fibrosis of the corpus songiosum.

Isolated hypospadias (hypospadias without micropenis and with normally descended testes in a normal scrotum), is rarely associated with an endocrine disorder. Surgeons should be asked to refer the following conditions for further investigation including karyotype testing.

• Perineal hypospadias.
• Hypospadias with micropenis.
• Hypospadias with cryptorchidism ± scrotal abnormality.

Testicular problems

Unilateral cryptorchidism

• Isolated unilateral cryptorchidism in an otherwise healthy child does not require endocrine investigation.
• Patient, skilful examination should distinguish between true cryptorchidism and a retractile testis.
• Definite and doubtful cases should be referred to a paediatric surgeon.
• Ultrasound or magnetic resonance imaging (MRI) of abdomen and inguinal areas is of value in identifying a cryptorchid testis, but failure to do so does not prove absence.

Bilateral cryptorchidism

In contrast, bilateral cryptorchidism always requires endocrine evaluation. This includes the following:
• Assessment of associated penile or scrotal abnormalities.
• Assessment of growth status, learning ability, dysmorphic features and general examination to exclude a syndrome, e.g. Noonan's.
• Ultrasound or MRI in an attempt to locate testes.
• In all cases, karyotype and basal gonadotrophins.
• In selected cases, LHRH and hCG tests.
• After discussion with a paediatric endocrinologist and surgeon it may be appropriate to give hCG twice weekly for 3 weeks in an attempt to descend the testes and facilitate surgery.

If one or both testes are impalpable, and cannot be identified by imaging, the child should be seen by a surgeon with expertise in laparoscopy.

Micro-orchidism

• Normal prepubertal testes may measure as little as 1.5 cm in length and 0.8 cm in width (volume <1 mL). Klinefelter's syndrome, cryptorchidism and irradiation may be associated with testes which are inappropriately small for pubertal stage, yet which show adequate Leydig cell function.
• If one or both testes are absolutely or relatively small consider:

   physiological prepubertal testes;
   normal degree of asymmetry in pubertal subjects;

gonadotrophin deficiency;

Klinefelter's syndrome;

previous cryptorchidism/irradiation; or

appropriately small testis with enlarged contralateral testis (e.g. Leydig cell tumour).

Macro-orchidism

Prepubertal testes measure less than 3.0 cm in length and 1.5 cm in width (volume <4 mL).

• If symmetrical macroorchidism in boy of prepubertal age, consider:

precocious puberty;

testotoxicosis; or

fragile X syndrome.

• If asymmetric testicular enlargement in boys of peripubertal/pubertal age, consider:

normal variation in testicular size;

one testis previously cryptorchid; or

neoplasia in larger testis (e.g. Leydig cell tumour, teratoma, seminoma).

• Boys with greatly enlarged testes may have an activating follicle-stimulating hormone (FSH) receptor defect and should be referred for full evaluation including molecular genetic testing.

Anorchia

Boys with testicular atrophy or removal, e.g. because of bilateral testicular torsion, need hormone replacement at and beyond puberty. The timing and need for insertion of testicular prostheses should be discussed with the boy and family. While insertion of prepubertal prostheses is possible, most families opt for surgery after pubertal induction.

Pubertal problems

Delayed/incomplete/arrested puberty and gynaecomastia are discussed in Chapter 5.

Disorders with no ambiguity: female phenotype

Internal genitalia

Hernia

Hernias are rare in girls. If a gonad is present in the hernial sac then complete androgen insensitivity is likely. If the gonad is palpable on examination the following investigations should be performed.

• Karyotype.

• Pelvic ultrasound.

• LH and FSH levels.

If the gonad is discovered at operation, a biopsy should be performed and the above investigations carried out postoperatively.

External genitalia

Fused labia

This is by far the most common genital anomaly seen in young girls and the impression of an absent vagina may cause considerable anxiety in the parents. The diagnosis is confirmed by clinical examination which shows fusion of the labia minora. Pelvic ultrasound will confirm the presence of a normal uterus.

Treatment is with ortho-gynest cream 0.01% applied twice daily to the fused area for 7 days. Once separation has occurred the use of a bland ointment such as petrolatum for 1–2 months may prevent fusion recurring. In cases where the labia remain fused, or where repeated courses of treatment are needed, and the child is experiencing problems such as urinary tract infections or a vaginal discharge, surgical referral is indicated.

Virilization

Enlargement of the clitoris with or without other signs of androgen excess, such as pubic hair, suggests androgen production by either the ovaries or adrenal glands. This is discussed in Chapter 5.

Pubertal problems

Delayed/incomplete/arrested puberty

This is discussed in Chapter 5.

Medical and surgical aspects of treatment

Medical aspects

Underdevelopment of male external genitalia

In prepubertal subjects, the size of the genitalia can be augmented by the following treatments:

• Intramuscular testosterone (e.g. Sustanon) in a dosage of 25–75 mg. Further injections may be given if necessary but the growth status and bone age must be carefully monitored.

• DHT cream, applied to the penis twice daily for a 6-week period. This usually results in penile development which may assist procedures such as hypospadias repair. This treatment is particularly effective in 5α-reductase deficiency.

• hCG 100 U/kg (1500 U max) twice weekly, intramuscularly for 3 weeks may promote testicular descent as well as developing the penis and scrotum.

These treatments should only be given following discussion with a specialist centre.

Female development

There is no place for oestrogen treatment in prepubertal girls as even small quantities may hasten epiphyseal closure (oestrogen induction of puberty is discussed in Chapter 5).

Surgical aspects

The surgical treatment of complex genital anomalies is controversial. Given that such problems are rare, surgery should be performed in a specialist centre. Early involvement of the paediatric surgeon is essential in cases where gender assignment is problematic, for surgery will be required whatever decision is taken. Specific surgical procedures include the following.

• Clitorophallic reduction towards the female gender. Modern techniques that preserve both the glans and neurovascular supply of the clitoris aim to preserve sexual function of the patient in adulthood. However, no long-term studies of their effectiveness are available. Most surgeons would therefore reserve this surgery for girls with more severe forms of cliteromegaly. If surgery is required there is general agreement that this should be performed before 1 year of age, partly for the parents' sake and also before the child has become aware of her body image.

• Hypospadias repair. In males with severe hypospadias, the best results are achieved with a two stage procedure which can be performed duirng the first 4 years of life. During the first stage of the procedure the penis is straightened by the release of the chordee present. Penile skin is then either rotated or grafted onto the ventral shaft. The second stage of the procedure involves creating a new urethra by 'tubularizing' this new skin to the tip of the glans penis.

• Vaginal reconstruction. This is a particularly controversial area. Early vaginal reconstruction, often with use of skin flaps to augment the introitus, can be performed at the age of 1 year. This is particularly desirable in infants with drainage problems of either the bladder or uterus early on. However, while early vaginoplasty may avoid the psychological trauma of genital surgery later in life, this approach carries a significant risk of stenosis requir-

ing further surgery at adolescence. For this reason some surgeons are preferring to delay vaginal reconstruction until puberty, followed by self dilation postoperatively.

• Gonadectomy. In 46,XY individuals who are to be raised as females, there is no reason to delay gonadectomy except in the instance of CAIS (complete androgen insensitivity syndrome). Currently there is no consensus as to the optimal age of gonadal removal in CAIS. Advocates of prepubertal removal feel that the risk of gonadal malignancy, however remote, is unacceptable. Advocates of gonadectomy following puberty believe that secondary sexual development is better with endogenous oestrogen production.

Psychological aspects of intersex

Counselling of parents

The scenario of ambiguous genitalia at birth with uncertainty as to gender assignment is associated with great parental anguish. The discovery, perhaps many years after birth, that the child has abnormal gonads and will be unable to have children without assistance, if at all, is also deeply wounding to many parents. It is important for the clinician to invest as much time as possible in counselling parents at the time that the intersex problem is discovered. It is unrealistic to expect all the information to be assimilated by the family in one sitting, and several sessions will be required. Equally, it is unrealistic to rely too much on printed information (e.g. parent booklets) in the early stages. Simple explanation, assisted by hand drawings, and tailored to the parents' psychological state, education and intellect require time, patience and experience. The continuing involvement of a psychologist or psychiatrist with an interest in intersex is highly desirable.

Counselling of patients

There is no place for withholding information from people with intersex. Children should receive a brief explanation of their problem as soon as they are able to understand. If the child is properly counselled by the paediatrician and parents during the prepubertal years it will then be possible to give a full and honest account of the problem in adolescence. The classic difficult scenario is explaining the condition to a girl with CAIS. It may be helpful to phrase the explanation thus: 'The great majority of girls and women have two X chromosomes and ovaries. A minority of otherwise normal women have XY chromosomes, testes in the abdomen instead of ovaries, but complete resistance to the male hormone (testosterone) made by the testes. In this situation the body is extremely sensitive to oestrogen, which is made from the testosterone, and this results in normal female development. However, there is no womb and therefore you will not be able to carry a child, nor will you be able to have periods.' If this degree of honesty seems unacceptable, then attendance at an androgen insensitivity syndrome support group is recommended. The anger and frustration felt by individuals in whom the diagnosis of intersex has been obscured or withheld makes a convincing case for honesty from childhood onwards.

Future developments

• Complex genital anomalies are uncommon, and children require help from a variety of health professionals. The development of a managed clinical network, with multidisciplinary clinics involving surgeons (adult and paediatric), endocrinologists, geneticists, psychologists, biochemists and radiologists will enhance both patient care and training. Several models for this approach have been established in the United Kingdom, and this trend is to be encouraged.
• Increased understanding of the molecular genetic basis for intersex disorders will clarify the aetiology in an increasing number of specific disorders.
• Long-term follow-up data are needed to help determine the optimal surgical management of complex genital anomalies, particularly congenital adrenal hyperplasia in females. Multi-centre studies organised jointly by paediatric endocrinologists and surgeons are required.
• The psychological management of parents, children and adolescents and adults affected by interesex disorders, including complex genital anomalies is improving but still requires considerable development.

Potential pitfalls

• Labial fusion, a common problem, may give the misleading impression of an absent vagina.
• Most boys referred with micropenis have simple obesity and a normal prepubertal phallus buried in surrounding fat.
• Incorrect assignment of male gender to masculinised females with 21-hydroxlase deficiency. The absence of palpable gonads in an apparent male with hypospadias should always arouse suspicion.

Controversial points

• When should clitoroplasty and vaginoplasty be performed in girls with congenital adrenal hyperplasia?
• Given the masculinizing effect of high androgen levels on the fetal brain, should severely virilized genetic females be raised as males, and should severely undermasculinised males still be raised as males?
• Should the gonads of individuals with CAIS be removed as soon as the diagnosis is made, or allowed to remain *in situ* until secondary sexual development is complete?

When to involve a specialist centre

• When a baby is born with complex genital anomaly.
• Severe hypospadias ± cryptorchidism.
• Complete androgen insensitivity syndrome.
• Gonadal dysgenesis.

CASE HISTORIES

Case 1
A newborn baby is of indeterminate gender with a clitorophallus, labioscrotal folds, single urogenital orifice and no gonad palpable. Pelvic ultrasound shows a uterus and vagina.

Question
What is the most likely diagnosis and what immediate investigations should be performed?

Answer
The most likely diagnosis is congenital adrenal hyperplasia in a genetic female. Essential investigations are the karyotype, which was 46,XX, and the 17-OHP level, which was 110 nmol/L [3663 ng/dL] on day 1

rising to above 300 nmol/L [10,000 ng/dL] on day 3. Although 17-OHP measurement should officially be deferred until day 3, a distinctly elevated level on day 1 in the context of a genital anomaly is diagnostic.

Case 2

A newborn baby has abnormal genitalia with a small gonad palpable in one labioscrotal fold and no gonad palpable on the other side. Pelvic ultrasound and genitography show a vagina and uterus. Karyotype is 45,X/46,XY. 17-OHP levels are normal.

Question

What is the diagnosis and how should the child be assigned?

Answer

The diagnosis is mixed gonadal dysgenesis with a dysplastic testis on one side and probably a streak gonad on the other. The presence of Mullerian structures indicates very poor AMH production by the dysplastic testis and it will probably be appropriate to raise this child as a female.

Case 3

A newborn baby has a small hypospadic phallus with bifid scrotum and both gonads palpable in the labioscrotal folds. Pelvic ultrasound shows no uterus and short vagina. Karyotype is 46,XY; 17-OHP levels are normal.

Question

What is the most likely diagnosis and how should the child be managed?

Answer

The suppression of female structures indicates that the gonads are testes which are producing AMH normally. The diagnosis lies between a biosynthetic defect in testosterone production (rare) or, more likely, a partial degree of androgen resistance. Plasma androgen should be measured before and following stimulation with hCG and, with PAIS, may show normal or high levels. In the absence of female structures a female gender assignment would be difficult surgically. The child should be brought up as a boy unless the amount of phallic tissue present is inadequate.

Further reading

Ahmed, S.F. & Hughes, I.A. (2002) The genetics of male undermasculinisation *Clinical Endocrinology* **56**, 1–18.

Ahmed, S.F., Khwaja, O. & Hughes, I.A. (2000) Clinical and gender assignment in cases of male undermasculinization: the role for a masculinization score. *British Journal of Urology* **85**, 120–124.

Grumbach, N.M. & Conte, F.A. (1998) Disorders of sex differentiation. In: *Williams' Textbook of Endocrinology* (eds J.D. Wilson, D. W. Foster, H.M. Kronenberg & P.R. Larsen), 9th edn, pp. 1303–1426. W.B. Saunders.

8 Adrenal disorders

Physiology

Adrenal anatomy and physiology

The adrenal glands are pyramidal structures which lie adjacent to the upper poles of the kidneys. The adrenal cortex is divided into three zones: the outer zona glomerulosa; middle zona fasciculata; and inner zona reticularis. The main types of steroid produced by the adrenal cortex are mineralocorticoids (principally aldosterone), glucocorticoids (principally cortisol) and androgens. Steroidogenesis in the zona fasciculata and reticularis is under hypothalamic–pituitary control; secretion of aldosterone from the zona glomerulosa is under the control of the renin–angiotensin system.

Hypothalamic–pituitary axis (Fig. 8.1)

Corticotrophin-releasing hormone (CRH) is synthesized in the hypothalamus and acts on the corticotrophs of the anterior pituitary to secrete the peptide pro-opiomelanocortin (POMC). POMC is the precursor of adrenocorticotrophic hormone (ACTH). ACTH binds to a melanocortin-2 receptor (MC-2R), a cell surface receptor in the cells of the adrenal cortex. ACTH also has affinity for the melanocortin-1 receptor (MC-1R) in the skin, so that ACTH excess results in hyperpigmentation. The MC-2R is G-protein coupled, and activation results in increased adenylate cyclase activity which in turn increases intracellular cyclic adenosine monophosphate (cAMP). Increased cAMP activity enhances the transport of cholesterol across the mitochondrial membrane by the steroidogenic acute regulatory (StAR) protein.

Cholesterol is metabolized into the three types of steroid: glucocorticoid, mineralocorticoid and androgen. Cortisol is vital for normal health; maintaining an adequate blood glucose level; and for combating stress. It follows a circadian rhythm, with high levels on waking and a nadir at midnight. Cortisol has a negative feedback influence on the hypothalamic–pituitary axis. Thus ACTH levels will be elevated in primary adrenal insufficiency and suppressed when cortisol excess is caused by autonomous adrenal lesions or exogenous glucocorticoids. In primary adrenal insufficiency, cortisol levels will depend on the severity of the defect. In severe deficiency cortisol is low despite massively raised ACTH, but in partial deficiency basal cortisol may be normal. However, since adrenal output is maximal in this situation, there will be no increase in response to stress—a dangerous state of affairs.

Steroid pathways

Adrenal steroidogenesis is under the control of the cytochrome P450 (CYP) and the hydroxysteroid dehydrogenase (HSD) enzymes. Pregnenolone may be converted along the mineralocorticoid pathway to aldosterone, along the glucocorticoid pathway to cortisol, or along the androgen pathway to testosterone (Fig. 8.2). Impairment of cortisol synthesis will result from disorders affecting the StAR protein and 3-β hydroxysteroid dehydrogenase (3-βHSD), CYP 21A2 (21-hydroxylase), CYP 11B1 (11-hydroxylase) and the CYP 17 (17-hydroxylase) enzymes. These enzyme disorders are collectively known as congenital adrenal hyperplasia (CAH), as cortisol deficiency causes increased ACTH secretion and thus enlargement

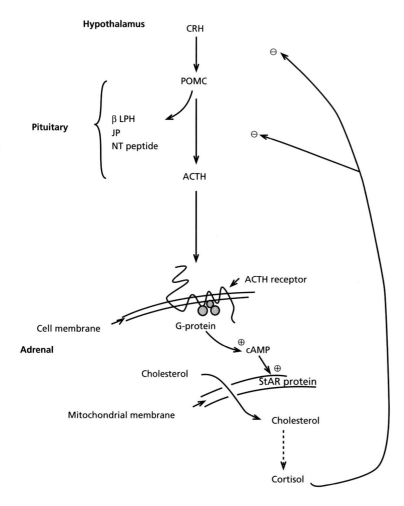

Fig. 8.1 Schematic diagram of hypotha-lamic–pituitary–adrenal axis. β LPH, β lipotrophic hormone; CRH, corticotro-phin-releasing hormone; JP, joining peptide; N-T peptide, N-terminal peptide; POMC, pro-opiomelanocortin; StAR protein, steroidogenic acute regulatory protein. +, positive effect; –, negative effect.

of the adrenal glands. Mineralocorticoid deficiency will result from StAR protein, 3-βHSD and CYP 21 deficiencies. In contrast, CYP 11B1 deficiency results in accu-mulation of the potent mineralocorticoid precursor deoxy-corticosterone (DOC), while 17-hydroxylase deficiency also causes mineralocorticoid excess. Finally, deficiency in the enzymes proximal to androgen synthesis—StAR protein, CYP 17 (17,20-desmolase) and 17-βHSD—result in androgen deficiency, although 3-βHSD deficiency paradoxically causes virilization in females as a result of increased synthesis of dehydroepiandosterone and its peripheral conversion to testosterone.

Mineralocorticoid synthesis

Aldosterone synthetase, encoded by the CYP 11B2 gene, converts DOC to aldosterone (Fig. 8.3). Renin, secreted from the juxtaglomerular apparatus in the kidney, causes cleavage of angiotensinogen into angiotensin 1. This in turn is cleaved by angiotensin-converting enzyme (ACE) into angiotensin 2, a potent stimulator of CYP 11B2 activity, promoting aldosterone secretion from the zona glomerulo-sa. Renin will thus be elevated when aldosterone synthesis is impaired, and suppressed with aldosterone excess. Al-dosterone enters the distal renal tubule cells, binds to its receptor and enters the nucleus causing transcription of messenger RNA and new protein synthesis. This protein contributes to enhanced $Na^+ K^+$ ATPase ('sodium pump') activity, causing sodium re-absorption in exchange for in-creased potassium excretion, while sodium for hydrogen ion exchange across the amiloride-sensitive epithelial sodium channel (ENaC) is also increased.

The following points should be noted:
• Cortisol has a similar affinity for the mineralocorticoid receptor as aldosterone, but is prevented from competing

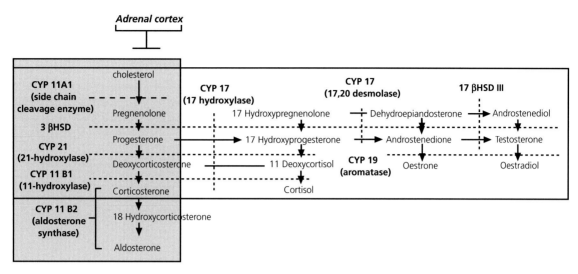

Fig. 8.2 Pathways of steroid synthesis in adrenal cortex. βHSD, β hydroxysteroid dehydrogenase. Shaded area indicates aldosterone synthesis in zona glomerulosa. Cortisol and androgen are synthesized in the zona fasciculata and zona reticularis.

by the enzyme 11-βHSD 2 which converts cortisol to cortisone. A deficiency of this enzyme causes apparent mineralocorticoid excess.

- Inactivating mutations of the ENaC result in failure of aldosterone action with elevated aldosterone levels—pseudohypoaldosteronism (PHA).
- Activating mutations of the ENaC result in apparent aldosterone excess despite low levels—Liddle's syndrome.
- Aldosterone excess causes sodium retention, with hypernatraemia, hypokalaemia, a metabolic alkalosis and hypertension.

Investigations of adrenocortical function

Biochemical

Glucocorticoid secretion (Table 8.1)

Glucocorticoid excess and deficiency states are often difficult to diagnose because cortisol levels normally fluctuate widely according to the time of day, state of arousal, and stress factors. Glucocorticoid excess results in normal or high random cortisol levels, loss of the normal circadian rhythm, an increase in urine-free cortisol and failure of plasma cortisol to suppress with low-dose dexamethasone.

Glucocorticoid deficiency is easy to diagnose if the defect is in the adrenal gland itself (primary adrenal insufficiency) because this will result in elevated ACTH levels and low cortisol levels with absent or impaired rise following synthetic ACTH (Synacthen) stimulation. Diagnosis is more difficult when the defect lies in the hypothalamus or pituitary gland (secondary adrenal insufficiency). In suspected secondary adrenal insufficiency the low-dose synthetic ACTH (Synacthen) test is helpful. The rationale for this test is that the adrenal glands, if understimulated for months or years, will respond subnormally to *quasi* physiological stimulation. If the pituitary axis is being assessed in the course of an insulin hypoglycaemia or clonidine test, the cortisol response to stress can be gauged.

Mineralocorticoid secretion (Table 8.2)

Mineralocorticoid deficiency is assessed by measurement of plasma electrolytes, renin and aldosterone.

Adrenal androgen secretion (Table 8.3)

Adrenal androgen status is assessed by urine steroid analysis and by assessment of serum steroids under basal and stimulated conditions. Salivary or capillary profiles collected at home for 17-hydroxyprogesterone (17-OHP) and androstenedione measurement are valuable in the monitoring of adrenal enzyme disorders, notably CAH resulting from 21-hydroxylase deficiency.

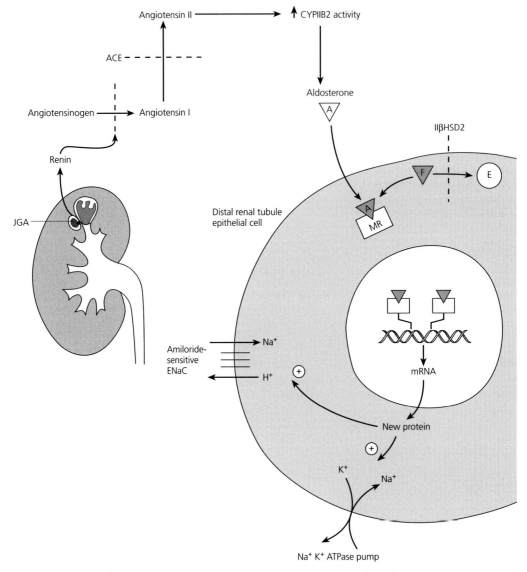

Fig. 8.3 Schematic diagram of aldosterone stimulation and action. A, aldosterone; ACE, angiotensin converting enzyme; E, cortisone; ENaC, epithelial sodium channel; F, cortisol; JGA, juxtaglomerular apparatus; MR, mineralocorticoid receptor.

Imaging

If a central cause for glucocorticoid excess or deficiency is discovered, imaging of the hypothalamic–pituitary axis by computed tomography (CT) or, preferably, magnetic resonance imaging (MRI) will be required. Adrenal ultrasound is a useful screening test for adrenal enlargement, but CT or MRI will be needed to identify small lesions.

Glucocorticoid excess

Cushing's syndrome

Cushing's syndrome, unless iatrogenic, is very rare in childhood (Fig. 8.4). However, its principal feature—obesity—is extremely common, so that the possibility of Cushing's syndrome is often raised.

Table 8.1 Investigation of glucocorticoid secretion.

Basal samples	Reference values
Plasma	
Fasting glucose	4–7 mmol/L
08.00 h ACTH	<20 mU/L
24.00 h (sleeping) cortisol	<50 nmol/L
08.00 h cortisol	200–700 nmol/L
Saliva	
08.00 h cortisol	6.5–28 nmol/L (usually 9–16) median 14.5
18.00 h cortisol	≤10 (mean 1.4)
Urine	
Urinary-free cortisol (random)	<25 μmol/mmol creatinine
Suppression tests	
Low-dose dexamethasone (0.5 mg 6-hourly ×8)	<50 nmol/L at 09.00 h 48 h after first dose
High-dose dexamethasone (2 mg 6-hourly ×8)	<50% basal value 48 h after first dose
Stimulation tests	
CRH (1 μg/kg IV)	Doubling of ACTH (usually to 8–25 mU/L)
	Cortisol peak ≥600 nmol/L with >20% increase over basal value
Standard short Synacthen (250 μg/m² IV)	Peak value >500 nmol/L ± doubling of basal value
Low-dose short Synacthen (500 ng/m² IV)	Peak value >500 nmol/L ± doubling of basal value
Insulin hypoglycaemia (min blood glucose <2.2 mmol/L)	Peak value >500 nmol/L
Metyrapone test	Doubling of plasma 11 deoxycortisol and urinary tetrahydrodeoxycortisol

Reference values are taken from the Institute of Biochemistry, Glasgow Royal Infirmary. Salivary cortisol data kindly provided by Dr J. Schulga are derived from 147 healthy children aged 5–15 years. Abbreviations: ACTH, adrenocorticotrophic hormone; CRH, corticotrophin-releasing hormone.

Causes

The causes of Cushing's syndrome in childhood are the following:

- Iatrogenic:
  oral steroids;
  skin preparations containing steroids;
  steroid nose drops; and
  inhaled steroids.
- Cushing's disease (ACTH-secreting pituitary tumour).
- Adrenal tumour (cortical adenoma or carcinoma).
- Primary adrenal hyperplasia:
  bilateral micronodular dysplasia (+/− Carney complex); and
  McCune–Albright syndrome.
- Ectopic ACTH syndrome.

Clinical diagnosis

Symptoms
- Obesity.
- Slow growth (overtaken by siblings and peers).
- Fatigue.
- Emotional lability.

Signs
- Cushingoid habitus with moon face, central obesity, buffalo hump.
- Facial plethora.
- Acne.
- Hirsutism.
- Striae.
- Hypertension.

Table 8.2 Investigation of mineralocorticoid secretion.

Electrolytes	Normal values	Mineralocorticoid excess	Mineralocorticoid deficiency
Sodium	Na 135–145 mmol/L	Normal or ↑	↓
Potassium	K 3.5–4.5 mmol/L	Normal or ↓	↑
Aldosterone (pmol/L)*			
Infants <1 month	1000–5500	↑ in hyperaldosteronism	↓ in hypoaldosteronism
Infants 1–6 months	500–4500	↓ in AME and Liddle's syndrome	↑↑ in PHA
Infants 6–12 months	160–3000		
Children 1–4 years	70–1000		
Children 5–15 years	30–600		
Adults	30–420		
Plasma renin activity (ng/ml/h)† (supine for 30 min)			
Infants (<1 year)	<31	Suppressed	↑
Children 1–4 years	<26		
Children 5–15 years	<9		
Adults	<2.6		

*Aldosterone data obtained using Diagnostic Products Corporation Coat-A-Count Aldosterone Kit. †Plasma renin activity data obtained using BioChem ImmunoSystems Renin Maia Kit (Code 129640). Abbreviations: AME, apparent mineralocorticoid excess; PHA, pseudohypoaldosteronism.

Auxology
- Height below mid-parental centile.
- Height velocity subnormal.
- Bone age usually delayed.

The crucial difference between obesity as a result of Cushing's syndrome and simple obesity is in the growth pattern. Cushing's syndrome is almost always associated with growth failure while simple obesity causes an increase in growth rate. Therefore, in simple obesity the child's height centile is above the midparental height centile, while in Cushing's syndrome it is below. Appreciation of this difference in auxology will largely protect children with simple obesity from being investigated for Cushing's syndrome although the occasional child with normal variant short stature and simple obesity may cause confusion.

Investigations

Where exogenous steroid excess is suspected a 09.00 hours plasma cortisol followed by a low-dose Synacthen test and ACTH measurement will confirm suppression of the pituitary–adrenal axis (Table 8.1). If the features of Cushing's syndrome are accompanied by virilization then an adrenal tumour is likely and an adrenal MRI (or CT) scan should be performed. If neither of the above apply and Cushing's syndrome is seriously suspected then careful evaluation is required.

Diagnosis of Cushing's syndrome
This suggested sequence can be carried out in a non-specialist centre.
- Measurement of midnight and 09.00 hours cortisol levels, looking for loss of the normal circadian rhythm.
- Measurement of three consecutive 24-hour urinary free cortisol estimations looking for elevated cortisol excretion.
- *Low-dose dexamethasone suppression test*, measuring 09.00 hours serum cortisol, then giving 0.5 mg dexamethasone at 09.00, 15.00, 21.00, 03.00 hours × 2, i.e. eight doses over 48 hours, then re-measuring 09.00 hours serum cortisol. Failure of cortisol to suppress below 50 nmol/L following low-dose dexamethasone confirms Cushing's syndrome.

Diagnosis of the **cause** *of Cushing's syndrome*
This can be difficult. Referral to a specialist centre is recommended.
- ACTH measurement at 09.00 hours—undetectable values suggests a primary adrenal lesion, detectable levels pituitary Cushing's and elevated levels ectopic ACTH syndrome.
- *High-dose dexamethasone suppression test*, measuring 09.00 hours serum cortisol, then giving dexamethasone 2 mg at 9.00, 15.00, 21.00 and 03.00 hours × 2, i.e. eight doses over 48 hours, then remeasuring 09.00 hours serum

Table 8.3 Investigation of adrenal steroid precursors and androgens.

17-hydroxyprogesterone
Plasma (nmol/L) of plasma

Normal neonates	<13	
Stressed / preterm neonates	<40	
Neonates with CAH	>100	
Adults		
Basal	<13	
60 min after 250 μm i.v. Synacthen	<20	
Blood spot (nmol/L of blood)	**Extraction assay**	**Direct assay**
Stressed / preterm neonates	<70	<140
Neonates with CAH	>180	>350
Saliva (nmol/L of saliva)		
Children 5–15 years 09.00 h	0.16–0.66 (median range 0.22–0.4)	

Androstenedione (mean ± SD)	**Male**	**Female**
Plasma (nmol/L)		
1–2 months	1.5 ± 0.45	0.66 ± 0.24
>6 months–adrenarche	<0.4	<0.4
Adult male	3.7 ± 0.9	
Adult female		
follicular phase		2.7 ± 1.0
luteal phase		5.2 ± 1.5
Saliva		
5–15 years 09.00 h	0.04–0.96 (median range 0.2–0.7)	

Testosterone (mean ± SD)	**Male**	**Female**
Plasma (nmol/L)		
First week	1.15 ± 0.15	0.45 ± 0.3
1–2 months	8.8 ± 2.7	0.28 ± 0.13
>6 months–prepubertal	<0.3	<0.3
Adult male	19.8 ± 4.7	
Adult female		
follicular phase		0.75 ± 0.2
luteal phase		1.28 ± 0.3

Dehydroepiandrosterone sulphate (μmol/L)	**Male**	**Female**
Infancy, pre-adrenarche	<2	<2
Adult	2–9	2–11

Blood spot 17-hydroxyprogesterone data are from A. M. Wallace *et al.* (1986). Salivary data are from Dr Schulga (see Table 8.1). Plasma androstenedione and testosterone data are from M. G. Forest (1993).

cortisol. A fall in cortisol to below more than 50% of the basal value is suggestive of pituitary Cushing's (Cushing's disease), while failure to suppress suggests a primary adrenal cause or ectopic ACTH syndrome.
• CRH test, giving CRH 1 μg/kg intravenously after overnight fast and measuring serum cortisol and ACTH at –15, 0, 15, 30, 45, 60, 90 and 120 minutes. A rise in serum cortisol to ≥600 nmol/L [≥17 micrograms/dL] suggests pituitary Cushing's; no rise in cortisol and undetectable ACTH suggests a primary adrenal lesion, and no rise in cortisol with elevated ACTH suggests ectopic ACTH secretion.

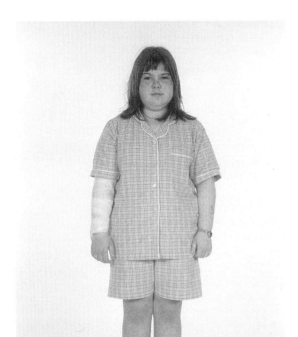

Fig. 8.4 A 10-year-old girl with Cushing's disease causing obesity and growth failure.

• High-resolution imaging of the pituitary gland with MRI scan may show a lesion in Cushing's disease in approximately 50% of cases.

The final step in the investigation of Cushing's disease is bilateral inferior petrosal sinus sampling via femoral vein catheters. This technique, which should only be carried out in a specialist center, is helpful in confirming that the ACTH secretion is of pituitary origin, and not from an ectopic lesion. It may also identify on which side of the pituitary gland the adenoma is located.

Treatment

Iatrogenic Cushing's syndrome must be managed by withdrawal of the steroid preparation or, if this is not possible, by minimizing the dosage given, or converting to an alternate day regimen. If severe adrenal suppression has occurred, hydrocortisone replacement may be required for months or even years following treatment. Treatment of an adrenal or pituitary tumour is by surgical resection,

followed by hydrocortisone replacement if the other adrenal gland is suppressed.

Cushing's disease is treated by trans-sphenoidal surgical exploration with removal of the microadenoma. If none is identified, but petrosal sinus sampling has suggested lateralization of ACTH secretion, then a hemi-hypophysectomy can be carried out. A postoperative cortisol level of <50 nmol/L [<1.4 micrograms/dL] indicates that the adenoma has been completely removed and the patient is cured. The treatment of choice for Cushing's disease following failed pituitary exploration is direct pituitary irradiation. The alternative, bilateral adrenalectomy, carries a risk of pituitary tumour development with hyperpigmentation—Nelson's syndrome.

The ectopic ACTH syndrome may be seen as part of an established malignancy. Occasionally, small carcinoid lesions (e.g. lungs, pancreas) may be responsible, requiring location by CT scanning with selective venous sampling where necessary, and surgical removal.

Cushing's syndrome caused by bilateral micronodular dysplasia with or without primary pigmentation (Carney's syndrome), or the McCune–Albright syndrome, should be treated medically if features are mild to moderate, otherwise by bilateral adrenalectomy. When surgical resection is impossible (e.g. with infiltrating carcinoma) or in pituitary Cushing's syndrome when there may be a delay of several months before remission occurs (e.g. following radiotherapy), then medical therapy must be given. Useful agents include metyrapone and ketoconazole. In adrenal carcinoma, the adrenal cytotoxic *o,p'*-dichlorodiphenyl-dichloroethane (*o,p'*-DDD) (mitotane) is of temporary benefit.

Follow-up

After definitive treatment of Cushing's syndrome patients should be seen 3-monthly to monitor growth rate, body composition and signs of recurrence.

Glucocorticoid deficiency

Adrenal insufficiency caused by hypothalamic-pituitary disease—secondary adrenal insufficiency

Causes

The causes of secondary adrenal insufficiency (SAI) are as follows:

Congenital:
• idiopathic congenital hypopituitarism;

- septo-optic dysplasia;
- other mid-line CNS disorders; or
- isolated ACTH deficiency.

Acquired:
- craniopharyngioma;
- cranial irradiation (e.g. for medulloblastoma);
- surgery to hypothalamic–pituitary area;
- steroid therapy; or
- rare causes of hypopituitarism (e.g. vascular insult, trauma, meningitis).

Clinical features

ACTH deficiency is usually seen in the context of panhypopituitarism. Severe ACTH deficiency at birth causes hypoglycaemia, poor feeding, convulsions and jaundice. The jaundice may be isolated or part of a neonatal hepatitis syndrome which resolves once hydrocortisone is started.

In older children, the symptoms of SAI are nonspecific. Cortisol deficiency is responsible for tiredness and lack of energy, while symptoms referable to the immune system are an increase in the frequency of intercurrent illnesses, and a longer recovery period from such illnesses.

Investigations

In the newborn infant, dynamic studies are difficult to perform. If congenital panhypopituitarism is strongly suspected (hypoglycaemia, jaundice, micropenis, low plasma thyroxine and random plasma cortisol levels of 50 nmol/L [<1.4 micrograms/dL] then replacement should be instituted without delay. In more doubtful cases where the child is reasonably stable 1 μg Synacthen can be given and the cortisol response assessed at 30, 60, 90 and 120 minutes under fasting conditions. Peak values of <500 nmol/L [<17 micrograms/dL] are suggestive of prenatal hypostimulation of the adrenal glands.

In children with suspected SAI, especially survivors of cancer, investigation depends on the severity of symptoms and the clinical context. Children who have received doses of >3000 cGy are particularly at risk. Cortisol secretion can be assessed by carrying out a low-dose Synacthen test, or a salivary cortisol profile. If the growth axis is also under investigation, the cortisol reponse to insulin-induced hypoglycaemia can be assessed.

Treatment

Hydrocortisone, 10 mg/m^2/day should be given either morning and evening or three times a day. Treatment during an intercurrent illness or during surgery is as for 21-hydroxylase deficiency (see below). Once the child is on glucocorticoid replacement, biochemical monitoring is not usually necessary.

Primary adrenal insufficiency

Causes

Congenital:
- Adrenal hypoplasia:
  X-linked (including DAX-1 mutation); or
  autosomal recessive.
- Congenital adrenal hyperplasia.
- Familial glucocorticoid deficiency (autosomal recessive).

Acquired (Addison's disease):
- Isolated autoimmune adrenalitis.
- Adrenalitis associated with other autoimmune endocrinopathies.
- Adrenoleukodystrophy (ALD).
- Tuberculosis.
- Bilateral adrenalectomy.
- Drugs (e.g. cyproterone).

Congenital adrenal hypoplasia

In the newborn period, cortisol deficiency will cause hypoglycaemia and jaundice while aldosterone deficiency will result in poor feeding, vomiting and failure to thrive. Symptoms usually start from day 10 onwards. Boys with the DAX-1 mutation may have bilateral cryptorchidism in infancy, manifesting gonadotrophin deficiency in adolescence. Investigations will show hyponatraemia, hyperkalaemia, elevated renin and ACTH, but low or normal 17-OHP.

Familial glucocorticoid deficiency

Familial glucocorticoid deficiency (FGD, also known as hereditary unresponsiveness to ACTH) is an autosomal recessive disorder in which the adrenal cortex is unable to respond to ACTH. In about 25% of cases a mutation on the ACTH receptor MC2-R can be identified. These children, who tend to be of tall stature, are classified as having FGD type I. FGD without an MC2-R mutation is termed FGD type 2. Recently mutations in a new gene encoding a protein called melanocortin 2 receptor accessory protein (MRAP) have been identified in some cases of FGD type 2. It is thought that MRAP may play a role in the processing, trafficking or function of the MC2-R.

FGD causes severe cortisol deficiency, presenting with jaundice, neonatal hepatitis syndrome, poor feeding, failure to thrive and hypoglycaemia in infancy. Older children may present with collapse and coma sometimes with fatal consequences so that the diagnosis is made *post mortem*. Investigation shows elevated ACTH, low cortisol with poor or no response to Synacthen, and normal renin levels. Plasma potassium is usually normal but a degree of hyponatraemia may be present. This is attributable to cortisol deficiency causing impaired water secretion at the renal tubule.

Treatment

Congenital adrenal hypoplasia should be treated similarly to 21-hydroxylase deficiency (see below). FGD should be treated with hydrocortisone but not fludrocortisone or salt.

Acquired adrenal insufficiency (Addison's disease)

Causes

Autoimmune adrenalitis is the most common cause of Addison's disease. Although seen in isolation it may also be associated with other autoimmune disorders, such as diabetes mellitus and Hashimoto's thyroiditis, and with the polyglandular autoimmune (PGA) syndromes. PGA I, also known as autoimmune polyendocrinopathy with cutaneous ectodermal dysplasia (APECED), is caused by a gene mutation of the AIRE gene on chromosome 21 and has its onset in childhood and adolescence. Components of APECED syndrome include the following:

Endocrine disorders:
- Addison's disease;
- hypoparathyroidism;
- primary ovarian failure
- diabetes mellitus; and
- Hashimoto's thyroiditis.

Non-endocrine disorders:
- vitiligo;
- alopecia;
- malabsorption;
- hepatitis; and
- keratitis.

Immune deficiency:
- increased prevalence of infections, particularly mucocutaneous candidiasis.

ALD is an X-linked disorder affecting both the central nervous system and the adrenal cortex. Onset may be in childhood or early adulthood The phenotype is highly variable, even within families, so that the presence and severity of neurological impairment and adrenal failure varies from case to case. Severely affected individuals suffer progressive neurological disability and ultimately death. The neurological symptoms may precede those of adrenal

insufficiency, or vice versa. Therefore, all males presenting with Addison's disease must be investigated for ALD.

Clinical features of Addison's disease

Symptoms include tiredness, weight loss, polyuria, increasing skin pigmentation (Plate 4, facing page 21) and, in the final stages, vomiting, drowsiness and coma. Examination shows increased pigmentation especially in the skin creases, old scars and buccal mucosa, with signs of recent weight loss, and low or normal blood pressure.

Investigations

ACTH is elevated (often >1000 mU/L) and plasma renin activity high. Fasting glucose is normal or low. Basal cortisol is low or normal with no rise following Synacthen administration and in some cases an actual fall in cortisol with symptoms of adrenal collapse. It is therefore important not to undertake a Synacthen test in suspected Addison's disease without full access to oxygen, intravenous glucose, and resuscitation equipment. In the Addisonian crisis, sodium is low, potassium is high and there may be severe hypoglycaemia.

In ALD, the diagnosis is established by measuring very long chain fatty acids (VLCFA) in the plasma. Given the association between Addison's disease, other endocrinopathies and ALD, the following further investigations are recommended:
- VLCFA in males;
- autoantibody screen (adrenal, thyroid, islet cell, parietal cell);
- calcium and phosphate;
- thyroid function;
- haemoglobin and film, vitamin B_{12} and folate; and
- liver function tests.

Thyroid function, haemoglobin and film, calcium and phosphate and liver function tests should be repeated annually to pre-empt the development of other autoimmune diseases.

Treatment

Addisonian crisis is managed by intravenous fluids with 0.9% saline and added 5% dextrose, hydrocortisone by intravenous bolus followed by infusion (see page 141) and conversion to oral hydrocortisone and fludrocortisone once recovery has occurred (Table 8.4).

Follow-up

Once a patient is on established treatment with hydrocortisone and fludrocortisone, clinical monitoring—adjusting the dosage as body surface area increases—is usually sufficient and there is no need for laboratory investigations.

Table 8.4 Dosage schedules for mineralocorticoid, glucocorticoid and salt therapy in adrenal disorders.

Disorder	Mineralocorticoid	Glucocorticoid	Salt
Hypothalamo–pituitary-adrenal insufficiency	Not required	Hydrocortisone 8–10 mg/m²/day	
Primary adrenal insufficiency (Addison's disease)	Fludrocortisone 100 μg/day from birth to adolescence, then 150 μg/day	Hydrocortisone 10–12 mg/m²/day	
Congenital adrenal hyperplasia	As for primary adrenal insufficiency	For first 6 months consider treatments as for CAH. (see pp. 140–1), then hydrocortisone 10–12 mg/m²/day	
FGD	Not required	As for Primary adrenal insufficiency (Addison's disease)	
CAH (21-hydroxylase deficiency)			
Salt-wasting	Fludrocortisone 100 μg/day from birth or 150 μg/m²/day, whichever is greater	For first 6 months of life see pp. 140–1 Oral hydrocortisone 10–15 mg/m²/day thereafter. Prednisolone 3–5 mg/m²/day in late pubertal girls	5 mmol/L/kg/day in three divided doses for first year Not required
Simple virilizing	As above if plasma renin activity ↑ at diagnosis	As above	
Pseudohypoaldosteronism	Not usually effective		Sodium chloride 10–40 mmol/kg/day + calcium resonium

Abbreviations: ACTH, adrenocorticotrophic hormone; CAH, congenital adrenal hyperplasia; FGD, familial glucocorticoid deficiency.

Mineralocorticoid excess

Apart from the secondary hyperaldosteronism, seen in cardiac and renal patients and in chronic volume depletion (leading to activation of the renin–angiotensin system), mineralocorticoid excess is very rare.

Causes
Secondary hyperaldosteronism.
Iatrogenic:
- fludrocortisone overdosage; or
- carbenoxolone therapy or liquorice ingestion.

Aldosterone-secreting adrenal adenoma/hyperplasia (Conn's syndrome).
Enzyme gene mutations:
- CYP 11B1 (11-hydroxylase) deficiency;
- CYP 17 (17-hydroxylase) deficiency;
- 11-βHSD 2 deficiency; or
- CYP 11B2 mutation.

Activating mutation of amiloride-sensitive epithelial sodium channel:
- Liddle's syndrome.

Secondary hyperaldosteronism does not normally present to the endocrinologist. Fludrocortisone overdosage may result in hypertension with or without hypokalaemia. Carbenoxolone is rarely used, but liquorice addiction can cause the syndrome of apparent mineralocorticoid excess (AME) brought about by 11-βHSD 2 inhibition (see below). Aldosterone-secreting adrenal adenomas are rare in childhood, and other causes of hyperaldosteronism must be ruled out before invasive procedures, such as selective adrenal vein sampling, are performed.

Two of the five enzyme disorders causing CAH—CYP 11B1 (11-hydroxylase) and CYP 17 (17-hydroxylase) deficiency—cause hypertension with hypokalaemia. 11-

hydroxylase deficiency causes virilization in girls and sexual precocity in boys from infancy but affected children are hypertensive because of the high levels of DOC, rather than salt losing as in 21-hydroxylase deficiency. 17-Hydroxylase deficiency causes cortisol and androgen blockade so that affected 46,XY individuals are phenotypically female and may present with pubertal failure in association with hypertension and hypokalaemia. Deficiency of the enzyme 11-βHSD 2 results in failure to metabolize cortisol to cortisone with consequent occupation of mineralocorticoid receptors by cortisol (Fig. 8.3). The clinical features are of mineralocorticoid excess but aldosterone levels are suppressed, hence the term *apparent mineralocorticoid excess* (AME).

Mutations of the CYP 11B2 gene may lead to a chimeric enzyme which is under ACTH control, resulting in glucocorticoid-suppressible hyperaldosteronism. This condition should be suspected in the hypertensive adolescent with or without hypokalaemia in whom there is a family history of hypertension and cerebral haemorrhage. Treatment is with dexamethasone or amiloride.

Liddle's syndrome is autosomal dominant and caused by an activating mutation of the ENaC leading to increased sodium absorption with aldosterone and renin suppression. Treatment is with amiloride.

Mineralocorticoid deficiency

Causes
Aldosterone deficiency:
- Congenital adrenal hypoplasia.
- Addison's disease.
- Enzyme disorders:
StAR protein deficiency;
3-βHSD deficiency;
CYP 21 (21-hydroxylase) deficiency; or
CYP 11B2 (aldosterone synthase) deficiency.
Aldosterone resistance (pseudohypoaldosteronism):
- Autosomal dominant or sporadic—affects renal tubule.
- Recessive—affects kidneys, colon, sweat and salivary glands.

Clinical features and investigation
Mineralocorticoid deficiency causes salt wasting with polyuria, vomiting, dehydration and hyperkalaemia which, if severe and untreated, leads to cardiac arrest. In older children, the salt-wasting tendency is partially offset by an instinctive increase in salt intake. Congenital

adrenal hypoplasia and Addison's disease are discussed above; the three types of CAH causing salt wasting are discussed below.

Pseudohypoaldosteronism may be associated with salt wasting and dangerous hyperkalaemia in the newborn period. Affected infants do not respond to large doses of fludrocortisone, and treatment consists of generous sodium replacement (Table 8.4), and calcium resonium to combat the hyperkalaemia. The dominant and sporadic forms are milder and resolve with age. The autosomal recessive variety, caused by inactivating mutations in the ENaC, is severe and runs a protracted course.

Sex steroid excess

Androgen excess

Adrenal causes of androgen excess
- Exaggerated adrenarche.
- Adrenocortical adenoma and carcinoma.
- Congenital adrenal hyperplasia:
CYP 21 (21-hydroxylase) deficiency; and
CYP 11B1 (11-hydroxylase) deficiency.
- 3-βHSD deficiency in females.
- 11-βHSD 1 deficiency.

The most common cause of mild androgenicity in boys and especially girls is an exaggerated form of the adrenal puberty (adrenarche) that occurs between the ages of 6 and 8 years (see Chapter 5). However, signs of severe androgenicity—with clitoral or phallic enlargement—in girls or prepubertal boys suggest an androgen-secreting tumour or an enzyme defect.

Adrenocortical tumour

Clinical features
Significant androgenic features develop over a period of weeks or months in a child of previously normal stature. In boys, the testes are prepubertal (Fig. 8.5). Height status, growth rate and bone age may be increased or normal, depending on the duration of the illness.

Investigations
These show elevation of one or more adrenal androgens, androstenedione and dehydroepiandrosterone (DHEAS), with low basal luteinizing hormone (LH) and follicle-stimulating hormone (FSH) and suppressed responses to luteinizing hormone-releasing hormone (LHRH). Urine steroid profile may show increased androgen secretion.

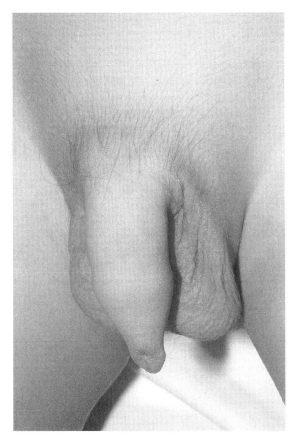

Fig. 8.5 Penile enlargement, pubic hair development and scrotal laxity with prepubertal (2 mL) testes in a 2-year-old boy. Investigation showed a small tumour in the right adrenal cortex.

Treatment

Treatment is by surgical removal wherever possible. Pathology usually shows an adrenal cortical cell adenoma, often with cellular pleomorphism and some worrying histological features including capsular invasion. However, if the tumour is well circumscribed and <5 cm in diameter the prognosis is good. Rarely, histology shows adrenal carcinoma in which case the prognosis is poor with death from locally invasive disease and metastases.

Adrenal enzyme defects

21-hydroxylase deficiency is by far the most common adrenal enzyme disorder and will be discussed in detail. 11- and 17-hydroxylase deficiency are discussed above (see page 137). 3-βHSD deficiency in females causes mild virilization because of high DHEAS levels. The very rare

11-βHSD 1 deficiency has been reported as causing virilization in adult females because of cortisol deficiency and increased ACTH drive.

21-hydroxylase deficiency

Incidence
The incidence varies between 1 in 2500 births in Yupik Eskimos to 1 in 30 000 in some countries; the overall incidence (including the UK) is approximately 1 in 15 000 births.

Pathogenesis and classification
21-hydroxylase deficiency results from mutations in the 21-B gene, which is situated on chromosome 6.

The phenotype of 21-hydroxylase deficiency correlates reasonably well with the genotype.
- Salt-wasting 21-hydroxylase deficiency (SW 21-OHD) results from a child inheriting two severe mutations, leading to complete or near-complete loss of 21-B function, with <1% of normal 21-hydroxylase activity.
- Simple virilizing 21-hydroxylase deficiency (SV 21-OHD) occurs if one of the two mutations (e.g. point mutation Ile 172Asn) is relatively mild with 1–5% preservation of 21-hydroxylase activity. Significant salt loss does not occur, although plasma renin activity is often elevated.
- Non-classical or late onset 21-hydroxylase deficiency (NC 21-OHD) results if one mutation is mild (e.g. Val 281Leu). The condition is seen in females from adolescence onwards and causes androgenicity with or without the polycystic ovary syndrome.

Clinical features
SW 21-OHD in females presents with virilization at birth. The clitoris (homologous with the glans penis) is enlarged, often to the size of a phallus; the labia majora (homologous with the scrotum) may be fused; and the labia minora (homologous with the shaft of the penis) may not be identifiable (Fig. 8.6). The vagina and urethra may enter a common urogenital sinus, which becomes increasingly narrow with the severity of virilization. Virilization can be graded in severity according to the Prader classification (Fig. 8.7).

Males with SW 21-OHD present from day 5 onwards, usually in the second week of life, with a salt-losing crisis featuring poor feeding, vomiting, poor weight gain and listlessness. Examination shows dehydration with pigmentation of the scrotum. Biochemistry reveals hyponatraemia, hyperkalaemia and, often, hypoglycaemia.

Boys with SV 21-OHD, and girls with SV 21-OHD in

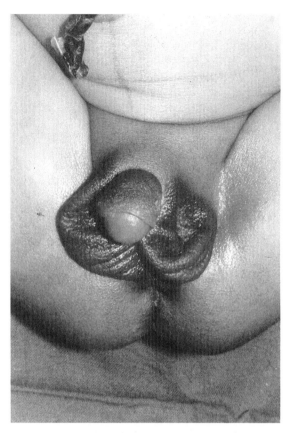

Fig. 8.6 Severe virilization with fusion and scrotalization of labia majora and gross clitoral enlargement in female infant with 21-hydroxylase deficiency.

whom virilization at birth has been mild and/or missed, will present later in childhood (usually 2–4 years) with the effects of androgen excess: enlarged penis or clitoris, pubic hair, greasy skin, long-standing tall stature and advanced bone age. Both girls and boys with SV 21-hydroxylase deficiency tend to develop true puberty early because of the early exposure of the hypothalamic–pituitary axis to sex hormones ('priming'). The combination of advanced bone age because of androgen excess, compounded by true puberty, leads to premature closure of the epiphyses and impaired adult final height.

NC 21-OHD is a rare but important cause of hyperandrogenism in adolescent and adult females and should be considered in the differential diagnosis of the polycystic ovary syndrome.

Diagnosis

SW 21-OHD is diagnosed in females with ambiguous genitalia, no palpable gonads, hyperpigmentation of the labia majora, and a uterus on ultrasound, and in boys with

a salt-wasting crisis. Biochemical confirmation is by 17-OHP measurement; values usually >100 nmol/L [>3300 ng/dL]. All infants should have urine taken for steroid analysis to confirm that the defect is 21-hydroxylase deficiency.

In SV and NC 21-OHD, 17-OHP elevation is milder. Levels should be measured between 08.00 and 09.00 hours under fasting conditions to capture the morning 17-OHP peak, followed by Synacthen stimulation which will demonstrate increased responses of 17-OHP, testosterone and androstenedione at 60 minutes.

Prenatal management

If a couple have a child affected with 21-OHD, the genotype of parents, affected child and healthy siblings can be determined. In future pregnancies, chorionic villus sampling at 9–10 weeks' gestation, or amniocentesis at 15–16 weeks, enables the sex and genotype of the fetus to be determined.

The main purpose of prenatal testing is to assist with maternal dexamethasone treatment. Pre-pregnancy counselling as to the pros and cons of this intervention is important. If prenatal treatment is to be given, it should be started at a dosage of 20 µg/kg/day as early as possible (preferably by 4–6 weeks' gestation) and continued throughout the pregnancy if the fetus is an affected female, but stopped if the fetus is male or an unaffected female. In future, it may be possible to avoid treating all male fetuses by detecting the male SRY gene in maternal serum early in pregnancy. The major benefits in reducing or preventing virilization in girls must be offset against the unknown effects of prenatal dexamethasone treatment on the fetus and, to a lesser extent, the side-effects of hypertension, weight gain and striae in the mother.

Prenatal treatment for 21-OHD should only be undertaken according to a strictly audited national protocol.

Neonatal management

Diagnosis and management of 21-OHD in newborn females is part of intersex management (see Chapter 7). The author recommends the following protocol:

1 Inform parents that there is doubt as to the gender of the child but that steps will be taken to make the decision within 48 hours if at all possible.

2 Urgent chromosome analysis, asking the laboratory to also screen for a Y chromosome using a Y-specific fluorescent marker.

3 Pelvic and adrenal ultrasound examination ± cystourethrovaginogram.

4 Surgical evaluation.

5 Plasma electrolyte and glucose measurement.

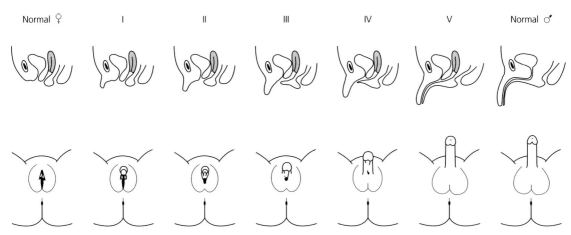

Normal ♀ I II III IV V Normal ♂

Fig. 8.7 Prader classification of five stages of virilization in the female infant.

6 2 mL heparinized blood for 17-OHP, ideally obtaining result on same day.

N.B. Blood taken before 72 hours of age may reflect placental 17-OHP levels, but a high value (100 nmol/L) [>3300 ng/dL] in the context of sexual ambiguity should be diagnostic, so a sample should be sent without delay.

Once the diagnosis has been confirmed, treatment must be started immediately. Treatment protocols vary. The author suggests the following protocol:

1 Fludrocortisone 100 µg/day.

2 Sodium chloride 5 mmol/kg/day in three divided doses given as either: 6% (1 mmol/mL); 15% (2.5 mmol/mL); or 30% (5 mmol/mL) solution. The solution may be added to milk feeds or given separately (e.g. if mother is breast-feeding).

3 Hydrocortisone 20 mg/m²/day in three divided doses.

In males presenting with salt-losing crisis and in missed/incorrectly assigned females the author recommends the following:

1 Measurement of electrolytes, glucose and 17-OHP.

2 Hydrocortisone phosphate 25 mg intravenously immediately.

3 Make up a mixture of hydrocortisone phosphate 50 mg in 50 mL 0.9% saline and infuse at 1 mL/h with saline drip.

4 Give 10–30 mL/kg of 0.9% saline over 1–3 hours depending on the degree of dehydration, then 0.9% saline at a rate sufficient to provide maintenance and correct any deficit over 24 h. Add potassium chloride when plasma K⁺ <4 mmol/L.

5 Give 10% dextrose, 2–4 mL/kg if capillary glucose is <3 mmol/L. Add dextrose to the 0.9% saline solution to make up a 10% dextrose mixture.

6 When plasma sodium is normal and infant is stable, start fludrocortisone, sodium chloride and hydrocortisone as above.

Management in infancy

Glucocorticoid therapy

Conventional treatment consists of oral hydrocortisone, approximately 20 mg/m²/day in three divided doses, e.g. 1.25, 1.25 and 2.5 mg. Suspensions are unreliable and 10-mg hydrocortisone tablets should be given halved or quartered, asking the pharmacy to prepare sachets if smaller doses are needed. By 6 months of age a total daily dosage of 5 mg hydrocortisone equates to approximately 14 mg/m²/day and can either be kept constant or increased, depending on the clinical and biochemical status of the baby.

In Glasgow a different approach is employed. Parents are taught to give intramuscular hydrocortisone and to measure capillary glucose before feeds twice daily to titrate the hydrocortisone dose. Daily injections of hydrocortisone 12.5 mg intramuscularly are given in the first week, followed by 12.5 mg on alternate days until 3 months of age. The advantages of this approach are that parents become proficient in giving emergency injections of hydrocortisone when the child is acutely unwell, and problems with oral hydrocortisone absorption in young infants are avoided. From 3 months onwards oral hydrocortisone is administered.

Fludrocortisone therapy

The author favours administering fludrocortisone 100 µg/day, provided that this is not associated with hypertension or hypokalaemia. Other centres prefer smaller dosage regimens, e.g. 25 µg twice daily. Suspensions are unreliable and should not be used.

Salt therapy

The dosage of 5 mmol/kg/day should be maintained for the first 3 months of life. Thereafter the salt intake can be kept at the same level. Salt is usually discontinued at, or shortly before, the first birthday.

Education and surveillance

A great deal of time must be invested in counselling the parents at diagnosis. Parent information leaflets are very useful. Contact with a family with an affected child of similar sex can also be very helpful. The infant should be reviewed weekly until the parents are comfortable with management, thereafter 1- to 2-monthly during infancy. Weight and length are measured on each occasion with blood pressure at least 3-monthly. Routine measurement of electrolytes is not indicated if the child is thriving. Quarterly measurement of steroids, renin and ACTH is optional and discussed below.

Management of acute illness

Infancy is a prime time for acute illness, including gastroenteritis. The key to successful management is correct parental instruction facilitated by provision of a CAH therapy card (similar to the asthma card). A CAH therapy card is shown in Appendix 3. If the following procedure is followed, children with CAH rarely need admission to hospital and duration of hospital stay will be minimized:

1 If the child has an intercurrent illness but is well, feeding and playing normally, then no change in dosage is required.

2 If the child is unwell, with fever, reduced activity, etc. then the oral total daily dosage of hydrocortisone is doubled and given in three divided doses.

3 If the child is particularly unwell, especially if there is vomiting, drowsiness, or diarrhoea—in which case oral hydrocortisone will not be reliably absorbed—give hydrocortisone phosphate intramuscularly in a dose of 12.5 mg for infants up to 6 months, 25 mg from 6 months to 5 years, 50 mg from 5 to 10 years, and 100 mg thereafter. If the parents are unable or unwilling to give intramuscular hydrocortisone then the child should be taken to hospital immediately.

4 If the child does not respond to the intramuscular injection, parents should bring the child immediately to hospital. Under these circumstances:

- take blood for glucose, electrolytes and full blood count;
- measure capillary glucose;
- give hydrocortisone intravenously if not given by parents (dosage as above);

- give 2–4 mL/kg 10% dextrose if capillary glucose <3 mmol/L [54 mg/dL];
- give 10–30 mL/kg 0.9% saline over 1–3 hours depending on the degree of dehydration, followed by 0.9% saline and 5% dextrose to provide maintenance and correct any deficit, adding potassium as indicated by electrolytes;
- give hydrocortisone infusion (50 mg in 50 mL 0.9% saline) 1 mL/h for infancy, 2 mL/h for preschool children, and 3 mL/h for older children until the child is able to tolerate oral medicines.

Genital surgery

Current practice is to perform clitoral recession by excising the shaft of the clitorophallus, carefully preserving the neurovascular supply to the tip. Surgery is usually between 6 and 12 months of age. Vaginoplasty may be performed at the same time but there is an argument in favour of leaving this procedure until much later in childhood to prevent stenosis. (see Intersex chapter for details)

Medical management of children undergoing surgery

1 On the day before surgery double the child's hydrocortisone therapy.

2 On the day of surgery the child should receive 25, 50 or 100 mg of hydrocortisone orally before becoming nil by mouth (Table 8.5). If this is not feasible, hydrocortisone can be given by injection with the premed.

3 For quick procedures, such as examination under anaesthetic, it is sufficient to give hydrocortisone as detailed above. The child should continue with the doubled oral dose for a further 2 days.

4 If surgery is to be carried out then a 1 mg/mL hydrocortisone infusion should be set up at induction giving 1, 2 or 3 mg/hour depending on body weight (Table 8.5). A 5% dextrose in 0.45% saline mixture should be given at a

Table 8.5 Preoperative hydrocortisone dosage and hydrocortisone infusion rates according to body weight in infants and children with adrenal insufficiency undergoing surgery.

Weight (kg)	Single dose of hydrocortisone preoperatively (mg)	Rate of infusion perioperatively (mg/h)
3–10	25	1
10–20	50	2
>20	100	3

maintenance rate during surgery to avoid hypoglycaemia (Table 8.5).

Management of linear growth

Standard treatment consists of daily or twice daily fludro-cortisone therapy to replace aldosterone, and twice or thrice daily hydrocortisone to suppress ACTH secretion and thus prevent virilization. The limitation of this ap-proach is that the glucocorticoid regime fails to mimic normal cortisol secretion. Moreover, if ACTH secretion is normalized, the presence of the enzyme block will still cause androgen excess in this situation. Therefore, to achieve satisfactory adrenal suppression, a slightly supra physiological dose of glucocorticoid is needed. Clearly, insufficient glucocorticoid dosage will result in androgen excess, early epiphyseal fusion and final height impairment.

It is also evident that frankly excessive glucocorticoid administration will result in cushingoid features, obesity and slow growth with final height impairment. What is less obvious is that lesser degrees of glucocorticoid over-dosage will cause hyperphagia resulting in obesity with normal or increased height velocity and advancing bone age, tempting the clinician to make a further increase in hydrocortisone dosage.

With these considerations in mind, the clinician needs to make a careful judgment as to the optimal glucocorti-coid dose, taking the clinical assessment, height velocity, bone age and biochemical profile into account, and being mindful that compliance problems are common, espe-cially during adolescence. The following approach may be helpful:

1 Treatment with either:
  - hydrocortisone 10–15 mg/m^2/day in two or three doses, titrating dosage to achieve a normal height velocity of 4–7 cm/year, or
  - prednisolone 4 mg/m^2/day in postpubertal girls.

The manner in which the daily glucocorticoid dose should be administered is controversial. We favour giv-ing a thrice-daily dose, equally divided, in pre-school children, then a twice-daily dose from school age (when compliance with a thrice-daily regime becomes problem-atic), giving a third of the dose in the morning and two-thirds in the evening (to suppress the morning 17-OHP surge).

2 Fludrocortisone 150 μg/m^2/day to suppress plasma renin to below the reference range.

3 Clinic visits 4-monthly for:
  - measurement of height, weight, height velocity and body mass index and (in older children) pubertal stage;

  - examination for features of overtreatment (Cush-ing's syndrome) and undertreatment (including pig-mentation and signs of androgen excess); and
  - measurement of blood pressure (to monitor fludro-cortisone dosage).

3 Annual bone age from 3 years onwards.

4 Annual measurement of fasting plasma renin activity, electrolytes, ACTH, testosterone, androstenedione and 17-OHP at 09.00 hours before the morning tablets.

5 Six-monthly 17-OHP and androstenedione capillary profiles before and 2 hours after the morning and evening hydrocortisone tablets.

Normalization of 17-OHP and androstenedione may reflect overtreatment with glucocorticoid and morning pretreatment and values of up to 100 and 10 nmol/L, respectively, can be acceptable. However, there is great in-dividual variation, some children showing normal growth and no cushingoid features with values of ≤10 and 3 nmol/L, respectively. Therefore it is necessary to establish the optimal hormone profile for the individual patient.

Morbidity

The sources of morbidity for parents and individuals with CAH are as follows.

Parents:

1 Shock of initial diagnosis;

2 In female infants, distress at the genital anomaly and uncertainty of gender at birth;

3 Anxiety over genital surgery and sequelae.

Patients:

1 Acute illness.

2 Learning disability in some salt-wasting patients.

3 Growth:
  - poor growth 0–2 years;
  - overgrowth 2–10 years;
  - impaired final height; and
  - early puberty;

4 Obesity;

5 Urogenital problems:
  - urinary tract infection;
  - incontinence; and
  - vaginal stenosis (haematocolpos, difficulty with tampon insertion and later with sexual intercourse);

6 Psychosexual:
  - self-esteem/confidence;
  - sexual activity;
  - sexual orientation; and
  - fertility.

The principal causes of morbidity are the complica-tions of surgery in girls, and of obesity in both sexes, particularly girls. Possible future strategies to minimize these problems include the use of prenatal dexamethasone, bilateral adrenalectomy during infancy in those with SW 21-OHD associated with severe genotype, and therapy with antiandrogens and aromatase inhibitors such as testolactone and anastrozole. However, none of these therapeutic options have become standard, despite having been under discussion for some years.

Oestrogen excess

Feminizing adrenal adenomas are exceptionally rare, but difficult to diagnose in that they mimic true precocious puberty in girls. The clue that the source of sexual precocity lies outside the hypothalamic–pituitary axis is the LHRH test which shows suppression of LH and FSH levels.

Sex steroid deficiency

Adrenal androgen deficiency

Causes
1 Adrenal hypoplasia.
2 Enzyme disorders:
   • StAR protein deficiency;
   • 3-βHSD deficiency;
   • 17-hydroxylase deficiency;
   • 17,20 desmolase deficiency; and
   • 17-βHSD deficiency.

The androgen deficiency of adrenal hypoplasia is insignificant if gonadal androgen synthesis is intact. However, severe enzyme deficiency affecting both adrenal and gonadal androgen synthesis results in undermasculinization with complete sex reversal in the more severe cases, and ambiguous genitalia in less severe cases. Management is discussed in Chapter 7.

Oestrogen deficiency

Oestrogens are responsible for closure of the epiphyses at adolescence. Gene mutations encoding the aromatase enzymes and the oestrogen receptors are associated with tall stature.

Adrenal medullary disorders

Phaeochromocytoma

Phaeochromocytoma is a chromaffin cell tumour which usually occurs as a single adrenal tumour but can be bilateral or extra-adrenal. It may be seen in isolation, either as a familial or nonfamilial disorder. Phaeochromocytoma may also occur in association with neurofibromatosis type 1, as part of the multiple endocrine neoplasia (MEN) syndromes; MEN type 2A (hyperparathyroidism, phaeochromocytoma, medullary thyroid carcinoma); MEN type 2B (phaeochromocytoma, medullary thyroid carcinoma, and tongue neuromas) and in von Hippel–Lindau syndrome, all of which are dominant in inheritance.

Although extremely uncommon in childhood, phaeochromocytoma is an important cause of hypertension. It is suggested by the combination of episodic pallor, sweating and headaches, with either sustained hypertension or raised blood pressure during a symptomatic episode. The diagnosis is made by examining urine catecholamine metabolites in children with hypertension and in children with symptoms suggestive of a phaeochromocytoma, even in the absence of hypertension.

Neuroblastoma

Neuroblastoma usually presents to the general paediatrician or oncologist. The diagnosis is suggested by hypertension in the context of malaise, sweating, pallor and an abdominal mass. There is an increase in catecholamine metabolites in the urine.

Future developments

• The molecular genetic basis for rare adrenal disorders is becoming more clear as progress continues in the field.
• Conventional therapy for 21-hydroxylase deficiency maybe overtaken by new strategies to reduce adrenal androgen production.
• Multicentre studies are needed in order to evaluate optimal surgical approach to female masculinization.
• The benefits and risks of prenatal dexamethasone will become more clear provided that treatment is administered in the context of structured national studies.

Potential pitfalls

• Gender mis-assignment as undermasculinized male in a female infant affected by 21-hydroxylase deficiency.
• Incorrect diagnosis of salt losing crisis in a male with hyponatraemia, caused by obstructive uropathy from urethral valves (modest elevation of 17-hydroxyprogesterone may occur in this situation).

- Incorrect diagnosis of congenital adrenal hyperplasia in child with adrenal tumour (note that urine steroid profile may be suggestive of CAH, possibly reflecting an enzyme deficiency in the tumour cells).
- Non-specific symptoms such as vomiting and hypoglycaemia in a patient with one endocrine disorder (such as diabetes) should alert the clinician to the possibility of a different endocrine problem (such as Addison's disease).

Controversial points

- Should pituitary surgery for Cushing's disease be performed in one or two designated national centres?

- What is the optimal treatment regimen for infants with 21-hydroxylase deficiency?
- Should dexamethasone be given antenatally to prevent virilization in fetuses at risk of 21-hydroxylase deficiency?

When to involve a specialist centre

- When Cushing's syndrome is either seriously suspected or confirmed.
- Primary and secondary adrenal insufficiency states.
- Conditions causing mineralocorticoid excess.
- Congenital adrenal hyperplasia.
N.B. Involvement of a specialist centre does not preclude a shared care arrangement.

CASE HISTORIES

Case 1

A 4-year-old boy with known asthma is admitted acutely with a convulsion and is found to be hypoglycaemic (blood glucose 0.8 mmol/l [14 mg/dL]). For the past year his asthma has been well controlled on fluticasone propionate 500 µg twice daily, but recently he has been lethargic and has had more than his fair share of intercurrent illnesses.

On examination (after glucose administration) his conscious level is normal. He looks slightly cushingoid with some increase in body hair especially over the back. Height is on the 3rd centile (midparental height 25th centile), weight on the 50th centile, blood pressure 120/50.

Random plasma is cortisol <24 nmol/L [<1 mg/dL]. Following low-dose Synacthen (500 ng/1.73 m^2) the peak value at 20 minutes is 50 nmol/L [1.4 mg/dL].

Question

How can this boy's cushingoid features be reconciled with his gross adrenal impairment?

Answer

This boy has an iatrogenic combination of Cushing's syndrome (causing the facial appearance, increase in body hair, and a degree of growth failure) together with adrenal suppression (lethargy, increased tendency to infections, hypoglycaemia). He is receiving over twice the licensed paediatric dose of fluticasone (400 µg daily). He will require hydrocortisone replacement while the respiratory team modify his therapy, and his adrenal status should be re-evaluated if and when the dose of inhaled steroid has been reduced.

Case 2

Four hours after delivery at 41 weeks' gestation, birth weight 3740 g, a baby boy becomes dusky while breast-feeding. True blood glucose 1.1 mmol/L. [<20 mg/dL].

On examination, the baby is noted to have a very small penis. He is started on a dextrose infusion and on day 5 undergoes stimulation with Synacthen (1 µg), LHRH (100 µg) and thyrotrophin-releasing hormone (TRH) (100 µg) giving 10% dextrose at the lowest rate needed to keep capillary glucose above 2 mmol/L. Plasma cortisol is <30 nmol/L rising to 50 nmol/L at 30 minutes; LH and FSH are unrecordable (<0.5 units/L) throughout; TSH is 2.5, 29.3 and 31.4 mU/L at 0, 30 and 60 minutes, respectively.

Question

What is the diagnosis, and what other system should be examined in detail?

Answer

This baby has panhypopituitarism with complete gonadotrophin deficiency leading to micropenis, ACTH deficiency resulting in hypoglycaemia, and hypothalamic hypothyroidism (the 60-minute TSH value exceeding that at 30 minutes).

On day 6 the baby is seen by an ophthalmologist who confirms that the optic discs are small with a 'double ring' sign, consistent with a diagnosis of septo-optic dysplasia.

Case 3

A 14-year-old boy is found to be hypertensive (blood pressure 170/130) when he attends his GP with headache. Investigations show normal electrolytes and renal imaging but aldosterone is elevated at 990 pmol/L [36 ng/dL], renin completely suppressed. There is a family history of hypertension with maternal uncle and grandmother dying young of stroke and the mother being hypertensive during pregnancy.

Question

What diagnostic possibilities should be considered and what further investigations should be performed?

Answer

The family history of hypertension in a boy with high aldosterone levels strongly suggests glucocorticoid-suppressible hyperaldosteronism. Molecular genetic studies confirmed a chimeric CYP 11B1/2 gene in both mother and son, and the boy's aldosterone suppressed quickly with dexamethasone. Detailed adrenal imaging in search of adenoma or hyperplasia was unnecessary in this case.

References and further reading

Consensus statement on management of 21-hydroxylase deficiency from the Lawson Wilkins Pediatric Endocrine Society and the European Society for Paediatric Endocrinology (2002) *Journal of Clinical Endocrinology and Metabolism* **97**(9), 4048–4053.

Forest, M.G. & Duncharme, J.R. (1993) Gonadotrophic and gonadal homones. In: *Paediatric Endocrinology* (eds J. Bertrand, B. Rappaport & P.C. Sizonenko), pp. 100–120. Williams & Wilkins, Baltimore.

Grumbach, M.M. & Conte, F.A. (1994) Disorders of sexual differentiation. In: *Williams Textbook of Endocrinology* (eds J.D. Wilson, D.W. Foster, H.M. Kronenberg & P.R. Larsen), 9th edn, pp. 1303–1426. W.B. Saunders.

Metherell, L.A., Chapple J.P., Cooray S. et al. (2005) Mutations in MRAP, encoding a new interacting partner of the ACTH receptor, cause familial glucocorticoid deficiency type 2. *Nature Genetics* **37**(2), 166.

Orth, D.N. & Kovacs, W.J. (1998) The adrenal cortex. In: *Williams' Textbook of Endocrinology* (eds J.D. Wilson, D.W. Foster, H.N. Kronenberg & P.R. Larsen), 9th edn, pp. 517–664. W.B. Saunders.

Savage, M.O. & Besser, G.M. (1996) Cushing's disease in childhood. *Trends in Endocrinology and Metabolism* **7**, 257–260.

Storr, H.L., Isidori, M., Monson, J.P. et al. (2004) Prepubertal Cushing's disease is more common in males, but there is no increase in severity at diagnosis. *Journal of Clinical Endocrinology and Metablolism* **89**(8), 3818–3820.

Wallace, A.M., Beastall, S.H., Cook, B. et al. (1986) Neonatal screening for congenital adrenal hyperplasia: a programme based on a novel direct radioimmunoassay for 17 hydroxyprogesterone in blood spots. *Journal of Endocrinology* **108**, 299–308.

Weber, A., Trainer, P.J., Grossman, A.B. et al. (1995) Investigation, management and therapeutic outcome in 12 cases of childhood and adolescent Cushing's syndrome. *Clinical Endocrinology* **43**, 19–28.

White, P.C. (1994) Disorders of aldosterone by synthesis in action. *New England Journal of Medicine* **331**, 250–258.

Zennaro, M.C. (1998) Syndromes of glucocorticoid and mineralocorticoid resistance. *European Journal of Endocrinology* **139**, 127–138.

9 Salt and water balance

Physiology and pathophysiology

Control of salt balance

Regulation of salt balance is achieved primarily through activation of the renin–angiotensin–aldosterone system and the release of atrial natriuretic peptide. Renin is secreted by the juxtaglomerular cells of the kidney in response to sodium depletion or extracellular fluid volume restriction. Renin converts angiotensinogen to angiotensin I which, in turn, is metabolized by angiotensin-converting enzyme to angiotensin II. Angiotensin II stimulates the production of aldosterone from the zona glomerulosa of the adrenal cortex. Aldosterone secretion can also be stimulated directly by adrenocorticotrophic hormone (ACTH) although the physiological importance of this mechanism is unclear. Potassium ions also facilitate the secretion of aldosterone. By contrast, the secretion of both renin and aldosterone may be inhibited by atrial natriuretic peptide.

Aldosterone binds to the mineralocorticoid receptor which increases the reabsorption of sodium in the kidney, sweat and salivary glands. Sodium ions are exchanged for potassium and hydrogen ions in the distal tubule. Cortisol also has a strong binding affinity for the mineralocorticoid receptor but is prevented from doing so as a result of metabolism to inactive cortisone by 11β-hydroxysteroid dehydrogenase 2 in aldosterone-selective tissues.

Control of water balance

Water balance is maintained as a result of the interrelation between thirst, renal function and the antidiuretic hormone arginine vasopressin (AVP). Vasopressin is synthesized in the supraoptic and paraventricular nuclei of the hypothalamus and transported along the supraoptic–hypophyseal tract to be stored in the posterior pituitary. Vasopressin release is regulated by osmoreceptors in the hypothalamus which detect changes in plasma osmolality from 280 to 295 mOsm/kg as may occur with loss of extracellular water. High concentrations of vasopressin may also be secreted following baroreceptor-detected reductions in blood volume or blood pressure of 5–10%. Baroreceptors are located in the carotid arch, aortic sinus and left atrium and modulate vasopressinergic neuronal function via vagus and glossopharyngeal stimulation of the brainstem.

Vasopressin binds to a V_2 receptor in the renal collecting tubule which regulates the insertion of water channel proteins (aquaporin 2) into the cell membrane. These allow water along an osmotic gradient into the cells lining the collecting duct and further aquaporins (aquaporin 4) allow this water to pass to the renal interstitium and circulation. This regulatory mechanism maintains plasma osmolality between 282 and 295 mOsm/kg. When the plasma osmolality exceeds 295 mOsm/kg, vasopressin secretion cannot be increased further and fluid balance is maintained by increased thirst leading to increased fluid intake. The vasopressin effect is under negative feedback modulation by locally generated prostaglandins in the medullary collecting duct cells. Glucocorticoids are also required for free water excretion.

Hyponatraemia

Aetiology

Hyponatraemia may occur as a result of either salt and water depletion in which salt loss exceeds water loss or following fluid overload with relatively more water than salt. The general mechanisms for the development of hyponatraemia are shown in Table 9.1.

Hyponatraemia associated with extracellular fluid loss is not always a direct consequence of the fluid loss, which is frequently hypotonic or isotonic by comparison with plasma, but may be caused by replacement of these fluid losses with hypotonic fluid (e.g. drinking of water alone or use of hypotonic intravenous fluids).

History and examination

When a child presents with hyponatraemia for which the cause is not immediately apparent, the following points should be highlighted in the history:

1 Features suggestive of salt loss:
  • the presence of symptoms causing excess fluid and sodium loss (e.g. vomiting, diarrhoea, polyuria) or a compensatory decrease in urine production which may occur when sodium loss has occurred from the skin or gut;
  • evidence that hyponatraemia is precipitated by intercurrent illness and associated with hyperkalaemia and hypoglycaemia which might suggest adrenal failure;
  • symptoms of malabsorption or recurrent chest infections or a tendency for hyponatraemia to develop during hot weather which may be indicative of cystic fibrosis;
  • the use of medication (e.g. diuretics) which predispose to hyponatraemia; and
  • family history of cystic fibrosis, congenital adrenal hyperplasia or hypoplasia or pseudohypoaldosteronism.

2 Features suggestive of water retention:
  • excess daily fluid intake;
  • symptoms suggestive of an underlying central nervous system or respiratory disorder (e.g. meningitis, raised intracranial pressure, pneumonia) associated with the syndrome of inappropriate antidiuretic hormone secretion (SIADH).
  • symptoms suggestive of heart failure, renal, liver or thyroid disease.

If sodium loss has occurred, clinical signs of volume depletion may be present as shown in Table 9.2. If such signs are absent, this may imply either previous fluid replacement with hypotonic fluids or the presence of water retention. In the latter circumstances, there may be evidence of oedema or rapid recent weight gain. The clinical signs of fluid overload are shown in Table 9.2. The rapid onset of a hypo-osmolar state may be associated with neurological manifestations including anorexia, apathy, confusion,

Table 9.1 Causes of hyponatraemia.

Mechanism	Examples
Salt loss	
Renal salt loss	Diuretic treatment
	Glucose or mannitol-induced diuresis
	Mineralocorticoid deficiency (e.g. congenital adrenal hyperplasia or congenital adrenal hypoplasia)
	Pseudohypoaldosteronism
	Salt-wasting nephropathy (e.g. renal dysplasia, obstructive uropathy, renal tubular acidosis)
Blood loss	Haemorrhage
Cutaneous loss	Excess sweat sodium loss (e.g. cystic fibrosis)
	Burns
Gastrointestinal loss	Diarrhoea
	Vomiting
	Excess salivary loss
	Pancreatitis
	Intestinal obstruction
Water retention	
Increased proximal renal tubule reabsorption	Congestive heart failure
	Cirrhosis
	Nephrotic syndrome
	Hypothyroidism
Decreased distal renal tubule dilution	SIADH
	Overtreatment with desmopressin
	Glucocorticoid deficiency
Excess water intake	Primary polydipsia
	Overtreatment with hypotonic intravenous solutions

Abbreviation: SIADH, syndrome of inappropriate antidiuretic hormone secretion.

headaches, weakness and muscle cramps. More severe symptoms may include vomiting, depressed deep tendon reflexes, bulbar or pseudobulbar palsy, Cheyne–Stokes breathing, psychotic behaviour, seizures, coma and death.

Evidence of growth impairment may suggest a long-standing cause of hyponatraemia resulting from sodium loss. Careful clinical examination should be undertaken of all systems for signs suggestive of intracranial or respiratory disease, cardiac, hepatic, renal or adrenal failure or hypothyroidism.

Investigations

• Serum and urine electrolytes and creatinine to calculate urinary sodium losses.

Table 9.2 Differences between sodium loss and water retention.

Sodium-losing states	SIADH
Fluid and weight loss	Water retention and weight gain
Clinical signs of hypovolaemia	Clinical signs of fluid overload
tachycardia	tachycardia or gallop rhythm
hypotension or occasionally hypertension	hypertension
caused by increased vasoconstriction	increased jugular venous pressure
poor peripheral perfusion (capillary refill	hepatomegaly
time greater than 2s)	oedema
decreased skin turgor	
sunken eyes	
impaired consciousness	
Increased urine osmolality	Increased urinary sodium loss
Urine sodium losses may be low or high	
depending on aetiology	

Abbreviation: SIADH, syndrome of inappropriate antidiuretic hormone secretion.

- Serum and urinary osmolalities.
- Plasma renin activity, aldosterone, 17-hydroxy progesterone and cortisol.
- Thyroid function tests.
- Other investigations as indicated for cardiac, respiratory, hepatic, renal or intracranial disease.
- If the patient is normo-osmolar, plasma proteins, lipids and glucose.

Differential diagnosis

Hyponatraemia can be spurious either as a result of contamination of the blood sample taken from an intravenous cannula with hypotonic intravenous fluids or because of interference with the flame photometer assay by excess serum lipids or proteins.

The key requirement in the assessment of a patient with hyponatraemia is to distinguish between causes associated with excess sodium loss and those associated with water retention caused by SIADH. The clinical distinction between these two states is summarized in Table 9.2.

If the cause of the hypo-osmolar state is not clear at presentation, urine osmolalities >100 mOsm/kg associated with urinary sodium concentrations >20 mmol/L suggest acute SIADH or renal, adrenal or cerebral salt-wasting. Urine osmolalities >100 mOsm/kg associated with urinary sodium concentrations <20 mmol/L suggest hypovolaemia or longer standing SIADH. Plasma renin is usually suppressed in SIADH but elevated in hypovolaemia. When it is uncertain whether SIADH is the cause of the hyponatraemia, a hypertonic saline infusion test (see below) may confirm SIADH by the demonstration of an exaggerated AVP response to the osmotic challenge.

Diagnosis

The causes of hyponatraemia are summarized in Table 9.1. Mineralocorticoid deficiency may be a consequence of idiopathic congenital adrenal hypoplasia or aplasia, biosynthetic defects of aldosterone synthesis (e.g. congenital adrenal hyperplasia) or acquired primary adrenal failure (e.g. Waterhouse–Friderichsen syndrome, autoimmune disease or following surgical removal). Resistance to aldosterone may also occur as a result of absence or abnormal function of the mineralocorticoid receptor. Hyponatraemia may also occur in hypopituitarism. Abnormalities of mineralocorticoid physiology are discussed in more detail in Chapter 8.

The various causes of SIADH are summarized in Table 9.3.

Treatment

Where hyponatraemia is a consequence of sodium loss and in the context of clinical signs of significant hypovolaemia, intravenous colloid or 0.9% saline should be given until there is clinical evidence of circulatory improvement. Adrenal insufficiency should be treated with fludrocortisone and glucocorticoids (see Chapter 8).

SIADH should be anticipated in individuals who have experienced significant head trauma or intracranial sur-

Table 9.3 Causes of syndrome of inappropriate antidiuretic hormone secretion (SIADH).

Cause	Examples
Central nervous system disorder	Meningitis, encephalitis
	Abscess, tumour
	Trauma, haemorrhage
	Hypoxia
	Guillain–Barré syndrome
	Ventricular shunt obstruction
	Acute intermittent porphyria
	Sinus thrombosis
Respiratory tract disease	Pneumonia
	Cavitation
	Tuberculosis
Tumours	Thymoma
	Lymphoma
	Ewing's sarcoma
Drugs	Stimulate AVP (phenothiazines, tricyclics, vincristine, narcotics)
	Potentiate AVP action (desmopressin, prostaglandin synthetase inhibitors)
	Others (chlorpropamide, cyclophosphamide, carbamazepine)

Abbreviation: AVP, arginine vasopressin.

gery and careful postoperative supervision of fluid balance is required. SIADH should be treated by fluid restriction which may on occasions amount to only 40% of normal intake. Where excessive thirst makes this impossible, demeclocycline may be used (in adults, 3–5 mg/kg has been given 8-hourly). Reversal of hyponatraemia by the use of hypertonic (3%) saline (0.1 mL/kg/minute for 2 hours should raise the plasma sodium concentration by about 10 mmol/L, to prevent hypervolaemia, furosemide with replacement of excreted urinary electrolytes may also need to be given) should be reserved for those with significant neurological symptoms following the relatively acute onset of SIADH, as there is a risk of lethal pontine myelinosis if serum sodium concentrations rise too rapidly (>10 mmol/L/day).

Endocrine hypertension

Aetiology
Hypertension in childhood as a result of endocrine pathology is usually a consequence of either glucocorticoid or catecholamine excess as shown in Table 9.4.

Table 9.4 Causes of endocrine hypertension.

Mechanism	Examples
Corticosteroid mediated	Iatrogenic
	Congenital adrenal hyperplasia
	11β-hydroxylase deficiency
	17α-hydroxylase deficiency
	Primary aldosteronism
	adrenal cortical hyperplasia
	adrenal tumour
	Cushing's syndrome
	Syndrome of apparent mineralocorticoid excess
	Liddle's syndrome
	Glucocorticoid-suppressible hyperaldosteronism
Catecholamine mediated	Neuroblastoma
	Phaeochromocytoma
	Ganglioma

History and examination
Key points to highlight in the history and on clinical examination include the following.
• A history of intermittent headaches, sweating, flushes, nausea or vomiting is suggestive of a phaeochromocytoma.
• Other affected family members: an autosomal recessive inheritance suggests congenital adrenal hyperplasia caused by 11β-hydroxylase or 17α-hydroxylase deficiency whereas an autosomal dominant pattern might suggest a phaeochromocytoma associated with a multiple endocrine neoplasia syndrome.
• Virilization in a girl might suggest congenital adrenal hyperplasia.
• Clinical signs of Cushing's syndrome (see Chapter 8).
• The presence of cutaneous signs suggestive of neurofibromatosis or of mucosal neuromas which are associated with von Hippel–Lindau disease may suggest the presence of a phaeochromocytoma which can be associated with these disorders.

Investigations
The following preliminary investigations should be considered if an endocrine cause of hypertension is suspected:
• Serum electrolytes and creatinine.
• Three 24-hour urinary-free cortisol collections.
• Urinary steroid metabolite profiling.
• Urinary catecholamine metabolites.

- Abdominal ultrasound.

If Cushing's syndrome seems likely, additional investigations to confirm the diagnosis and treatment are described in Chapter 8. If the urinary excretion of catecholamine metabolites is increased, then a blood sample should be taken for the measurement of catecholamines. Two-thirds of phaeochromocytomas are located in the adrenal medulla but may also be found anywhere in the sympathetic chain, most commonly close to the renal hilum or aortic bifurcation. Abdominal imaging with magnetic resonance imaging (MRI), computerized tomography (CT), ^{123}I metaiodobenzylguanidine (MIBG) scanning and, possibly, selective venous catecholamine sampling by catheterization may be necessary to locate the site(s).

Diagnosis

The various causes of endocrine hypertension are shown in Table 9.4. In 11β-hydroxylase- and 17α-hydroxylase-deficient congenital adrenal hyperplasia, deoxycorticosterone which has mineralocorticoid activity accumulates, resulting in hypertension caused by sodium and water retention with suppression of renin and aldosterone. 11β-Hydroxylase deficiency is also associated with excess androgen production and virilization whereas 17α-hydroxylase deficiency causes glucocorticoid and androgen deficiency with inadequate masculinization of the male.

Primary aldosteronism is associated with hypernatraemia, increased plasma volume and hyporeninaemia. Hypertension is common in childhood Cushing's syndrome. The syndrome of apparent mineralocorticoid excess is characterized by low plasma renin and aldosterone concentrations and is associated with a deficiency of 11β-hydroxysteroid dehydrogenase 2 which is responsible for metabolizing cortisol to cortisone to prevent high concentrations of cortisol from binding to the mineralocorticoid receptor.

Liddle's syndrome arises from an abnormality of renal tubular transport caused by an activating mutation of the amiloride-sensitive sodium channel which results in increased sodium reabsorption and potassium loss with a biochemical and clinical picture similar to that of apparent mineralocorticoid excess. Glucocorticoid-suppressible hyperaldosteronism is a rare disorder in which primary aldosteronism is regulated by ACTH rather than renin–angiotensin because of fusion of regulatory sequences of the 11β-hydroxylase gene to coding sequences of the aldosterone synthase gene.

Treatment

In 11β-hydroxylase- and 17α-hydroxylase-deficient congenital adrenal hyperplasia, hypertension responds to glucocorticoid therapy which suppresses ACTH secretion and thus deoxycorticosterone production. The treatment of Cushing's syndrome is discussed in detail in Chapter 8.

A phaeochromocytoma requires surgical removal. Pre- and perioperative control of blood pressure must be achieved by the use of adequate β-blockade using phenoxybenzamine. As this is achieved, salt intake may need to be increased to assist in extracellular fluid expansion. β-Blockers may also be necessary to treat α-blocker-induced tachycardia. The perioperative medical management of these patients requires skilled and experienced anaesthetic and surgical support and should only be undertaken in specialist centres. When a neuroblastoma causes catecholamine-induced hypertension, similar medical management will be necessary in the preoperative period.

Diabetes insipidus

Aetiology

Diabetes insipidus may occur either as a result of inadequate secretion of AVP (cranial diabetes insipidus) or when there is resistance to the antidiuretic effect of AVP (nephrogenic diabetes insipidus). Cranial diabetes insipidus may be a consequence of cerebral malformations (e.g. septo-optic dysplasia), caused by acquired disease (e.g. craniopharyngioma, histiocytosis or surgery) of the hypothalamo–pituitary axis or familial (Table 9.5). Autosomal dominant cranial diabetes insipidus may be caused by a mutation of the AVP-neurophysin II gene which leads to impaired processing of the AVP hormone precursor causing progressive damage to the neurosecretory neurones of the hypothalamus and the development of increasingly severe symptoms of diabetes insipidus with increasing age. Nephrogenic diabetes insipidus may occur as a consequence of mutations affecting the V_2 receptor gene (X-linked) or aquaporin 2 gene (autosomal recessive) or because of disorders of the kidney which impair other components of the urinary concentrating mechanism (Table 9.6).

History and examination

Diabetes insipidus causes polyuria and polydipsia. Additional clinical features may include constipation, fever, vomiting, loss of weight, failure to thrive and dehydration. The following points should be highlighted in the history and clinical examination:

Table 9.5 Causes of cranial diabetes insipidus.

Congenital	
Familial	Autosomal dominant
	DIDMOAD syndrome
Cerebral anomaly	Septo-optic dysplasia
	Empty sella syndrome
	Laurence–Moon–Biedl syndrome
Acquired	
Trauma	Neurosurgery
	Head injury
Tumours	Craniopharyngioma
	Germinoma
	Optic glioma
Infiltrative	Histiocytosis
	Leukaemia
	Sarcoidosis
Vascular	Haemorrhage
	Hypoxia
	Sickle cell disease
	Severe infection
	Anomaly
Others	Autoimmune
	Inflammatory
	Idiopathic
	Drugs (narcotic agonists)

Abbreviation: DIDMOAD, Diabetes insipidus, diabetes mellitus, optic atrophy and deafness syndrome.

Table 9.6 Causes of nephrogenic diabetes insipidus.

Congenital	X-linked
	Autosomal recessive
Acquired	Metabolic (hypokalaemia, hypercalcaemia)
	Nephrocalcinosis
	Osmotic (diabetes mellitus)
	Polycystic disease
	Sickle cell disease
	Drugs (demeclocycline, lithium)
	Urinary tract obstruction
	Chronic renal disease

• The severity of the polyuria and polydipsia. Excess consumption of flavoured liquids only as opposed to water suggests habitual excess drinking. Drinking from unusual places, such as from the toilet or bath, or unusual fluids, such as shampoo, suggests an underlying organic disorder.

• Whether the symptoms were present from birth, suggesting a congenital abnormality, or developed later in life, suggesting an acquired disorder.
• Associated neurological symptoms (e.g. blindness, neurodevelopmental delay, headache) and signs (e.g. optic atrophy) or history of a recent neurological disorder suggesting risk factors for hypothalamo–pituitary dysfunction.
• Past medical history of renal disease.
• Other symptoms or signs suggestive of diabetes mellitus or hypercalcaemia.
• Medication.
• Family history of similarly affected cases.
• Congenital abnormalities of the mid-line of the face or signs of Laurence–Moon–Biedl syndrome (see Chapter 11).
• Blood pressure or presence of enlarged kidneys.
• Height and weight.

Investigations

Habitual excess drinking can be diagnosed by demonstrating that when the parents stop flavoured fluids but allow the child unrestricted access to water, the polydipsia resolves. If symptoms persist, the child should be admitted for observation and the severity of the polyuria and polydipsia should be confirmed by measurement of the 24-hour fluid intake and urinary losses. A fasting blood sample should be taken for the measurement of plasma glucose and serum sodium, potassium, calcium and creatinine concentrations and a urine sample screened for glycosuria and proteinuria.

In a significantly symptomatic individual, an early morning blood and urine sample should be taken for the measurement of serum electrolytes and osmolality and urinary osmolality. Diabetes insipidus may be confirmed by the presence of a hyperosmolar state (i.e. serum osmolality >295 mOsm/kg) with inappropriately dilute urine (urine <750 mOsm/kg) and the plasma or urine sample should then be sent for the measurement of AVP to confirm whether the cause is cranial or nephrogenic. In these circumstances, a water deprivation test would be dangerous and is contraindicated. Furthermore, a water deprivation test is not required when there is a clear history of polydipsia and polyuria in the context of underlying disease or treatment (e.g. craniopharyngioma or histiocytosis or following surgical removal of a craniopharyngioma) known to cause cranial diabetes insipidus.

Water deprivation test

If the early morning blood sample is normal, which may

occur if a patient has consumed fluid overnight to prevent the development of a hyperosmolar state, the investigation of choice is a water deprivation test. This should be undertaken with great care in young children. The following protocol can be used:

1 Allow the child to consume their normal overnight fluid intake.

2 Weigh child at 08.00 hours at start of the fluid deprivation and measure plasma and urinary osmolalities.

3 Repeat weight, blood and urine samples every 2 hours and monitor the child carefully to prevent fluid intake.

4 For most children, an 8-hour fast is adequate and the test should be discontinued before then if more than 5% of body weight is lost or the thirst cannot be tolerated longer.

5 At the end of the fluid deprivation, administer desmopressin [DDAVP] either as an injection of 0.3 µg (subcutaneously, intramuscularly or intravenously) or 5 µg by the intranasal route and collect simultaneous urine and blood samples for osmolality measurements about 4 hours later. During the 4 hours following desmopressin, the child can be allowed to drink up to 1.5 times the volume of any urine voided.

Hypertonic saline infusion test

In children in whom the water deprivation test has given equivocal results and who are old enough to tolerate two intravenous cannulae and adequate blood samples for AVP measurements, a hypertonic saline infusion test may clarify the diagnosis. This requires the infusion of 0.05 mL/kg/min of 5% saline for 2 hours, or less if a plasma osmolality >300 mOsm/kg is achieved before then. Blood samples should be taken every 30 minutes from 30 minutes before the start of the test for the measurement of plasma osmolality and AVP concentrations which can be interpreted from Fig. 9.1. Urine samples should be collected from before the start of the test and approximately every hour thereafter for the measurement of sodium and osmolality. Thirst and blood pressure should be documented every 30 minutes.

Central nervous system imaging and other investigations

If a diagnosis of cranial diabetes insipidus is made, MRI of the hypothalamo–pituitary axis should be performed as there may be a pituitary tumour or stalk abnormality. If the MRI demonstrates thickening of the pituitary stalk, repeat scans should be organized over the next few years to monitor the development of infiltrative disorders such

as histiocytosis X or a germinoma, especially if symptoms such as headache or additional pituitary hormone deficiencies develop.

Tests of anterior pituitary function may also be indicated. Diabetes insipidus may be masked by concurrent adrenal insufficiency. If adrenal failure is present, glucocorticoid treatment should be instituted before diagnostic tests for diabetes insipidus are performed.

Diagnosis

If during the water deprivation test, the plasma osmolality remains between 282 and 295 mOsm/kg and the urine osmolality increases to >750 mOsm/kg, the patient does not have diabetes insipidus and the possibility of primary polydipsia because of abnormal drinking habits should be considered.

A diagnosis of cranial diabetes insipidus is suggested by the development of increased plasma osmolality >295 mOsm/kg in the presence of a urine osmolality <300 mOsm/kg which is then increased to >750 mOsm/kg following the administration of desmopressin. Failure of the urine to respond to desmopressin is indicative of nephrogenic diabetes insipidus. A partial urinary response (300–750 mOsm/kg) to water deprivation or

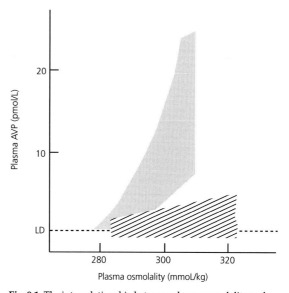

Fig. 9.1 The interrelationship between plasma osmolality and AVP concentration. Measurements which fall within the grey area suggest normal osmoregulation. Values which plot above and to the left of this area suggest nephrogenic diabetes insipidus whereas values below and to the right (in the striped area) are suggestive of cranial diabetes insipidus.

desmopressin suggests partial cranial or nephrogenic diabetes insipidus. In these circumstances, the plasma AVP response to the hypertonic saline infusion test should clarify the diagnosis (see Fig. 9.1).

Treatment

Cranial diabetes insipidus should be treated with the long-acting AVP analogue desmopressin. Widely varying regimens may be required, usually in two or three divided doses. Desmopressin may be given intranasally in a dosage of 2–40 μg/day (except in neonates who may require as little as 0.5 μg/day). A 10-μg per metered nasal spray may be used or, in children requiring a smaller dose, a 2.5-μg per spray product or intranasal solution in a dropper bottle with a catheter for nasal administration. In those individuals taking desmopressin by the nasal route, an increase in the dosage of medication may be required during upper respiratory tract illnesses which may cause congestion of the nasal mucosa and impaired drug absorption. If patients will not tolerate nasal administration, desmopressin may be given orally in dosage ranging from 100 to 1000 μg/day or parenterally in dosage of 0.4–4.0 μg/day.

Patients with cranial diabetes insipidus may be very sensitive to desmopressin and so treatment should start with small doses and gradually increase according to the clinical and biochemical response. The initial response to therapy should be monitored closely by measurement of the serum electrolytes and osmolality every few days at the start of therapy. Overtreatment may be recognized by an abnormally low serum sodium concentration and osmolality. Once stabilized on treatment, patients should be reviewed in clinic at least 3-monthly as seasonal changes in temperature may alter their requirements for desmopressin. Patients who are experienced in the management of their diabetes insipidus may be allowed to adjust their own doses of desmopressin if they detect recurrence of polyuria. However, it is advisable to allow a short period of diuresis during the day to allow the patient to excrete any excess water load which may have occurred after excess fluid intake. Although it is not normally necessary to prescribe a fluid intake, this step may be necessary in those individuals who have both diabetes insipidus and impaired thirst sensation who may be especially difficult to treat.

Nephrogenic diabetes insipidus should be managed by treatment of any underlying metabolic cause. In the absence of this, treatment with indometacin (0.5–1.0 mg/kg twice daily) and/or a thiazide diuretic (e.g. hydrochlorothiazide 0.5–1.0 mg/kg twice daily from birth to 12 years of age, or 12.5–25 mg twice daily in older children) together with a potassium-sparing diuretic such as amiloride (5–10 μg/1.73 m² twice daily) can be tried. Unfortunately, patients with nephrogenic diabetes insipidus often respond poorly to treatment and must be allowed adequate access to liberal amounts of fluid intake as required.

When to involve a specialist centre

- If the investigation and diagnosis of individuals with disturbances of their salt and water balance is proving difficult (e.g. in determining whether hyponatraemia is caused by salt loss or water retention, whether diabetes insipidus is cranial or nephrogenic or in cases of suspected diabetes insipidus in infants).
- Endocrine causes of hypertension which usually require specialist investigations and expertise (e.g. endocrine surgeons).
- Diabetes insipidus, particularly when associated with impaired thirst sensation which can be difficult to manage.
- If patients fail to thrive following the introduction of apparently appropriate treatment for salt or water loss.
- Patients with oncological causes of their salt and water imbalance.
- Multiple hormone dysfunction.

Future developments

- The management of nephrogenic diabetes insipidus remains difficult and further research is required to understand the mechanisms more clearly so that more effective treatments can be developed.
- Excessive urine output and natriuresis leading to hyponatraemia is a recognized complication of a serious central nervous system insult (so-called 'cerebral salt wasting') which is distinct from SIADH. Clarification of whether this is a consequence of inappropriate atrial natriuretic peptide secretion and appropriate treatment options are required.
- Recent research has suggested that the endocrine control of blood pressure in fetal and early postnatal life may be responsible for the 'programming' of blood pressure in adult life. This hypothesis requires further examination.

Controversial points

• Should intranasal or oral desmopressin be used as the treatment of first choice?

• To what extent should the hypertonic saline infusion test replace the water deprivation test as the investigation of first choice in patients with possible diabetes insipidus?
• What is the most appropriate treatment for nephrogenic diabetes insipidus?

Potential pitfalls

• Inappropriate and potentially life-threatening management of hyponatraemia due to failure to undertake a sufficiently careful history and clinical examination to distinguish between causes due to salt loss and those due to water retention.
• An inconclusive water deprivation test result due to inadequate supervision of the patient who surreptitiously obtained water to drink (e.g. from the tap in the toilet while producing a urine sample for measurement of osmolality) or failure to extend the test for a sufficient length of time.
• Symptomatic hyponatraemia following administration of desmopressin at the end of the water deprivation test due to failure to prevent the thirsty child consuming excess water.
• Symptomatic hyponatraemia in a child with cranial diabetes insipidus receiving regular desmopressin due to failure to allow a short period of diuresis each day to excrete any excess fluid intake or due to inadequately frequent out-patient review and adjustment of desmopressin dose to take into account changing fluid requirements through the seasons.
• Failure to plan and frequently adjust the fluid intake in a child with cranial diabetes insipidus and adipsia.
• Inadequately aggressive management of nephrogenic diabetes insipidus leading to failure to thrive.

CASE HISTORIES

Case 1
A 2-week-old boy was admitted with hyponatraemia following an 11-day history of vomiting, constipation and failure to regain his birthweight. On examination, he appeared underweight, with no other abnormal signs. The mother's brother was known to have developed a similar problem in infancy and was receiving long-term treatment for this. Initial investigations demonstrated the following:

sodium	114 mmol/L
potassium	8.1 mmol/L
cortisol	241`nmol/L
[8.7 micrograms/dL]	
17-hydroxy progesterone	5.4 nmol/L
[179 mg/dL]	

Questions
1 What is the most likely diagnosis?
2 What additional investigations are indicated?
3 What treatment should the baby be given?

Answers
1 In the context of severe hyponatremia, the cortisol is inappropriately low. The low 17-hydroxy progesterone excludes 21-hydroxylase-deficient congenital adrenal hyperplasia and the family history suggests a likely diagnosis of X-linked congenital adrenal hypoplasia.
2 A blood sample for the measurement of plasma glucose, renin, aldosterone, ACTH, luteinizing hormone (LH), follicle-stimulating hormone (FSH), testosterone and glycerol (gonadotrophin and glycerol kinase deficiency are associated with X-linked congenital adrenal hypoplasia). A urine sample for the measurement of steroid metabolites or a Synacthen stimulation test will help confirm the diagnosis if there is any doubt.
3 Once the initial blood sample for investigations has been taken, the baby should be treated with intravenous fluids containing 0.9% saline with additional dextrose to provide a concentration of 10% dextrose. He requires intravenous hydrocortisone at a dosage of approximately 60 mg/m^2/day subdivided 8-hourly which can be reduced to 10–15 mg/m^2/day orally once the patient has recovered from the presenting illness (see Chapter 8). Once the vomiting has ceased,

oral fludrocortisone can be added at a dosage of 150 mg/m²/day.

Case 2

An 11-year-old boy presented with an 8-week history of polyuria and polydipsia. He was otherwise well apart from recent headaches. Investigations in clinic demonstrated the following:

serum sodium	142 mmol/L	
serum potassium	3.7 mmol/L	
serum urea	2.3 mmol/L	[6.5 mg/dL]
serum creatinine	52 μmol/L	[0.6 mg/dL]
plasma osmolality	305 mOsm/kg	
plasma glucose	6.2 mmol/L	
urine sodium	16 mmol/L	[112 mg/dL]
urine osmolality	78 mOsm/kg	

Questions

1 What further investigation is required to clarify the diagnosis?
2 What additional investigations are then required?

Answers

1 Given that this child is spontaneously hyperosmolar, a formal water deprivation test is contraindicated. However, it is not clear whether this child has cranial or nephrogenic diabetes insipidus and the response to desmopressin needs evaluating. His urinary osmolality increased from 75 to 530 mOsm/kg and there was a dramatic reduction in his urine output suggesting that he has cranial diabetes insipidus.
2 Given a diagnosis of cranial diabetes insipidus and a history of headaches, a full assessment of pituitary function and cranial imaging are indicated. His hypothalamo–pituitary axis was normal on MRI. A basal blood sample demonstrated normal thyroid function and cortisol concentrations. However, after 6 months he demonstrated poor growth despite a dramatic resolution of his symptoms with regular desmopressin. In response to insulin-induced hypoglycaemia, his maximum serum growth hormone concentration was 4.7 mU/L (normal >20). Repeat MRI demonstrated the presence of a tumour which was shown to be a germinoma.

Further reading

Baylis, P.H. & Cheetham, T. (1998) Diabetes insipidus. *Archives of Disease in Childhood* **79**, 84–89.

Deal, J.E., Sever, P.S., Barratt, T.M. & Dillon, M.J. (1990) Phaeochromocytoma: investigation and management of 10 cases. *Archives of Disease in Childhood* **65**, 269–274.

Gruskin, A.B. & Sarnaik, A. (1992) Hyponatraemia: pathophysiology and treatment, a paediatric perspective. *Paediatric Nephrology* **6**, 280–286.

Ishikawa, S. & Schrier, R.W. (2003) Pathophysiological roles of arginine vasopressin and aquaporin-2 in impaired water excretion. *Clinical Endocrinology* **58**, 1–17.

Maghnie, M., Cosi, G., Genovese, E. *et al.* (2003) Central diabetes insipidus in children and young adults. *New England Journal of Medicine* **343**, 998–1007.

Mohn, A., Acerini, C.L., Cheetham, T.D. *et al.* (1998) Hypertonic saline test for the investigation of posterior pituitary function. *Archives of Disease in Childhood* **79**, 431–434.

Sakarcan, A. & Bocchini, J. (1998) The role of fludrocortisone in a child with cerebral salt wasting. *Paediatric Nephrology* **12**, 769–771.

10 Calcium and bone

Physiology

Introduction

About 99% of the total body calcium is found in the skeleton bound to phosphate and hydroxyl ions in the form of hydroxyapatite. The normal total serum calcium concentration at all ages ranges from 2.2 to 2.6 mmol/L and consists of physiologically active ionized calcium (about 50%), with the remainder being either bound to albumin or globulins (about 40%) or circulating complexed to citrate, phosphate or other constituents in the serum (about 10%). Calcium in intracellular and extracellular fluid is involved in many metabolic processes, including many enzymatic reactions, hormone secretion and blood coagulation. Serum calcium concentrations are influenced by:
- intestinal calcium absorption;
- calcium deposition in bone and mobilization of calcium following bone resorption; and
- renal tubular calcium reabsorption.

Approximately 85% of body phosphate is contained within bone hydroxyapatite. Many cellular reactions require either organic or inorganic phosphate. Normal inorganic serum phosphate concentrations drop from 1.3–2.3 mmol/L in infancy to 0.8–1.5 mmol/L at the end of puberty. About 15% of circulating phosphate is protein-bound. Free phosphate is required together with ionized calcium for normal bone mineralization. Calcium metabolism is regulated primarily by vitamin D, parathyroid hormone (PTH) and calcitonin.

Vitamin D

Vitamin D is either ingested in the diet or synthesized in the skin following ultraviolet irradiation from sunlight. Circulating vitamin D (Fig. 10.1) is metabolized in the liver to 25-hydroxyvitamin D and then in the kidneys to either a metabolically active form (1,25-dihydroxyvitamin D) or an inactive form (24,25-dihydroxyvitamin D). 1,25-Dihydroxyvitamin D synthesis is stimulated by hypocalcaemia, PTH and hypophosphataemia.

Circulating vitamin D exerts its target organ effect by binding to an intracellular vitamin D receptor. Vitamin D stimulates the activity of osteoclast-like cells but suppresses that of osteoblast-like cells and, in the presence of PTH, mobilizes calcium from bone. 1,25-Dihydroxyvitamin D stimulates intestinal calcium absorption but whether it influences renal handling of calcium and phosphate is less clear. Vitamin D receptors have been located in many other tissues in the body, suggesting a wider role for vitamin D than just regulation of calcium metabolism.

Parathyroid hormone

The PTH gene has been localized to the short arm of chromosome 11. PTH is synthesized as a pre-pro-hormone in the four parathyroid glands. Pre-pro-PTH is converted to pro-PTH as it is transported across the rough endoplasmic reticulum and is stored in secretory granules in the form of the mature 84 amino-acid peptide PTH. PTH release is stimulated by hypocalcaemia and inhibited by hypercalcaemia acting through a specific calcium-sensing receptor on the plasma membrane of the parathyroid cell.

The primary function of PTH is to prevent hypocalcaemia. Within minutes changes in PTH secretion affect renal tubular function, increasing calcium absorption and phosphate excretion, and osteoclastic bone resorption. Over a period of 1–2 days, by stimulating the synthesis of 1,25-dihydroxyvitamin D, PTH also increases intestinal calcium absorption.

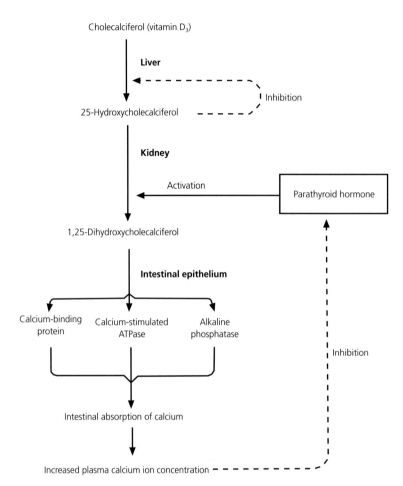

Fig. 10.1 Vitamin D metabolism.

PTH produces its target cell effect by binding to a membrane-bound receptor which stimulates guanine nucleotide-binding protein (G protein) mediated production of cyclic adenosine monophosphate (cAMP) from adenosine triphosphate (ATP). This in turn stimulates activation of protein kinase A and phosphorylation of intracellular enzymes leading to the physiological action of PTH.

Calcitonin

Calcitonin is produced in the 'C' or parafollicular cells of the thyroid gland. Calcitonin is encoded by a gene also located on the short arm of chromosome 11 and is synthesized in the form of a large precursor molecule. Tissue-specific processing may lead to an alternative calcitonin gene product, calcitonin gene-related peptide, which is a potent vasodilator.

Calcitonin secretion is stimulated by calcium and some gastrointestinal hormones (gastrin, cholecystokinin and glucagon). The primary function of calcitonin is unclear as it appears to have a relatively minor role in calcium metabolism. It reduces serum calcium concentrations by direct inhibition of PTH and 1,25-dihydroxyvitamin D mediated osteoclastic bone resorption. Calcitonin also increases the urinary excretion of calcium and phosphate but facilitates the absorption of nutrition-derived calcium into blood.

Bone metabolism

Bone has two main functions, forming the rigid skeleton and having a central role in calcium and phosphate homeostasis. Macroscopically, there are two types of bone:
1 Trabecular (cancellous, spongy) bone is found in the metaphyseal areas of long bones, vertebrae and most flat

bones. It accounts for about 20% of the skeleton and is metabolically very active, having an important role in calcium and phosphate metabolism.

2 Cortical bone is found in the diaphyses of the long bones and is relatively metabolically inactive.

Bone consists of:
- an organic matrix—mostly collagen;
- an inorganic mineral phase—hydroxyapatite;
- osteoblasts which synthesize and mineralize the organic bone matrix;
- osteoclasts which resorb bone and are then replaced by osteoblasts which produce new bone; and
- osteocytes which are osteoblasts which have become embedded within mineralized bone and which may play a part in sensing mechanical strain or controlling rapid mineral exchange between bone and serum without bone matrix degradation.

Bone growth and re-shaping takes place throughout childhood and adolescence. Longitudinal growth of the long bones occurs by enchondral bone formation (Fig. 10.2). In this process, cartilage cells (chondrocytes) proliferate in columns and undergo hypertrophic differentiation within the growth plate. Chondrocyte proliferation is regulated locally by the interaction of fibroblast growth factor with the fibroblast growth factor receptor 3 (FGFR3). Activating mutations of the FGFR3 are responsible for achondroplasia and hypochondroplasia. Hypertrophic differentiation of the chondrocyte is regulated by a negative feedback loop involving the cytokine parathyroid hormone-related peptide (PTHrP) and a signalling molecule known as 'Indian hedgehog'. The hypertrophic chondrocytes become surrounded by a matrix in which calcium is laid down. Newly calcified cartilage then condenses to become surrounded by osteoblasts which produce calcified osteoid. This calcified tissue is resorbed and replaced by bone trabeculae. By contrast, growth in width and thickness occurs by the process of intramembraneous bone formation. This process occurs at the periosteal surface, without a cartilage matrix and with bone resorption taking place at the endosteal surface.

By contrast, bone remodelling is the lifelong process by which skeletal tissue is being continuously resorbed and replaced to maintain skeletal integrity, shape and mass. In healthy individuals, the balance between bone formation and bone resorption is finely tuned. Bone mass increases progressively through childhood and adolescence until the maximum is attained in young adult life (so-called 'peak bone mass') during the third decade. Thereafter, a net loss of bone mass occurs as bone resorption exceeds the synthesis of new bone in later life. The amount of peak bone mass is a major risk factor for fractures in old age and is influenced by genetic factors, hormones, nutrition and mechanical strain (Table 10.1).

Hypocalcaemia

Aetiology
The causes of hypocalcaemia may be subdivided into those which present in infancy and those which present in older children as shown in Table 10.2. PTH-deficient

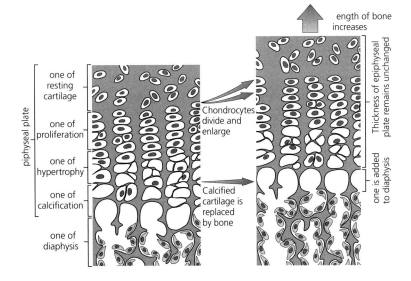

Fig. 10.2 Longitudinal growth of the long bones by enchondral bone formation.

Table 10.1 Factors which influence peak bone mass.

Influence	Increased bone mass	Decreased bone mass
Genetic	Afro-Caribbeans	Caucasians
		Orientals
Hormones	Calcitonin	Parathyroid hormone
	Oestrogen	Vitamin D
	Growth hormone	Glucocorticoids
Cytokines	Transforming	Interleukin 1
	growth factor β	Tumour necrosis factor α
Nutrition	Calcium	Anorexia
	Obesity	Malabsorption
Mechanical	Exercise	Inactivity

Table 10.2 Causes of hypocalcaemia.

Infancy	Childhood
Prematurity	Vitamin D deficiency
Asphyxia	Vitamin D-dependent rickets
Gestational diabetes	(types 1 and 2)
Transient or permanent	Chronic renal failure
hypoparathyroidism	Hypoparathyroidism
High milk phosphate load	Pseudohypoparathyroidism
Hypomagnesaemia	
Parenteral nutrition	
Exchange transfusion	
Chronic alkalosis or	
bicarbonate therapy	
Maternal hyperparathyroidism	

hypoparathyroidism may be familial (autosomal dominant, recessive or X-linked recessive) and associated with other abnormalities, such as Addison's disease or deafness. Non-familial PTH-deficient hypoparathyroidism may present in infancy and be transient or persistent (e.g. in association with DiGeorge's syndrome). In older children it may be idiopathic or secondary (e.g. following surgical removal of the parathyroids or hypomagnesaemia).

Pseudohypoparathyroidism is caused by resistance to the action of PTH. This is known as Albright's hereditary osteodystrophy (AHO) when associated with the dysmorphic features described in Table 11.5 and Fig. 11.4. The PTH resistance of AHO is most commonly associated with decreased G-protein activity in cell membranes (type 1a) which may also affect other G-protein coupled receptors (e.g. adenocorticotrophic hormone (ACTH),

thyroid-stimulating hormone (TSH), luteinizing hormone (LH), follicle-stimulating hormone (FSH) and glucagon).

History and examination

When assessing a child with hypocalcaemia, the following points should be highlighted in the clinical history:
• Symptoms suggestive of hypocalcaemia (e.g. paraesthesia, muscle cramps or tetany, seizures and diarrhoea);
• Predisposing risk factors (e.g. intestinal or renal tubular disease) for hypomagnesaemia;
• Evidence of endocrine disease affecting other G-protein coupled receptors (e.g. previous thyroxine treatment for a low normal serum T_4 concentration with mildly elevated serum TSH concentration);
• Symptoms of autoimmune disease;
• Previous surgical risk factors (e.g. thyroidectomy or parathyroidectomy);
• A family history of hypoparathyroidism.

If an older child is suspected to have hypocalcaemia, latent tetany may be detected from positive Chvostek's sign (facial twitching in response to tapping of the facial nerve in front of the ear) and Trousseau's sign (carpal spasm within 3 min of inflating a blood pressure cuff above systolic blood pressure; Fig. 10.3) or stridor. Extrapyramidal signs from basal ganglia calcification, cataracts, papilloedema, dry skin, coarse hair, brittle nails and enamel hypoplasia with dental caries are signs suggestive of chronic hypocalcaemia. In contrast with the older child, hypocalcaemia in infancy is associated with relatively nonspecific symptoms including tremor, apnoea, cyanosis and lethargy. Clinical signs suggestive of autoimmune hypoparathyroidism or pseudohypoparathyroidism are shown in Table 10.3 with details of the dysmorphic features of pseudohypoparathyroidism shown in Table 11.5 and Fig. 11.4.

Investigations

If hypocalcaemia is suspected, a blood sample should be taken for the measurement of:
• calcium;
• phosphate;
• alkaline phosphatase;
• PTH;
• 25-hydroxyvitamin D; and
• a sample stored for possible measurement of 1,25-dihydroxyvitamin D concentration later, should this be indicated.

The differential diagnosis of biochemical abnormalities of calcium metabolism is shown in Table 10.4.

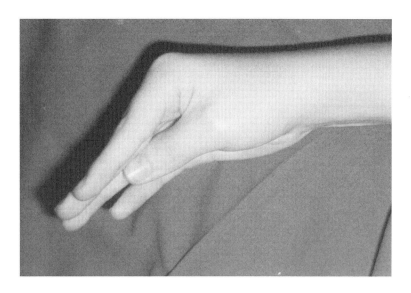

Fig. 10.3 Trousseau's sign.

Treatment

Acute hypocalcaemia when complicated by tetany should be treated with a slow intravenous injection over 5–10 minutes of 0.3 mL/kg body weight of 10% calcium gluconate followed by a maintenance infusion of 0.2 mL/kg/ hours which may be necessary for a few days. Care must be taken when intravenous calcium is administered as extravasation of calcium into subcutaneous tissues around the injection site can lead to tissue necrosis. In the absence of acute neurological symptoms, 50 mg/kg/day of calcium can be given orally subdivided into four doses.

Long-term maintenance treatment of hypocalcaemia requires vitamin D given as cholecalciferol (50 μg (2000 IU)/kg), or alfacalcidol (25–50 ng/kg) or calcitriol (25–50 ng/kg). The latter two are recommended because of their shorter half-life and rapid cessation of action should toxicity occur. Vitamin D may need to be given in combination with calcium (20 mg/kg/day). Frequent monitoring of serum calcium concentrations is required shortly after starting treatment—weekly if there is concern about the response to therapy. Once the patient has demonstrated a satisfactory response, serum calcium concentration and the urinary calcium:creatinine ratio should be measured every 3 months thereafter with regular renal ultrasounds to monitor for calcification.

In children with hypoparathyroidism, the aim of therapy is to achieve low normal serum calcium concentrations (2.0–2.25 mmol/L) [8.0–9.0 mg/dL] while avoiding urinary calcium:creatinine ratios greater than 0.7 mmol/L [0.16 mg/dL]. In those with pseudohypoparathyroidism, the resistance to PTH primarily affects the proximal renal tubule. Therefore, to avoid adverse bone sequelae, treatment should suppress PTH levels to the normal range which may require maintenance of serum calcium concentrations towards the upper end of the normal range (2.25–2.5 mmol/L) [9.0–10.0 mg/dL].

Rickets

Aetiology

Rickets is caused by delayed matrix mineralization at the growth plate resulting in excessive accumulation of uncalcified cartilage and bone (osteoid) matrix. The most common causes of rickets are those associated with vitamin D deficiency. They present most frequently at times of rapid growth which may occur in infancy or in puberty, particularly in Asian children. Vitamin D deficiency may be a result of dietary insufficiency, malabsorption (e.g. coeliac disease) or inadequate exposure to sunlight. There is a need for a greater clinical awareness of vitamin D deficient rickets in Western industrialized societies as the current prevalence, particularly in infancy and adolescence seems higher than is often appreciated, even in relatively sunny countries. To prevent rickets, it is recommended in the USA that food be supplemented with 200 units of vitamin D daily for all children and in the UK, 340 units for infants under six months and 280 units for children under four years of age. Rickets of prematurity is thought to be

Table 10.3 Clinical signs to look for on examination.

Clinical sign	Possible diagnosis

Candidiasis
Dental enamel and
   nail dystrophy
Alopecia
Vitiligo
Signs of Addison's disease
   or hypothyroidism
	Autoimmune
	   hypoparathyroidism
	   (polyglandular
	   autoimmune
	   disease type 1)

Short stature Subcutaneous calcification Dysmorphic features	Pseudohypoparathyroidism

Swollen wrists
Prominent costochondral
   junctions (rachitic rosary)
   and Harrison's sulci
Bow-leg or knock-knee
Craniotabes
Delayed dental eruption and
   enamel hypoplasia
Muscle weakness and tetany
	Vitamin D-deficient rickets

Poor growth Bowing of the legs	Hypophosphataemic rickets
Blue sclerae Abnormal dentition Hyperextensible joints Deafness	Osteogenesis imperfecta

Broad and prominent forehead
Short turned-up nose with flat
   nasal bridge
Overhanging upper lip
Late dental eruption
Supravalvular aortic stenosis
Peripheral pulmonary stenosis
Learning difficulties with
   emotional lability
Mild short stature
	Williams syndrome

caused by calcium and/or phosphate deficiency rather than vitamin D deficiency.

Hypophosphataemic rickets is an X-linked dominant disorder which is associated with a failure of phosphate resorption in the proximal renal tubule. Vitamin D-dependent rickets is very rare and is caused either by deficiency of 1α-hydroxylation of 25-hydroxyvitamin D (type 1) or resistance to 1,25-dihydroxyvitamin D (type 2). The classification of the different forms of rickets and their biochemical characteristics are shown in Table 10.4.

In severe renal failure, 1,25-dihydroxyvitamin D synthesis is impaired which, in conjunction with increasing serum phosphate concentrations, leads to hypocalcaemia and secondary hyperparathyroidism with bone disease (renal osteodystrophy).

Both rickets and osteomalacia (defective mineralization of osteoid tissue) are common in the many causes of Fanconi's syndrome and type 2 renal tubular acidosis. The metabolic bone disease is caused by a combination of phosphaturia-induced hypophosphataemia, hypercalciuria, abnormal vitamin D metabolism and renal insufficiency.

History and examination

If a child presents with rickets, then the following details should be elicited:

• Symptoms suggestive of associated disease (e.g. renal failure, malabsorption).

• Dietary history of food intake, such as dairy products which are rich in calcium and vitamin D.

• Risk factors for inadequate exposure to sunlight.

• Family history of rickets.

The child should undergo careful clinical examination, including documentation of growth and pubertal status. The clinical signs to look for on examination are shown in Table 10.3.

Investigations

Rickets causes abnormal bone mineralization which may be evident on X-ray. Additional radiological features commonly include a characteristic widening of the growth plate with cupping, splaying and fraying of an irregularly margined metaphysis (Fig. 10.4). The characteristic clinical signs of vitamin D-deficient and hypophosphataemic rickets are detailed in Table 10.3 and Figs 10.5 and 10.6.

The lowered renal threshold for resorption of phosphate which is associated with hypophosphataemic rickets can be calculated from simultaneous serum and urinary biochemical measurements by reference to Kruse *et al.* (1982) or Shaw *et al.* (1990) which also contain details of age-appropriate reference ranges. The presence of glycosuria, amino-aciduria or a metabolic acidosis with inappropriately alkaline urine is suggestive of a wider defect of tubular function, such as Fanconi's syndrome or renal tubular acidosis.

Table 10.4 Differential diagnosis of disorders of vitamin D and parathyroid hormone (PTH) metabolism.

Diagnosis	Ca$_2$	PO$_4$	PTH	25-OHD	1,25-(OH)$_2$D
Vitamin D-deficient rickets	LN	L	H	L	L,N,H
Vitamin D-dependent rickets					
type 1 (deficiency of 1α-hydroxylation)	L	L	H	N,L	L
type 2 (resistance to 1,25-(OH)$_2$D)	L	L	H	N,L	N,H
X-linked hypophosphataemic rickets	N	L	N	N	L,N
Hypophosphataemic rickets with hypercalciuria	N	L	N	N	H
Tumour-induced rickets	N	L	N	N	L
Renal osteodystrophy	N,L	H	H		N,L
Primary hyperparathyroidism	H	L	H	N	N,H
Hypoparathyroidism	L	H	L	N	L,N
Pseudohypoparathyroidism	L	H	H	N	L,N
Vitamin D intoxication	H	N	L	H	N,H
Hypercalcaemia in granulomatous disorders	H	N	L	N	H

Abbreviations: Ca$_2$, calcium; PO$_4$, phosphate; 25-OHD, 25-hydroxyvitamin D; 1,25-(OH)$_2$D, 1,25-dihydroxyvitamin D; H, high; N, normal; L, low; LN, low–normal.

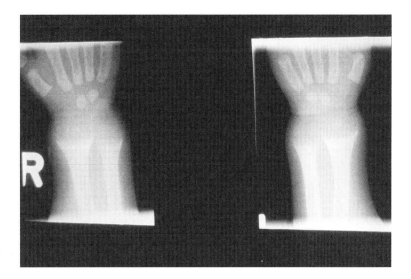

Fig. 10.4 X-ray of the wrist of a child with rickets caused by vitamin D deficiency.

Treatment

Depending on the cause of the rickets, different preparations of vitamin D are required for effective treatment as shown in Table 10.5. Where renal dysfunction is associated with metabolic bone disease, treatment of the wider systemic metabolic abnormality is required. Detailed guidance for this is beyond the scope of this volume and the reader is advised to consult appropriate textbooks on paediatric nephrology. Children with Fanconi's syndrome may require phosphate therapy whereas those with renal tubular acidosis require treatment with bicarbonate.

Osteoporosis

Aetiology

Unlike in adults, osteoporosis in childhood is not clearly defined but is caused by reduced bone mass per unit volume with a normal ratio of mineral to matrix. The possibility of osteoporosis should be considered in a child who presents with fractures following minimal trauma in whom there is also evidence of decreased bone mineral density (usually more than three standard deviations below the mean for age, size and puberty). This may occur as a result of an imbalance between bone formation and bone resorption because of a variety of reasons or as a result of abnormalities of type 1 collagen synthesis (e.g. osteogenesis imperfecta). The causes of decreased bone mineral density which may predispose to osteoporosis and present in childhood, are shown in Table 10.6.

History and examination

Osteoporosis may present with obvious signs of a long bone fracture following minimal trauma or with back pain and deformity because of underlying vertebral compression fractures (Fig. 10.7). Clinical assessment and investigations should aim to exclude the causes of

decreased bone mineral density shown in Table 10.6. If a child presents with osteopenia, then the following details should be elicited:

• Symptoms suggestive of associated disease (e.g. renal disease, malabsorption, inflammatory bowel disease);
• Features suggestive of growth failure or pubertal delay;
• Past medical history of fractures in the absence of significant underlying trauma;
• Medication (e.g. steroids);
• Family history of osteoporosis or fractures.

Clinical examination should include a careful assessment of growth, nutritional state, pubertal development and the clinical signs of osteogenesis imperfecta listed in Table 10.3. The presence of unexplained bone tenderness and pain, particularly in the spinal region, and in association with a spinal deformity, such as a kyphosis or

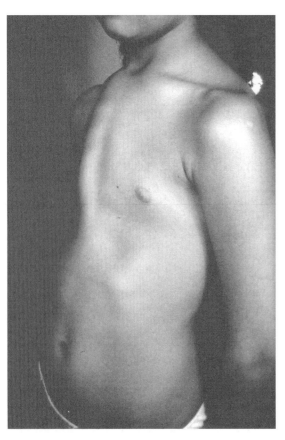

Fig. 10.5 Rachitic rosary.

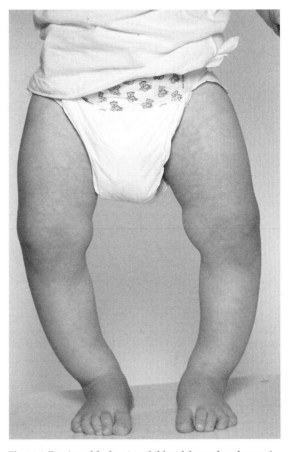

Fig. 10.6 Bowing of the legs in a child with hypophosphataemic rickets.

Table 10.5 Treatment of rickets.

Aetiology	Treatment
Vitamin D-deficient rickets	Vitamin D, 50–150 μg/day for 2 weeks reduced thereafter to 10 μg daily *or* ergocholecalciferol, 15 000 μg single intramuscular dose
Rickets of prematurity as a result of calcium deficiency	Calcium, 700 mg/day orally if bottle-fed or 30 mg/kg/day orally if breast-fed (prevention: 200 mg/kg/day orally or 20–60 mg/dL in parenteral nutrition)
Rickets of prematurity as a result of phosphate deficiency	Phosphate, 115–120 mg/kg/day orally if bottle-fed, 25 mg/kg/day if breast-fed or 15–47 mg/dL in parenteral nutrition
Vitamin D-dependent rickets (type 1)	Calcitriol, 0.25–2 μg/day
Vitamin D-dependent rickets (type 2)	Calcitriol, large doses (up to 50 μg/day) and long-term high-dose oral or intravenous calcium
Hypophosphataemic rickets	Phosphate, 50–70 mg/kg/day (increase from a starting dosage of 20–40 mg/kg and subdivide into four to six daily doses to limit gastrointestinal side-effects) Calcitriol, start with 15–20 ng/kg/day and increase to 30–60 ng/kg/day subdivided into one or two daily doses

scoliosis, might suggest previously unsuspected fractures. These may occur with severe osteoporosis or osteogenesis imperfecta.

Distinguishing between osteogenesis imperfecta and idiopathic juvenile osteoporosis may prove difficult. Osteogenesis imperfecta should be considered in the presence of the clinical signs listed in Table 10.3. A skull X-ray for the presence of wormian bones and a skin biopsy for fibroblast culture to assess abnormalities in the synthesis of type 1 collagen may assist in the diagnosis of osteogenesis imperfecta. Idiopathic juvenile osteoporosis may be suggested by X-ray evidence of metaphyseal compression fractures at the knee. Histomorphometric examination of bone biopsy material may also help distinguish between these two conditions.

Investigations

Bone mineral density may be measured by dual energy X-ray absorptiometry scanning of the lumbar spine or hip (Fig. 10.8). This method involves minimal radiation exposure and is based on the measurement of the attenuation of X-rays of differing energy intensity as they pass through bone. However, these characteristics are influenced by the width of bone through which the X-rays pass which in children may vary as a consequence of age, body size or puberty in addition to illness. Interpretation of the data needs to take these factors into account (Warner *et al.* 1998). It is recommended that bone mineral density should only be measured in children with risk factors for low bone density associated with low trauma or recurrent fractures, back pain,

spinal deformity or loss of height, change in mobility status or malnutrition.

Treatment

The following measures may help in the treatment of osteoporosis.

- Adequate analgesia for fractures;
- Physiotherapy, splints and orthopaedic intervention and occupational therapy where necessary;
- Optimal dietary calcium and vitamin D intake with supplements where necessary;
- Effective treatment of underlying disease;
- If osteoporosis is steroid-induced, reduce daily glucocorticoid dosage as much as possible, consider alternate day therapy or use those with minimal side-effects (e.g. deflazacort);
- Induction of puberty with low-dose testosterone or oestrogen if pubertal delay present (see Chapter 5);
- Calcitonin has been suggested in a few small studies to be beneficial in children with osteopenia;
- Bisphosphanates (e.g. pamidronate) have been used in childhood, mostly to treat osteogenesis imperfecta. Despite residual uncertainty about their long-term safety, there is growing evidence that they benefit children by reducing the pain associated with fractures, increasing bone mineral density and facilitating physical rehabilitation and mobility. There seem to be few side-effects in the short to medium term though it is advised to optimize dietary calcium and vitamin D intake during therapy to reduce to a minimum, the risks of developing hypocalcaemia.

Table 10.6 Causes of osteoporosis and other disorders which may lead to decreased bone mineral density.

Pathogenetic basis	Examples
Primary bone disease	Idiopathic juvenile osteoporosis
	Osteogenesis imperfecta
	Osteoporosis pseudoglioma syndrome
Inflammatory	Inflammatory bowel disease
	Rheumatoid arthritis
Endocrine	Cushing's syndrome
Drugs	Glucocorticoids
Others	Immobility
	Acute lymphoblastic leukaemia
	Thalassaemia
	Homocystinuria
	Post transplant
Causes of decreased bone mineral content (osteopenia) not necessarily severe enough to cause osteoporosis	Anorexia
	Coeliac disease
	Hypopituitarism
	Hypogonadism (e.g. Turner's or Klinefelter's syndromes)
	Hyperparathroidism
	Renal failure
	Chronic liver disease
	Thyrotoxicosis
	Burns
	Methotrexate

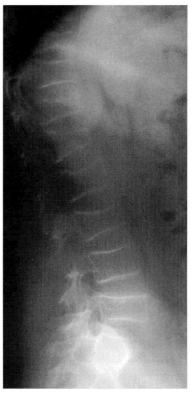

Fig. 10.7 X-rays showing vertebral compression in a child with osteoporosis.

Hypercalcaemia

Aetiology

Hypercalcaemia occurs when the serum calcium concentration exceeds 2.65 mmol/L. The causes of hypercalcaemia are shown in Table 10.7.

Mild idiopathic hypercalcaemia of infancy presents with symptoms between the ages of 2 and 9 months but resolves spontaneously by the age of 4 years. When severe, it may present in the neonatal period in association with the dysmorphic features of Williams syndrome (Table 10.3 and Fig. 10.9). Hypercalcaemia is associated with granulomatous disease (e.g. sarcoidosis and tuberculosis) as a result of the conversion of 25-hydroxyvitamin D to 1,25-dihydroxyvitamin D in granulomatous cells.

Neonatal hypercalcaemia

Neonatal primary hyperparathyroidism is a serious disorder of unknown aetiology which causes anorexia, hypotonia, chest deformities and respiratory distress. It is associated with a high mortality in the neonatal period and, to be successfully treated, requires urgent parathyroidectomy. This disorder is caused by homozygous mutations of the calcium-sensing receptor gene, the product of which regulates PTH secretion. Similar heterozygous mutations are responsible for autosomal dominant familial hypocalciuric hypercalcaemia.

Hypercalcaemia in childhood

Primary hyperparathyroidism may also occur in association with pituitary adenomas and gastrinomas or other pancreatic tumours (multiple endocrine neoplasia type 1) or in association with medullary thyroid cancer and phaeochromocytoma (multiple endocrine neoplasia type 2A). These two groups of disorders are inherited in an autosomal dominant fashion and all offspring of affected

University Hospital of Wales.

k = 1.208 d0 = 117.9(1.000H)

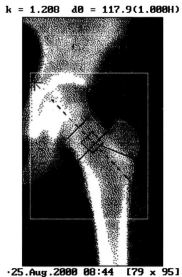

·25.Aug.2000 08:44 [79 x 95]
Hologic QDR-1000/W (S/N 1043 P)
Left Hip V4.76P

Y05059904   Wed 05.May.1999 10:08
Name: EXAMPLE
Comment: Osteope nia
I.D.:   Sex: F
S.S.#: .   - -   Ethnic: W
ZIPCode: Height: 135.10 cm
Scan Code: EAJ Weight: 48.80 kg
BirthDate: 01.Jan.90   Age: 9
Physician:
Image not for diagnostic use

TOTAL BMD CV 1.0%
C.F.   1.008   1.088   1.000

Region	Area (cm²)	BMC (grams)	BMD (gms/cm²)
Neck	4.08	2.10	0.514
Troch	4.64	1.48	0.318
Inter	12.41	7.06	0.569
TOTAL	21.13	10.64	0.503
Ward's	1.10	0.44	0.402

Midline (82, 98)-(136, 44)
  Neck   -44 x 16 at [23, 13]
  Troch   14 x 29 AXIS 9.049 cm
  Ward's -11 x 11 at [6, 5]

HOLOGIC

University Hospital of Wales.

P Left Hip
Reference Database .

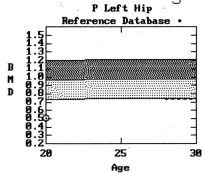

BMD(Total[L]) = 0.503 g/cm²

Y05059904   Wed 05.May.1999 10:08
Name: EXAMPLE
Comment:
I.D.:   Sex: F
S.S.#:   - -   Ethnic: W
ZIPCode: Height: 135.10 cm
Scan Code: EAJ Weight: 48.80 kg
BirthDate: 01.Jan.90   Age: 9
Physician:

Region	BMD	T	Z
Neck	0.514	-3.81 57% (22.0)	
Troch	0.318	-4.48 44% (30.0)	
Inter	0.569	-4.13 50% (29.0)	
TOTAL	0.503	-3.93 52% (28.0)	
Ward's	0.402	-3.58 50% (20.0)	

♦ Age and sex matched
T = peak bone mass
Z = age matched   TK   25 Oct 91

HOLOGIC

Fig. 10.8 Dual-energy X-ray scan report of the hip and lumbar spine.

University Hospital of Wales.

k = 1.204 d0 = 113.3(1.000H)

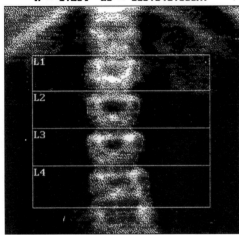

·25.Aug.2000 08:40 [119 x 99]
Hologic QDR-1000/W (S/N 1043 P)
Lumbar Spine V4.76P

Y05059903   Wed 05.May.1999 09:56
Name: EXAMPLE
Comment: Osteope nia
I.D.:   Sex: F
S.S.#:   - -   Ethnic: W
ZIPCode: Height: 135.10 cm
Scan Code: EAJ Weight: 48.80 kg
BirthDate: 01.Jan.90   Age: 9
Physician:
Image not for diagnostic use

TOTAL BMD CV FOR L1 - L4 1.0%

C.F.   1.000   1.000   1.000

Region	Area (cm^2)	BMC (grams)	BMD (gms/cm^2)
L1	6.73	2.87	0.426
L2	7.05	2.90	0.411
L3	7.49	3.51	0.469
L4	9.79	4.15	0.424
TOTAL	31.07	13.43	0.432

University Hospital of Wales.

P Lumbar Spine
Reference Database ♦

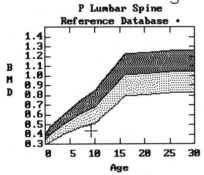

Y05059903   Wed 05.May.1999 09:56
Name: EXAMPLE
Comment:
I.D.:   Sex: F
S.S.#:   - -   Ethnic: W
ZIPCode: Height: 135.10 cm
Scan Code: EAJ Weight: 48.80 kg
BirthDate: 01.Jan.90   Age: 9
Physician:

BMD(L1-L4) = 0.432 g/cm^2

Region	BMD	T(30.0)		Z	
L1	0.426	-4.54	46%		
L2	0.411	-5.60	40%		
L3	0.469	-5.59	43%		
L4	0.424	-6.29	38%		
L1-L4	0.432	-5.59	41%	-2.81	65%

♦ Age and sex matched
T = peak bone mass
Z = age matched   TK   04 Nov 91

Fig. 10.8 *Continued*

Table 10.7 Causes of hypercalcaemia.

Gestational maternal hypocalcaemia
Idiopathic hypercalcaemia of infancy
Williams syndrome
Neonatal primary hyperparathyroidism
Preterm or intrauterine growth retarded-associated
  phosphate depletion
Vitamin D intoxication
Parathyroid adenoma
Isolated familial hyperparathyroidism
Multiple endocrine neoplasia type 1
Multiple endocrine neoplasia type 2A
Familial hypocalciuric hypercalcaemia
Hypercalcaemia in granulomatous disorders
Acute lymphoblastic leukaemia
Immobilization

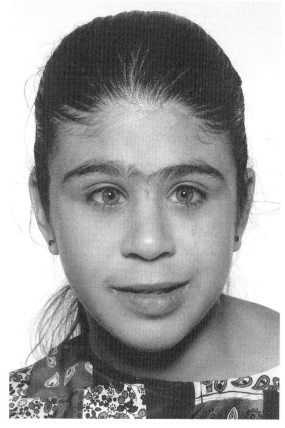

Fig. 10.9 Williams syndrome.

individuals should be screened for these endocrinopathies. The presence of elevated serum concentrations of PTH will distinguish hyperparathyroidism from hypercalcaemia caused by vitamin D intoxication, idiopathic infantile hypercalcaemia, granulomatous disease and malignancy.

History and examination

When assessing a child with possible hypercalcaemia, the following points should be highlighted in the clinical history:
• Symptoms suggestive of hypercalcaemia (e.g. weakness, anorexia, nausea and vomiting, constipation, polyuria and polydipsia);
• Symptoms suggestive of tuberculosis or sarcoidosis;
• Vitamin D therapy;
• A family history of multiple endocrine neoplasia.

Investigations

If hypercalcaemia is suspected, a blood sample should be taken for the measurement of:
• calcium;
• phosphate;
• PTH;
• 25-hydroxyvitamin D; and
• a sample stored for possible measurement of 1,25-dihydroxyvitamin D concentration later, should this be indicated.
  The differential diagnosis of biochemical abnormalities of calcium metabolism is shown in Table 10.4.

Treatment

The treatment of hypercalcaemia involves stopping vitamin D and calcium supplementation where relevant. Patients should be encouraged to drink plenty of fluids. The introduction of intravenous saline with or without frusemide and prednisolone may be necessary. A parathyroid adenoma may be located by careful ultrasound examination and treated by surgical removal of the affected gland. Hyperparathyroidism caused by diffuse hyperplasia requires surgical removal of all four glands.

When to involve a specialist centre

- Hypoparathyroidism.
- Hypophosphataemic rickets.
- Osteoporosis which is of sufficient severity that treatment with bisphosphanates is to be considered.
- Osteoporosis secondary to other underlying disorders (e.g. inflammatory bowel disease, rheumatoid arthritis or Cushing's syndrome) should have the treatment of their underlying disease discussed with the relevant specialists.
- Hyperparathyroidism.

Future developments

- Administration of sufficiently high doses of phosphate to children with hypophosphataemic rickets remains problematical and alternative therapeutic strategies are required to prevent the development of bone deformity in these children.
- The cause of idiopathic juvenile osteoporosis remains to be established. A diagnostic test for both this and osteogenesis imperfecta is much needed to assist clinicians in the investigation and management of children presenting with fractures associated with severe osteoporosis.
- More information is required about the long-term safety of bisphosphanate treatment and on alternative strategies for the treatment of severe childhood osteoporosis.
- Clarification of the molecular basis of primary hyperparathyroidism will enable earlier detection of this disorder and of multiple endocrine neoplasia type 1. The discovery of the calcium-sensing receptor offers the promise of alternative therapeutic strategies for the treatment of hyperparathyroidism.

Controversial points

- Does the severity of osteopenia in the growing child predict the future fracture risk as in postmenopausal women?
- Do girls with Turner's syndrome have an increased risk of osteopenia over and above that caused by inadequately treated hypogonadism?

- Do androgens have a direct effect on bone mineralization which is independent of their conversion to oestrogens?
- Is bisphosphanate treatment indicated for the treatment of osteopenia in the absence of fractures?
- Is bisphosphanate treatment in young children without risk to future bone health?
- The frequency and aetiology of fractures in infancy which are not due to non-accidental injury?

Potential pitfalls

- Diagnostic confusion between vitamin D deficiency and hypoparathyroidism as the cause of hypocalcaemia in infancy: careful interpretation of serum concentrations of phosphate, PTH and vitamin D should help distinguish between the two conditions.
- Over aggressive treatment of hypoparathyroidism increasing the risks of nephrocalcinosis.
- Unnecessary measurement of bone mineral density in a child at relatively low risk of developing osteoporosis.
- Incorrect diagnosis of osteoporosis based only on X-ray findings reportedly suggestive of osteopenia or from failure to take into account a child's small size when interpreting a dual energy X-ray measurement of bone mineral density.
- Failure clinically to suspect vertebral compression fractures. These should be considered in any child with osteoporosis who complains of back ache or stiffness or who has evidence of even relatively minor spinal shape deformity.
- Diagnostic confusion between osteogenesis imperfecta and non-accidental injury as the cause of fractures in a young child: where the diagnosis is unclear, these children should be referred for further evaluation by clinicians with expertise in child protection and bone disease.
- Failure to appreciate that most causes of hypercalcaemia in infancy are benign, self-limiting and respond well to conservative management.

CASE HISTORIES

Case 1

A 2-year-old boy was referred for further assessment of his increasingly bow legs. His mother was known to have hypophosphataemic rickets. X-rays show bowing of the femoral shafts but no radiological evidence of rickets. The following blood measurements were obtained:

calcium	2.37 mmol/L	[9.50 mg/dL]
phosphate	1.13 mmol/L	[3.50 mg/dL]
alkaline phosphatase	805 IU/L (reference range 100–400)	
PTH	1.3 pmol/L	[12.35 pg/mL] (reference range 0.9–5.5).

Questions

1 Is this child likely to have X-linked hypophosphataemic rickets?

2 What additional investigations may clarify the diagnosis?

Answers

1 This boy has a 50% chance of inheriting rickets from his mother. With an X-linked dominant disorder, he would be expected to be more severely affected than his mother. In the presence of his bone deformity, the absence of biochemical evidence of hypophosphataemia is surprising.

2 A simultaneous blood and urine sample should be obtained for the measurement of phosphate and creatinine so that the renal threshold phosphate concentration can be calculated (Kruse *et al.* 1982; Shaw *et al.* 1990). In this patient, the diagnosis of X-linked hypophosphataemic rickets was confirmed by the demonstration of a markedly decreased tubular reabsorption of phosphate (55%) and a renal threshold phosphate concentration of 1.4 mmol/L.

Case 2

A 9-year-old girl was admitted with severe back pain after she had fallen over her dog. She had sustained a previous fracture of her wrist following significant trauma. Her weight was above the 99th centile, height on the 50th centile and she had early breast development. X-rays demonstrated multiple wedge collapse fractures of several thoracic and lumbar vertebrae and widespread osteopenia. Initial investigations demonstrated the following:

calcium	2.45 mmol/L	[9.82 mg/dL]
phosphate	1.32 mmol/L	[4.10 mg/dL]
alkaline phosphatase	264 IU/L (reference range 100–400)	
PTH	4.2 pmol/L	[40 pg/mL] (reference range 0.9–5.5)
25-hydroxyvitamin D	12.4 ng/mL	[39.9 pg/mL] (reference range 8–50)
C-reactive protein	<1 mg/L.	

Normal renal, liver and thyroid function tests and antiendomysial antibody concentrations.

Questions

1 What further clinical observations would be of interest?

2 What additional investigations are required?

3 What is the differential diagnosis?

Answers

1 It would be helpful to know if she had evidence of blue-coloured sclerae, joint hyperextensibility or abnormal hearing which might suggest osteogenesis imperfecta. Given her obesity, it might also be important to assess for other signs suggestive of Cushing's syndrome.

2 A dual-energy X-ray absorptiometry scan confirmed the severity of the osteopenia with a lumbar spine bone mineral content of –2.79SD and femoral neck –3.65SD. Three 24-hour urine collections demonstrated normal cortisol excretion rates which excluded Cushing's syndrome.

3 This girl is most likely to have either idiopathic juvenile osteoporosis or, possibly, osteogenesis imperfecta.

References and further reading

Al Zahrani, A. & Levine, M.A. (1997) Primary hyperparathyroidism. *Lancet* **349**, 1233–1238.

Fewtrell, M.S., on behalf of the British Paediatric and Adolescent Bone Group. (2003) Bone densitometry in children assessed by dual x ray absorptiometry: uses and pitfalls. *Archives of Disease in Childhood* **88**, 795–798.

Kruse, K. (1992) Vitamin D and parathyroid. In: *Functional Endocrinologic Diagnostics in Children and Adolescents* (ed. M.B. Ranke), 1st edn, pp. 153–167. J & J Verlag, Mannheim.

Kruse, K., Kracht, U. & Göpfert, G. (1982) Renal threshold phosphate concentration (TmPO$_4$/GFR). *Archives of Disease in Childhood* **57**, 217–223.

Marini, J.C. (2003) Do bisphosphanates make children's bones brittle or better? *New England Journal of Medicine* **349**, 423–426.

Reid, I.R. (ed.) (1997) *Baillière's Clinical Endocrinology and Metabolism: Metabolic Bone Disease*. Ballière Tindall, London.

Shaw, N.J., Wheeldon, J. & Brocklebank, J.T. (1990) Indices of intact serum parathyroid hormone and renal excretion of calcium, phosphate and magnesium. *Archives of Disease in Childhood* **65**, 1208–1211.

Singh, J., Moghal, N., Pearce, S.H.S. & Cheetham, T. (2003) The investigation of hypocalcaemia and rickets. *Archives of Disease in Childhood* **88**, 403–407.

Warner, J.T., Cowan, F.J., Dunstan, F.D.J. *et al.* (1998) Measured and predicted bone mineral content in healthy boys and girls aged 6–18 years: adjustment for body size and puberty. *Acta Paediatrica* **87**, 244–249.

Wharton, B. & Bishop, N. (2003) Rickets. *Lancet* **362**, 1389–1400.

11 Obesity

Physiology

Definition

In childhood, obesity may be assessed in different ways. Measurement of weight alone is inadequate given the influence of height on weight. Although obesity may be clinically obvious if the child's weight centile is greater than the height centile, the severity of obesity is better defined by the use of the body mass index (BMI) in which

BMI = weight (kg) / height (m)^2.

Alternatively, body fatness can be assessed from direct measurements of subcutaneous skinfold thicknesses using skinfold thickness calipers or from measurement of waist circumference. Given the normal variation of BMI, skinfold thicknesses and waist circumference through childhood, reference to centile charts is required for interpretation of the data. The utility of skinfold thickness and waist circumference measurements is limited by the practical difficulties of obtaining these measurements accurately and so measurement of BMI is currently the best clinical method for identifying and monitoring obesity in childhood.

There are no widely agreed definitions of obesity in childhood as there are few data correlating specific definitions with future health risks. In practice in the United Kingdom, children with a BMI above the age and sex-specific 91st centile can be defined as overweight and those above the 98th centile as obese (see Appendix 2 for United Kingdom 1990 sex-specific BMI centile reference charts). Throughout the industrialized world, there is clear evidence of a recent, rapid increase in the prevalence of obesity in children and adults, with older children more affected than infants. In the United States, more than 30% of children have a body mass index that exceeds the 95th centile.

Aetiology

An increased risk of obesity is associated with genetic, environmental (Table 11.1) and pathological factors (Table 11.2). It is likely that a combination of an increasingly sedentary lifestyle combined with an excessive calorie intake for need is principally responsible for the rapid increase in prevalence of obesity noted over the last decade.

Obese children under 3 years of age without obese parents are at low risk of obesity in adulthood. However, in older children the presence of obesity becomes an increasingly important predictor of adult obesity, regardless of whether the parents are obese, with more than two-thirds of children who are obese aged 10 years or older becoming obese adults. Parental obesity more than doubles the risk of adult obesity in young children. Twin studies have suggested a heritability of fat mass of 40–70%.

Regulation of body fat

The normal amounts of body fat change through childhood, as can be seen from either the BMI centile charts (Appendix 2). Infants gain fat, as a consequence of increasing adipose cell size, relatively rapidly until the age of 1 year, but then slim down until the age of approximately 6 years as adipose cells reduce in size. From this point onwards, there is a steady increase in body fat into young adult life (the so-called 'adiposity rebound') associated with increases in adipose cell numbers. There is little difference in the amount of body fat in infant girls and boys. However, after infancy subcutaneous fat increases more

173

Table 11.1 Non-pathological risk factors for obesity.

Risk factor	Examples
Genetic	Obesity in either or both parents
	Early adiposity rebound
Environmental	Socioeconomic deprivation
	Single child
	Single parent
Diet-related	Bottle-fed in infancy
	High fat diet
	Disorganized eating patterns
Activity-related	Physical inactivity
	Increased television watching
	Short sleep duration

Table 11.2 Pathological causes of obesity.

Cause	Examples
Syndromes	Laurence–Moon–Biedl syndrome
	Down's syndrome
	Prader–Willi syndrome (Fig. 11.2)
Single gene mutations	Melanocortin-4 receptor
	Proopiomelanocortin
	Leptin
	Leptin receptor
	Pseudohypoparathyroidism
Hypothalamic damage	Trauma
	Tumours, e.g. craniopharyngioma
	Post encephalitis
Endocrine abnormalities	Growth hormone deficiency
	Hypothyroidism
	Cushing's syndrome
	Hyperinsulinism
Immobility	Spina bifida
	Cerebral palsy
Impaired skeletal growth	Achondroplasia
Drugs	Insulin
	Steroids
	Antithyroid drugs
	Sodium valproate

Table 11.3 Factors which influence the hypothalamic regulation of energy intake.

Factors which increase food intake	Factors which decrease food intake
Noradrenaline	Serotonin
Opioids	Dopamine
Ghrelin	Cholecystokinin
Galanin	Corticotrophin-releasing factor
Neuropeptide Y	Neurotensin
Melanin-concentrating	Bombesin
hormone	Calcitonin gene-related peptide
	Amylin
	Adrenomedullin
	Peptide YY3-36
	Leptin
	Glucagon
	Glucagon-like peptide 1

rapidly in girls, particularly during puberty when males demonstrate greater centralization of body fat stores.

Obesity occurs when energy intake chronically exceeds energy expenditure. In obese children there are wide variations in energy intake and not all obese children eat excessively. The high calorie density and fat content of the modern diet is associated with an increased risk of obesity.

The hypothalamus has a central role in the regulation of energy balance, integrating neuronal, hormonal and nutrient messages from within the body and transmitting signals which lead to the sensations of hunger or satiety (Fig. 11.1). The hypothalamus also influences energy expenditure via autonomic nerve function and the regulation of pituitary hormone release. Many hypothalamic neurotransmitters have been shown to influence energy intake (Table 11.3).

Energy expenditure consists of three components:

1 Resting metabolic rate is the energy expended at rest for the maintenance of basic cellular activities, excluding maintenance of body temperature, and accounts for 60–70% of total energy expenditure. Fat-free mass is metabolically more active than fat mass. Obese individuals have increased amounts of both body fat and fat-free mass and therefore most obese individuals have increases in their *absolute* resting metabolic rates because of their increased fat-free mass.

2 Thermogenesis is the energy expended in response to digestion and absorption of food, temperature changes, emotional influences or drugs which influence the physiological responses to such stimuli. It accounts for about 10% of total energy expenditure. It is unlikely that variations in thermogenesis are clinically important in the energy balance of the obese individual.

3 Energy expended in physical activity in children varies widely both on an individual daily basis and between

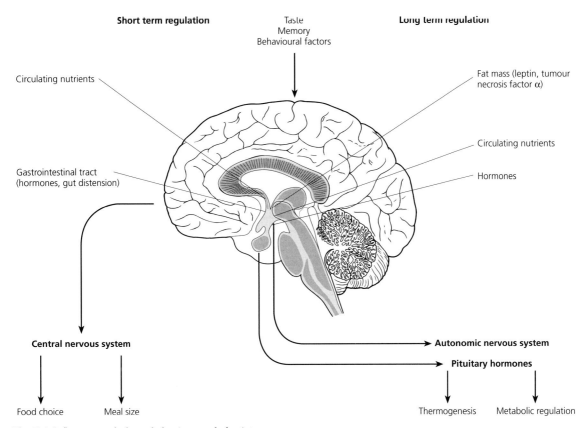

Fig. 11.1 Influences on the hypothalamic control of satiety.

individuals and accounts for 20–30% of total energy expenditure. Although obese children may be relatively physically inactive, they have an increase in the energy cost of weight-bearing activities and therefore do not demonstrate marked reductions in this component of energy expenditure when compared to normal-weight children.

As a consequence of these influences on energy expenditure, in most obese children, *absolute* total energy expenditure is increased. However, there is evidence that a low *relative* metabolic rate (i.e. adjusted for body size) predisposes to weight gain.

Complex interactions exist between signaling pathways that control energy intake and satiety and those that regulate fat mass. Adipose tissue may influence the hypothalamic regulation of energy balance through the secretion of leptin, a hormone which crosses the blood–brain barrier and suppresses the production of neuropeptide Y within the hypothalamus leading to reduced appetite and increased energy expenditure. However, most obese children have increased leptin concentrations in proportion to their increased body fat. Disorders of leptin synthesis or action are very rare and account for few cases of obesity.

Preliminary examination and investigation

History

Most children with obesity do not have an underlying pathological cause and have so-called 'simple obesity'. Such children usually demonstrate rapid growth and physical development. By contrast, children who are obese, short and growing slowly are much more likely to have an endocrine abnormality or, if associated with dysmorphic features and intellectual impairment, a syndromic cause to their obesity. A careful history and

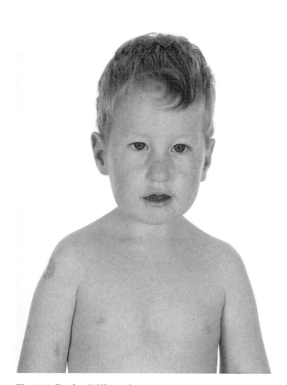

Fig. 11.2 Prader–Willi syndrome.

Table 11.4 Clinical signs to look for on examination.

Clinical sign	Possible diagnosis
Acanthosis nigricans (Plate 1)	Type 2 diabetes (insulin resistance)
Hypertension	Syndrome X
Dysmorphic features (see Table 11.5)	Laurence–Moon–Biedl syndrome (Fig. 11.3)
	Prader–Willi syndrome (Fig. 11.2)
	Pseudohypoparathyroidism (Fig. 11.4)
	Beckwith–Wiedemann syndrome
Impaired visual fields	Intracranial tumour, e.g. craniopharyngioma
Papilloedema or optic atrophy	
Tall stature or increased height velocity	Simple obesity
	Hyperinsulinism
Short stature or decreased height velocity	Growth hormone deficiency
	Hypothyroidism
	Laurence–Moon–Biedl syndrome
	Prader–Willi syndrome
	Pseudohypoparathyroidism
Cranial midline defects (e.g. cleft lip and palate)	Growth hormone deficiency
Truncal obesity	
Goitre	Hypothyroidism
Prolonged ankle tendon reflexes	
Proximal myopathy	Cushing's syndrome
Hypertension	
Truncal obesity	
Abnormal gait	Spina bifida
	Cerebral palsy

examination is required to distinguish the few children with significant underlying pathology causing their obesity from those who have 'simple obesity'. The history should include the following details:

• Birth weight. If increased this suggests an underlying mechanism, such as hyperinsulinism, which may have started *in utero*.

• Age of onset of obesity as early onset of obesity before the age of 2 years or while exclusively breast fed is more suggestive of a genetic or syndromic cause.

• Presence of congenital abnormalities or symptoms suggestive of a syndrome (e.g. initial feeding problems requiring nasogastric tube feeds and hypotonia with certain dysmorphic features might suggest Prader–Willi syndrome; Fig. 11.2).

• Detailed feeding and dietary history. It is often useful to go through a typical day's diet.

• Information about levels of physical activity.

• The extent to which the obesity may be having adverse effects—particularly psychosocial or related to school—on the child, the desire of the child and parents for the child to lose weight and the extent and success of previous interventions to achieve weight control.

• Medication.

• Symptoms of hypothalamo–pituitary pathology (e.g. headache, visual symptoms or previous history of trauma or encephalitis).

• Symptoms suggestive of endocrine abnormality (Table 11.2).

• Presence of polydipsia and polyuria (indicative of type 2 diabetes).

• Family history of obesity.

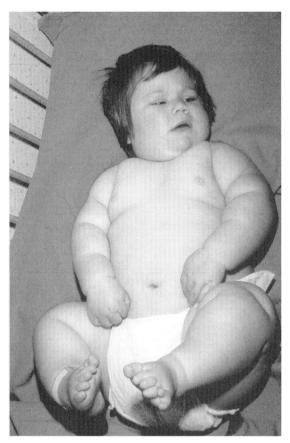

Fig. 11.3 Polydactyly in a child with Laurence–Moon–Biedl syndrome.

Examination

On examination, the child should undergo an accurate assessment of height and weight with measurements plotted on height, weight and BMI centile charts. Height measurements should be compared with the target height range derived from the mid-parental height centile as those who are relatively short for their genetic background are more likely to have a syndromic or endocrine cause for their obesity, whereas those who are relatively tall are more likely to suffer from simple obesity. Further assessment of the severity of the obesity can be made from the measurement of waist circumference or triceps and subscapular skinfold thicknesses although these measurement techniques require training and are difficult to perform in very obese individuals. Not all pathological causes of obesity will be self-evident and careful clinical examination is required to identify signs suggestive of certain disorders or complications of obesity. It is particularly important to note the presence of acanthosis nigricans (Plate 1) most commonly seen in the axillae or neck as this may indicate evolving insulin resistance and an increased risk of developing type 2 diabetes. Key signs to note on clinical examination are shown in Table 11.4. The clinical features of syndromes which may present with obesity are summarized in Table 11.5.

Complications

The main adverse effects of obesity are summarized in Table 11.6. In childhood, acute medical complications of simple obesity are few and minor. The combination of insulin resistance, hypertension, hypertriglyceridaemia and a low concentration of high-density lipoprotein cholesterol (so-called Syndrome X or the multimetabolic syndrome) used to be rarely seen in childhood though in the

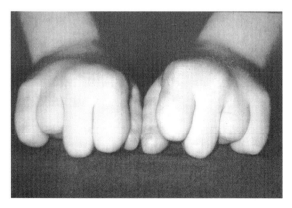

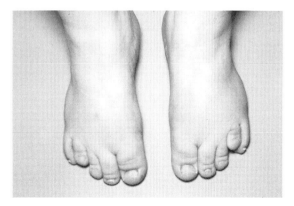

Fig. 11.4 Shortening of the fourth metacarpal and metatarsal in pseudohypoparathyroidism.

Table 11.5 Clinical features of common syndromic causes of obesity (Figs 11.2, 11.3 and 11.4).

System	Prader–Willi syndrome	Laurence–Moon–Biedl syndrome	Pseudohypo-parathyroidism
Facial	Narrow forehead Olive-shaped eyes Antimongoloid slant Epicanthic folds Squint Carp mouth Micrognathia Abnormal ear lobes	Squint	Round facies Short neck
Skeletal	Short stature Small hands and feet Clinodactyly Syndactyly Scoliosis Dislocated hips	Short stature Polydactyly Clinodactyly	Short stature Shortened fourth metacarpals and metatarsals
Neuromuscular	↓IQ Hypotonia and feeding problems in infancy Insatiable appetite Uncontrollable rage	↓IQ Retinitis pigmentosa	↓IQ
Endocrine	Hypogonadotrophic hypogonadism Type 2 diabetes	Hypogonadotrophic hypogonadism Diabetes insipidus	PTH-resistant hypocalcaemia
Other		Renal anomalies	Subcutaneous calcifications

United States, one in four overweight children in the age group 6–12 years now has inpaired glucose tolerance and 60% of these have at least one risk factor for heart disease. More commonly, obese children are tall for their age and have advanced skeletal development with an advanced bone age. A few may undergo precocious puberty with potentially adverse consequences for their final adult height. Why excess body fat has this effect is unclear. Obese children may also have an impaired self-image and for boys this may be complicated by a marked suprapubic fat pad leading to the penis being buried in fat and, as a result, appearing very small.

Investigations

The following investigations should be considered in those in whom there is clinical concern regarding an underlying pathological cause or a possible metabolic complication of obesity.
- An assessment of glucose tolerance, e.g. urinalysis for glycosuria, fasting blood glucose or, occasionally, an oral glucose tolerance test.
- Increased fasting serum insulin and decreased sex-

Table 11.6 Complications of simple obesity.

System	Adverse effect
Metabolic and endocrine	Hyperinsulinaemia Impaired glucose tolerance Type 2 diabetes Hyperlipidaemia Syndrome X (multimetabolic syndrome) Advanced pubertal development Polycystic ovarian disease Steatohepatitis
Cardiovascular	Hypertension
Respiratory	Breathless on exertion Obstructive sleep apnoea Pickwickian syndrome
Skeletal	Knock knee or bow legs Slipped capital femoral epiphysis
Psychological	Poor self-image Bullying Behavioural problems

hormone-binding globulin concentrations may confirm the presence of insulin resistance.
- Lipid profile.
- Thyroid function tests (serum T4 and thyroid-stimulating hormone (TSH) concentrations).
- Liver function tests.
- Three 24-hour urinary cortisol estimations.
- Bone age.
- Serum LH, FSH, oestradiol, 17-hydroxy progesterone, androstenedione and testosterone concentrations and a pelvic ultrasound in a girl with hirsuitism or menstrual irregularity thought to be at risk of having polycystic ovarian disease.

The need for additional investigations will depend on the level of clinical concern.
- In cases of suspected or proven hypothyroidism, Cushing's syndrome, hyperinsulinism or growth hormone deficiency, consult the relevant chapter for further investigations.
- If Laurence–Moon–Biedl syndrome is suspected, referral to a geneticist may be of help in identifying the relevant dysmorphic features and referral to an ophthalmologist for detailed retinal examination including electroretinography is important.
- Children with Prader–Willi syndrome caused by a deletion of chromosome 15(q11–13) or unimaternal disomy may be diagnosed by a combination of fluorescent *in situ* hybridization (FISH) probing and DNA testing.
- If pseudohypoparathyroidism is suspected, measure serum calcium, phosphate and parathyroid hormone concentrations. In the case of a low serum calcium and elevated phosphate and parathyroid hormone (PTH), the diagnosis may be confirmed by demonstration of deactivating mutations of the gene encoding the G protein stimulatory α subunit which is located on the long arm of chromosome 20.
- In syndromes associated with hypogonadism, investigation of the pituitary–gonadal axis should be considered in those who have genital hypoplasia, markedly delayed puberty or inadequate development of secondary sex characteristics (see Chapter 5).

Treatment

Young infants frequently appear obese and a spontaneous reduction in body fat occurs as part of the normal changes in body composition with increasing age. In general therefore, it is rare that a slimming regimen needs to be considered in the young child. However, investigations to exclude a pathological cause of obesity should be undertaken in all infants with severe, early onset obesity. If calorie restriction is deemed necessary in infancy, the aim should be maintenance of body weight rather than weight loss, as the latter may lead to specific dietary (e.g. vitamin) deficiencies or growth failure.

For many obese children, weight loss down to an 'ideal body weight for height' is probably unrealistic. Nevertheless, more modest weight reduction, or even prevention of further weight gain, may produce significant longer term health benefits. Such goals, which are more likely to be achievable, should be considered when planning individual therapeutic regimens. Unfortunately, there is almost no published evidence for any effective treatment for childhood obesity.

Older children with simple obesity should be encouraged to try and control their weight gain by:
- education about the nature of obesity and its longer term consequences;
- realistic assessment of the ease and likely benefits of slimming regimens;
- healthy eating (e.g. regular family meal times, avoidance of excessive 'snacking', fried foods, added fats and sugars and high energy drinks while encouraging foods with high fibre content) with modest calorie restriction and advice from a dietitian where necessary;
- increasing habitual physical activity (e.g. walking rather than taking transport to school, participation in games or sports that the child enjoys, restricting television or computer games); and
- psychological support (e.g. regular attendance at a dedicated clinic with dietetic support, group therapy (e.g. Weight Watchers) with the emphasis on mutual support and promotion of positive self-esteem).

Once a child has developed significant obesity, weight loss and long-term maintenance of an improved body weight are both difficult to achieve. Encouragement for children with simple obesity is best provided by frequent visits (e.g. 3-monthly) by the patient to a clinic or support service with motivated and interested staff. Multidisciplinary services involving community paediatricians, general practitioners, dietitians, psychologists or psychiatrists may help to improve the outcome. However, there is no point in continuing to encourage attendance in obese patients who fail to comply with suggested interventions and who fail to achieve significant weight loss, although intermittent clinical follow-up to monitor for early signs of the complications of obesity may still be necessary.

Although medical therapy, including inhibitors of

nutrient absorption from the gut (e.g. acarbose, guar gum and pancreatic lipase inhibitors), appetite suppressants (e.g. amphetamine derivatives and serotoninergic agents) and agents which increase energy expenditure (e.g. thyroxine and adrenergic agonists), have been used in the treatment of obesity in adults there is little experience of their use and efficacy in childhood. Side-effects may be problematical and their use is not currently recommended in children. There is increasing interest in the value of surgical interventions, such as laparoscopic gastric banding or the Roux-en-Y gastric bypass procedure in extremely obese children. When undertaken in children, dramatic amounts of weight loss can be achieved though such children will require careful monitoring for side-effects.

Where obesity is the consequence of an underlying endocrinopathy, treatment of hormone deficiency with the relevant hormone replacement (e.g. growth hormone or thyroxine) should result in a decrease in body fat. There is evidence that Prader-Willi syndrome is associated with hypothalamic dysfunction, including impaired growth hormone secretion. Growth hormone therapy (0.25 mg/kg/week to a maximum of 2.7 mg daily) is now indicated for the improvement of growth and body composition in children with Prader-Willi syndrome, providing there is no evidence of upper airway obstruction or severe obesity (weight exceeding 200% of ideal for height) and pre-treatment sleep studies do not demonstrate any evidence of sleep apnoea. Specific medical or surgical interventions for hyperinsulinism or Cushing's syndrome will also lead to significant weight loss.

When to involve a specialist centre

• Children with suspected hypothalamic tumours or endocrine causes of obesity should be managed in consultation with centres with expertise in the relevant neurosurgical investigations and paediatric endocrinology.
• Children with obesity of such severity that significant adverse cardiorespiratory consequences are suspected may need referral to a specialist unit for a detailed cardiorespiratory assessment, including sleep studies.
• Children with sufficiently severe obesity that drug treatment or surgery is to be considered should be referred to a specialist centre for further evaluation.

Future developments

• High-quality randomized controlled trials of lifestyle interventions which aim to prevent or treat obesity in childhood by altering eating behaviour or patterns of physical activity are required.
• An evaluation of the possible benefits of metformin or inhibitors of pancreatic lipase action in the gut to promote weight loss and insulin sensitivity in obese children is needed.
• An evaluation of the risks and benefits of surgery to treat childhood obesity.
• Further research should clarify the role and relationship between the multiple neurotransmitters known to influence hypothalamic function in the hope that a compound will be discovered which may have a significant effect on satiety without adverse side-effects.
• An alternative therapeutic approach may arise from improvements in our understanding of the control of energy expenditure, such as the recent discovery of uncoupling proteins in humans. These proteins disrupt the connection between food breakdown and energy production, resulting in increased heat production rather than 'useful' energy (i.e. inefficient utilization of energy).

Controversial points

• How extensively should tall, obese children with no dysmorphic features be investigated?
• How relatively important are genetic and environmental risk factors for obesity in childhood?
• What is the future risk of obesity in adult life for an obese young child?
• Is childhood-onset obesity more dangerous in adult life than adult-onset obesity?
• Are children who become obese less active than those who do not?
• Do children from obese families, who are at increased risk of obesity, have an inherited decrease in their metabolic rates?

Potential pitfalls

- Failure to recognize the diagnostic importance of distinguishing between obese children who are relatively tall and those who are short.
- Excessive and unrealistic expectations of the likely success of interventions to treat childhood obesity, especially when both parents are already obese.
- Over-investigation for a non-existant pathological cause of obesity in an otherwise well, normally growing relatively tall child.

- Encouraging obese children to achieve dramatic short-term weight loss is unlikely to be successful in achieving satisfactory regulation of longer term weight.
- Excessive weight loss may lead to impaired growth.
- Delayed diagnosis of type 2 diabetes or its misdiagnosis as type 1 diabetes in an obese child with minimal symptoms and absence of ketonuria when hyperglycaemia is finally documented.

CASE HISTORIES

Case 1

A 12-year-old boy presented with obesity. He had been floppy and a poor feeder as an infant with recurrent fits until the age of 7 years. On examination he had developmental delay and special educational needs. His height was on the 50th centile and weight well above the 97th centile. The following measurements were obtained on a basal blood sample:

calcium	1.95 mmol/L	[7.82 mg/dL]
albumin	41 g/L	[4.1 g/L]
phosphate	1.90 mmol/L	[5.9 mg/dL]
creatinine	78 μmol/L	[0.9 mg/dL]
alkaline phosphatase	202 IU/L (reference range 100–400)	
PTH	14.5 pmol/L (reference range 0.9–5.5)	[138 pg/ml (reference range 10–65)]
25-OH-cholecalciferol	16.1 ng/mL (reference range 8–50)	
free T_4	11 pmol/L (reference range 9.8–23.1)	[0.88 ng/dL (reference range 0.8–2.4)]
TSH	5.7 mU/L (reference range 0.35–5.5).	

Questions

1 What do these results demonstrate?
2 What is the most likely diagnosis?
3 What additional investigations may clarify the diagnosis?

Answers

1 Hypocalcaemia with hyperphosphataemia, raised PTH concentration and borderline thyroid function test results.
2 Pseudohypoparathyroidism is the most likely diagnosis.
3 The presence of PTH resistance may be confirmed by demonstrating absence of a urinary cyclic adenosine monophosphate (cAMP) response to an infusion of PTH. DNA analysis may confirm the underlying genetic defect. If hypothyroidism is suspected clinically, repeat thyroid function testing or a thyrotrophin-releasing hormone (TRH) stimulation test may be helpful to assess for possible associated TSH resistance.

Case 2

A 1-year-old girl was referred with massive obesity. She had been the product of a normal delivery at 41 weeks' gestation, birth weight 4.28 kg. She was noted to have polydactyly of both hands and a bifid left fifth toe. She was breast-fed from birth, with solids introduced at 9 months. There was no evidence of retinal pigmentation. Her general intelligence quotient (excluding locomotor skills) was 89. Initial serum biochemical investigations demonstrated the following:

urea, electrolytes and glucose	normal	
calcium	2.24 mmol/L	[9.0 mg/dL]
phosphate	1.33 mmol/L	[4.1 mg/dL]
free T_4	14.9 pmol/L	[1.2 ng/dL]
TSH	1.82 mU/L	
IGF-1	5.7 nmol/L (normal range 5.0–33.6).	[44 ng/dL (38–257)]

Questions
1 What is the most likely diagnosis?
2 What additional investigations may be of assistance?

Answers
1 Laurence-Moon–Biedl syndrome is the most likely diagnosis.

2 Further evaluation of her retinal function demonstrated no visual evoked potential or electroretinogram response to flash. An abdominal ultrasound examination did not demonstrate any associated renal abnormalities.

Further reading

Auwerx, J. & Staels, B. (1998) Leptin. *Lancet* **351**, 737–742.

Berger, A., Brand, M. & O'Rahilly, S. (1998) Uncoupling proteins: the unravelling of obesity? Increased understanding of mechanisms may lead, in time, to better drugs. *British Medical Journal* **317**, 1607–1608.

Gortmaker, S.L., Must, A., Perrin, J.M. *et al.* (1993) Social and economic consequences of overweight in adolescence and young adulthood. *New England Journal of Medicine* **329**, 1008–1012.

Leibel, R.L. (1997) And finally, genes for human obesity. *Nature Genetics* **16**, 218–220.

Miller, J., Rosenbloom, A. & Silverstein, J. (2004) Childhood obesity. *Journal of Clinical Endocrinology & Metabolism* **89**, 4211–4218.

Rudolf, M.C.J. (2004) The obese child. *Archives of Disease in Childhood* **89**, ep57–ep62.

Whitaker, R.C., Wright, J.A., Pepe, M.S. *et al.* (1997) Predicting obesity in young adulthood from childhood and parental obesity. *New England Journal of Medicine* **337**, 869–873.

Wilding, J. (1997) Obesity treatment. *British Medical Journal* **315**, 997–1000.

12 Endocrine effects of cancer treatment

Pathophysiology

There has been a remarkable increase in the survival rates of children with most malignancies during the past 30 years. This improvement has resulted from the use of sophisticated regimens of multi-agent chemotherapy, frequently combined with new radiotherapy and surgical techniques. Treatment of childhood cancer is intensive and associated with effects on a number of organs, of which the endocrine system is particularly vulnerable. The risk of late endocrine effects in survivors is related more to the treatment received than to the nature of the underlying malignancy. Organs related to endocrine function or growth which are susceptible to the effects of cancer treatment are shown in Table 12.1.

Chemotherapy

Cytotoxic chemotherapy may damage normal developing cells and the damage is dependent on the type and dose of chemotherapeutic agent used. The germinal epithelium in the testis is highly susceptible to alkylating agents, such as cyclophosphamide. Similarly, the potential for normal ovarian function may be impaired with intensive chemotherapy. Direct damage to the growth plate is currently being studied as a mechanism of chemotherapy-induced growth impairment.

Radiotherapy

Radiotherapy, used either alone or in combination with chemotherapy or surgery, is effective in treating a number of childhood cancers. However, there is frequently a cost in terms of endocrine function and growth. The potential for damage is related to the dose of radiotherapy deliv-

ered, the protocol of delivery and the site of the primary lesion. Damage to the hypothalamo–pituitary axis is relatively common following irradiation of tumours of the brain, face, orbit and adjacent areas. The thyroid is susceptible to head and neck irradiation and the growing spine is vulnerable to direct or indirect radiotherapy. Similarly, the prepubertal testis—often the site of relapse in leukaemia—is susceptible to direct treatment.

Investigation and management of late endocrine effects

The combined oncology–endocrine clinic

The establishment of a combined oncology–endocrine clinic, or alternatively an oncology late effects clinic with an endocrinologist in attendance, has been shown to be of benefit to patient management (Fig. 12.1). Paediatricians and paediatric endocrinologists should be encouraged to work closely with oncologists to establish a joint clinic aimed at identification, investigation and management of late endocrine effects. The principal aim of the oncologist is to treat and monitor the status of the patient's primary disorder. The endocrinologist can support this process by contributing knowledge and experience of potential and actual endocrine and growth dysfunction. Auxological monitoring is an essential function of this clinic.

Referral to the oncology–endocrine clinic

Late referral to this clinic can lead to considerable delay in diagnosis of treatable endocrine effects. Consequently, *all patients* who have received radiotherapy in childhood *to any organ* should be referred 1 year after completion of treatment. In this way auxological monitoring can identify early growth failure and potential abnormalities of puberty can be studied. Patients treated by chemotherapy, which can cause potential endocrine dysfunction, should also be referred. Any oncology patient with concerns about growth, puberty or changes in body composition, e.g. obesity, can benefit from early referral to this clinic.

Investigation and monitoring of patients
Procedures which may be undertaken either in or associated with the joint clinic are shown in Table 12.2.

Table 12.1 Organs related to endocrine function or growth which are susceptible to damage from cancer treatment.

Hypothalamic–pituitary axis
Growth hormone
Adrenocorticotrophic hormone
Luteinizing hormone/follicle-stimulating hormone
Thyroid-stimulating hormone
Thyroid
Testis
Ovary
Spine
Long bones
Growth plate
Breast tissue
Fat mass

Specific endocrine and growth abnormalities associated with cancer treatment

Cancer treatment may affect the function of a number of specific endocrine organs and tissues related to growth. Frequently, several organ systems are affected in the same patient. The major endocrine and growth abnormalities are described individually.

Abnormal linear growth
Growth can be impaired by:
- direct effect of radiotherapy on the spine;
- damage to the hypothalamic–pituitary axis with resulting growth hormone (GH) deficiency;
- gonadal damage with sex steroid deficiency, resulting in impaired pubertal growth; and
- effect of radiotherapy and chemotherapy on growth plates.

Spinal irradiation
Spinal irradiation, as given for conditions such as medulloblastoma (Fig. 12.2) and germinoma, will seriously affect subsequent spinal growth. The effect is particularly severe in early childhood. Spinal growth is an essential component of the adolescent growth spurt. Consequently, short stature with disproportion because of shortness of the trunk is frequently seen in these patients.

Growth hormone deficiency
Damage to the hypothalamic–pituitary axis resulting

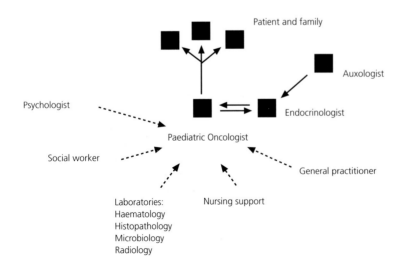

Fig. 12.1 Suggested model for a joint paediatric oncology–endocrinology clinic.

Table 12.2 Procedures in or associated with the joint oncology-endocrine clinic.

Clinic attendance — every 4–6 months
Auxology monitoring
 Height
 Height velocity
 Sitting height
 Weight
 Bone age
 Body mass index
Puberty development staging (including testicular volume)
Hormone measurements
 Basal levels
 T4, TSH, cortisol, testosterone, oestradiol, LH, FSH, prolactin, IGF-I
 Dynamic tests
 Growth hormone (and ACTH) stimulation, e.g. glucagon,
  insulin, clonidine tests, overnight growth hormone profile
 LHRH test
 TRH test
 hCG stimulation
Thyroid ultrasound
Pelvic ultrasound
DEXA scan for bone mineral density and body composition

Abbreviations: ACTH, adrenocorticotrophic hormone; FSH, follicle-stimulating hormone; hCG, human chorionic gonadotrophin; IGF-I, insulin-like growth factor I; LH, luteinizing hormone; LHRH, LH-releasing hormone; T4, thyroxine; TRH, thyrotrophin-releasing hormone; TSH, thyroid-stimulating hormone.

in GH deficiency can occur following radiotherapy given in:

• high doses (>3000 cGy) as curative therapy for brain, orbit, adjacent tissue tumours;
• doses of 1800–2400 cGy as prophylaxis for CNS leukaemia; and
• doses of 750–1600 cGy as total body irradiation.

The prevalence and severity of GH deficiency is related to the total dosage of radiotherapy and the fractionation schedule. The same total dosage given in a larger number of smaller fractions is likely to be less damaging. Radiotherapy regimens for brain tumours and tumours of the face and orbit, which deliver doses >3000 cGy to the hypothalamic–pituitary axis, will almost always result in GH deficiency. This is usually present by 2 years after treatment.

The frequency of GH deficiency following prophylactic CNS irradiation and after total body irradiation is variable. However, several studies have reported a prevalence of up to 50%. A more subtle form of GH deficiency may be seen where the GH response to pharmacological stimulation may be normal; however, physiological GH secretion and the normal increment in GH secretion occurring at puberty is impaired.

Diagnosis
A high index of suspicion is important when children at risk of GH deficiency are seen in the oncology–endocrine clinic. Children should undergo GH stimulation testing at the earliest suspicion of a subnormal height velocity. For interpretation of the results see Chapter 3. The puberty status must always be assessed and considered when interpreting the auxological findings. Puberty will stimulate growth, which can mask underlying GH deficiency.

Treatment
The same principles apply to the treatment of irradiation-induced GH deficiency as with other aetiologies. There is no evidence that normal human GH (hGH) therapy increases the risk of recurrence of malignancy after remission has been induced. Although it is recognized that in these patients the basic defect may be in hypothalamic growth hormone-releasing hormone (GHRH) secretion, therapy with hGH is indicated and, as always, early diagnosis will lead to the best long-term result.

Sex steroid deficiency and direct damage to growth plate and long bones

Sex steroid deficiency will be discussed in the section on gonadal damage. Growth failure in the absence of direct spinal irradiation or GH deficiency has been described. The mechanism of this apparent effect of chemotherapy is not clear. It is possible that the growth plates in the spine and long bones are susceptible to damage from intensive chemotherapy.

Abnormal pituitary function

The growth hormone axis is most vulnerable to damage by radiotherapy. Other anterior pituitary hormones are relatively resistant. Gonadotrophin and adrenocorticotrophic hormone (ACTH) deficiencies may occur at a longer interval of approximately 10 years after treatment, followed by thyroid-stimulating hormone (TSH) deficiency, which appears to be even more infrequent.

Early puberty following cranial irradiation

This phenomenon was first reported in the 1980s and is

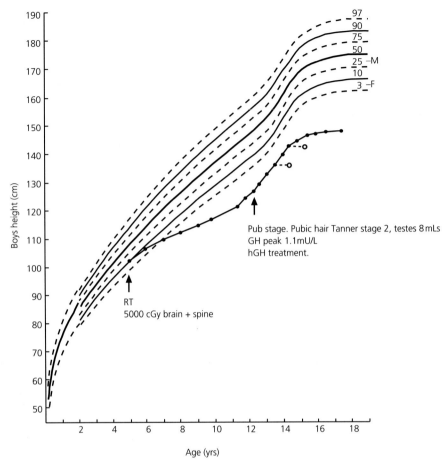

Fig. 12.2 Growth following radiotherapy to brain and spine for medulloblastoma. Note the severe height loss because of spinal irradiation, the rather early puberty and the severely restricted final height.

now a recognized complication, particularly in girls. Children who received cranial irradiation, particularly at a young age, have a significantly earlier onset of puberty with respect to chronological age and bone age.

The combination of GH deficiency and early puberty severely reduces growth potential. In this situation, puberty should be suppressed using gonadotrophin-releasing hormone (GnRH) analogue therapy to allow maximum benefit from hGH replacement.

Gonadal damage

Gonadal damage in childhood can occur following chemotherapy or radiotherapy. There are specific differences affecting the testis and ovary, so each will be described separately.

The testis

Chemotherapy

The use of chemotherapeutic regimens which include alkylating agents, such as cyclophosphamide, chlorambucil and the nitrosureas, in addition to procarbazine, vinblastine, cytosine arabinoside and possibly *cis*-platinum, are likely to cause damage to germinal epithelium resulting in azoospermia and infertility in adult life. This has been reported particularly in leukaemia and Hodgkin's disease. With this established knowledge, chemotherapeutic regimens are now being modified with the aim of minimizing this complication. Elevation of basal follicle-stimulating hormone (FSH) is a useful guide to damage of germinal epithelium. Testosterone production from Leydig cells is not generally affected.

Radiotherapy

The testis is vulnerable to radiation damage, which in turn depends on the total dosage and dose per fraction. Following total body irradiation (dose 1200–1500 cGy) to prepubertal children for leukaemia, Leydig cell function was not affected; however, azoospermia occurred. After direct testicular irradiation, testosterone production was severely reduced and infertility resulted.

Consequently, it is important to assess testicular size and function, by human chorionic gonadotrophin (hCG) stimulation if necessary and measurement of basal gonadotrophins, in order to define the need for testosterone replacement. Long-term androgen therapy may be indicated to ensure satisfactory pubertal development and normal testosterone levels in adult life.

The ovary

Chemotherapy

The ovary is apparently more resistant to damage than the testis. Normal fertility and endocrine function can be expected in adult survivors of childhood leukaemia treatment. Intensive chemotherapeutic regimens for conditions such as Hodgkin's disease may confer more risk of ovarian dysfunction. Elevation of basal FSH may indicate ovarian damage.

Radiotherapy

The ovary is susceptible to damage from radiotherapy. Direct, or indirect radiotherapy as in total body irradiation, can cause ovarian failure with impairment of ovulation and possible subnormal sex steroid secretion. Vulnerable patients need to be carefully assessed by the endocrinologist and normal pubertal development ensured.

Thyroid abnormalities

Thyroid abnormalities are likely to occur after radiotherapy which has included the thyroid area. There are three main types of potential thyroid dysfunction: hypothyroidism, benign thyroid nodules and thyroid cancer. The children most at-risk are those treated for Hodgkin's disease who receive 3000–5000 cGy to the neck. In these patients approximately 25% develop hypothyroidism during the first few years after treatment. The first sign is usually elevation of TSH, which should be promptly treated with thyroxine replacement. The frequency increases to >50% after 6 years.

Total body irradiation and cranial irradiation are also associated with hypothyroidism, which should be excluded by regular thyroid function tests performed in the joint oncology–endocrine clinic. Thyroid nodules may develop after a longer interval. They can be detected clinically or on ultrasound.

Thyroid cancer is also usually a late complication of neck irradiation. Any suspected thyroid neoplasm should be investigated by ultrasound. Elevation of TSH for long periods of time is said to confer greater risk of malignancy in the irradiated gland.

Adrenal abnormalities

Abnormal adrenal function is rare in children treated for cancer. ACTH deficiency may be a late complication of high-dose (>3000 cGy) cranial irradiation and should be considered if other anterior pituitary hormones are deficient.

Abnormalities of body composition

It is becoming recognized that survivors of childhood leukaemia and brain tumours may become obese. There is currently no good explanation for this. Impaired bone mineralization may also occur during childhood and can be demonstrated on DEXA scanning. Chronic illness, reduced exercise, steroid therapy, direct effects of other chemotherapeutic agents on osteoblasts, GH deficiency and impaired sex steroid secretion at puberty are all potential factors contributing to this finding. The prompt and accurate diagnosis and treatment of endocrine deficiencies will help to normalize bone mineralization, hence diminishing the risk of osteoporosis in adult life.

When to involve a specialist centre

- All long-term survivors of childhood cancer should be under review by a specialist oncology department. Where appropriate, these patients should attend the joint oncology–endocrine follow-up clinic.

Future developments

- The challenge for oncologists is to develop future treatments which are effective for the treatment of the primary neoplasm but cause minimal late effects.
- More specific and targeted radiotherapy techniques are being developed.

• Cryopreservation of gonadal tissue prior to cancer therapy is being explored within ethical limits.

Controversial points

• Ethical issues and practicalities of harvesting and cryo-preservation of gametes prior to treatment causing gonadal damage.
• Possible protection of gonads from chemotherapeutic or radiotherapeutic damage by endocrine therapy, i.e. GnRH suppression of pituitary–gonadal axis.
• Management of prevention of menstruation in patients likely to develop heavy bleeding.

Potential pitfalls

• Failure to appreciate that a suboptimal growth response to GH in children with GHD previously treated with cranio-spinal radiotherapy may reflect radiotherapy-induced growth plate damage.
• Importance of clinically staging puberty to ensure that GHD coexistent with precocious puberty is not missed.
• Failure soon after radiotherapy to identify evolving endocrine deficiency which becomes increasingly likely the longer the time after treatment. Hence the need for long-term follow-up in patients who received cranial irradiation in excess of 1800 or 2400 Gy.

CASE HISTORY

A 3-year-old boy was diagnosed to have a rhabdomyosarcoma of the left maxillary antrum. He received radiotherapy to the tumour (5046 cGy) and chemotherapy. There has been no recurrence of the tumour. At the age of 5 years his growth started to slow down. He was not referred to the joint oncology–endocrine clinic until the age of 7.4 years by which time his height was far below the 3rd centile and his height velocity was 3.6 cm/year.

Questions
1 What investigations are indicated?
2 What is the likely diagnosis and what tests would you do?
3 How do you interpret this test?
4 Does he have gonadotrophin deficiency in addition to his GH and TSH defiencies?

Answers
1 Detailed auxology and basal hormone measurements were performed (Table 12.2). Biochemistry was normal. A dynamic GH stimulation test (glucagon 15 µg/kg intramuscularly) was performed and his peak GH level was 1.4 mU/L. He therefore had severe GH deficiency. He was started on GH therapy in a standard dosage of 14 IU/m^2/week. His height velocity increased to 8.4 cm/year.

At the age of 14 years his T_4 was 58 nmol/L (normal range 57–170) and his TSH was 1.6 mU/L (normal range 0.4–5.0). This is suggestive of central hypothyroidism.
2 The results suggest central hypothyrodism. A TRH test was performed with TRH 200 µg intravenously. The results were as shown in Table 12.3.
3 This is an abnormal test. The 20-minute level should be higher than the 60-minute level. He has central hypothyroidism and was started on treatment with thyroxine 100 µg/day.

At the age of 15 years he was still prepubertal.
4 This is very difficult to say and to diagnose at this age. No test is specific. The most important step is to treat his delayed puberty. He was started on testosterone enantate 125 mg monthly.

Overall diagnosis: multiple pituitary hormone deficiencies secondary to irradiation of a rhabdomyosarcoma in close proximity to the hypothalamic–pituitary axis.

Table 12.3 Results of thyrotrophin-releasing hormone test.

Time (min)	TSH (mU/L)
0	1.6
20	6.8
60	8.9

Abbreviation: TSH, thyroid-stimulating hormone.

References and further reading

Bath, L.E., Wallace, H.B. & Kelnar, C.J.H. (1998) Disorders of growth and development in the child treated for cancer. In: *Growth Disorders: Pathophysiology and Treatment* (eds C.J.H. Kelnar, M.O. Savage, H.F. Stirling & P. Saenger), pp. 640–641. Chapman & Hall Medical, London.

Wallace, W.H. Thomson, A.B. (2003) Preservation of fertility in children treated for cancer. *Archives of Disease in Childhood* **88**, 493–496.

United Kingdom and North American patient support groups

Diabetes UK
10 Parkway
London NW1 7AA
UK
Tel: 020 7424 1000
Fax: 020 7424 1001
Website: www.diabetes.org.uk

Child Growth Foundation
2 Mayfield Avenue
Chiswick
London W4 1PW
UK
Tel: 020 8995 0257
Fax: 020 8995 9075
Website: www.heightmatters.org.uk

The Turner Syndrome Support Society
12 Irving Quadrant
Hardgate
Clydebank G81 6AZ
UK
Tel: 01389 380385
Fax: 01389 380384
Email: Turner.Syndrome@tss.org.uk
Website: www.tss.org.uk

Premature Sexual Maturation Group
This group works under the umbrella
of the Child Growth Foundation (see above).

Restricted Growth Association (RGA)
PO Box 4744
Dorchester DT2 9FA
UK
Tel: 01308 898445
Website: www.restrictedgrowth.co.uk

Prader Willi Syndrome Association UK (PWSA UK)
125a London Road
Derby DE1 2QQ
UK
Tel: 01332 365676
Fax: 01332 360401
Website: www.pwsa-uk.demon.co.uk

The British Thyroid Foundation
PO Box 97
Clifford
Wetherby
West Yorkshire LS23 6XD
UK
Tel/fax: 0870 7707933
Website: www.btf-thyroid.org

Laurence-Moon-Bardet-Biedl Society (LMBBS)
10 High Cross Road
Rogerstone
Newport NP10 9AD
UK
Tel: 01633 718415
Website: www.lmbbs.org.uk

The Congenital Adrenal Hyperplasia Support Group
2 Windrush Close
Flintwick
Bedfordshire MK45 1PX
UK
Tel: 01525 717536
Website: www.cah.org.uk

Androgen Insensitivity Syndrome Group UK
PO Box 429
Oldham
Lancs OL4 4ZT
UK
Website: www.medhelp.org/www/ais

Juvenile Diabetes Research Foundation International (JDRF)
120 Wall Street
New York, NY 10005-4001
USA
Tel. 1-800-533-CURE (2873)
Email: info@jdrf.org
Website:www.jdf.org/

The MAGIC Foundation (short stature and other endo-crine disorders)
6645 W. North Avenue
Oak Park, IL 60302
USA
Tel. 1-800-00.362.4423 (1.800.3 MAGIC 3)
Website: www.magicfoundation.org

Human Growth Foundation
997 Glen Cove Avenue, Suite 5
Glen Head, NY 11545
USA
Tel. 1-800-451-6434
Fax 1-516-671-4055
Email: hgf1@hgfound.org
Website: www.hgfound.org

Turner Syndrome Society of the United States
14450 TC Jester, Suite 260
Houston, TX 77014
USA
Tel. 1-800-365-9944;
Email: tssus@turner-syndrome-us.org
Website: www.turner-syndrome-us.org

CARES Foundation, Inc.for CAH
189 Main Street, 2nd flr.,
Millburn, NJ 07041
USA
Tel. 1-973-912-3895, 1-866-227-3737 (toll free)
Fax: 973-912-8990
Website: www.caresfoundation.org

2 Growth and BMI charts

• Please place a sticker (if available) otherwise write in space provided.

Surname

First names

NHS no: Local no

G.P.   Code

H.V.   Code

GIRLS
GROWTH CHART
(BIRTH - 18 YEARS)

United Kingdom cross-sectional reference data : 1996/1

D.O.B. ...... : ...... : ...... WEEKS GESTATION ....

HOSPITAL COMPUTER No. ....

pre-term

for a girl born before 37 completed weeks, draw a vertical "pre-term" line at the appropriate week and plot measurements from this line for at least twelve months. For all later deliveries plot from the EDD (Estimated Delivery Date) line.

measurements

weight: an infant or toddler should always be weighed naked on a self-calibrating or regularly calibrated scale. An older child should be weighed with the minimum of clothing.

head circumference: head circumference measurements should be taken from midway between the eyebrows and the hairline at the front of the head and the occipital prominence at the back. Appropriate thin plastic or metal tape should be used: sewing tape or paper tape is not recommended for this purpose.

supine length: an infant:- a child up to approximately 18 months - should be measured supinely (on her back) by two people with equipment featuring both a headboard and moveable footboard. Whilst one person holds the head against the headboard, with the head facing upwards in the Frankfurt plane*, a second person measures the length by bringing the footboard up to the heels. The downward pressure on the child's knees to ensure that the legs are flat will not endanger hip dislocation.

standing height: standing height should be measured against an appropriate vertical measure, door or wall free from radiators, pipes or large skirting board. The feet should be together with the heels, buttocks and shoulder blades touching the vertical and the head positioned in the Frankfurt plane*. To ensure that the maximum height is taken, upward pressure to the mastoid processes should be considered.

*The Frankfurt plane is an imaginary line from the centre of the ear hole to the lower border of the eye socket.

guidelines for recording, plotting and referral

Record the measurement using the boxes on this chart immediately you have taken it. Enter the date, specify the measurement in the box with the asterisk (i.e. **H/C** = head circumference, **H** = height, **L** = length, **W** = weight) and name your entry. You might find it helpful to enter her current age in the appropriate column. Plot each measurement on the grid with a well defined dot. Trace the growth curve with a line but leave the dots clearly visible. A normal growth curve is one that always runs roughly on/parallel to one of the printed centile lines. If it doesn't, consider these guidelines:-

Refer a girl whose height falls above the 99.6th or below the 0.4th centile line or outside her Target Centile Range (TCR). Refer her also if, pre-school, her growth curve veers upwards/downwards over the period 12-18 months by the width of one centile band or, post school entry, by $2/3$ of a band, if, prior to school entry, the curve veers by only $2/3$ of a band or, subsequently, by $1/2$ a band, flag the child for recall in 12 months and refer if the trend continues. Respond to parental concern about a child's growth, irrespective of the current centile, by monitoring height over a period of at least nine months and follow the criteria above. *(Source: BSPED September 1996)*

Date	Age	*	Measurement	Name
24 : 09 : 92	ⁿ/₁₂	L	72 : 5 cm	Mary Brown
24 : 09 : 92	ⁿ/₁₂	H/C	44 : 3 cm	Mary Brown
24 : 09 : 92	ⁿ/₁₂	W	9 : kg	Mary Brown
: :	:		: :	

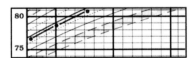

adult height potential

The table and illustrations below show how the adult height potential of a girl is calculated. They show that she is following her genetic pattern and that her growth curve should border the 50th centile to reach 164cm as an adult - **mid-parental height (MPH)**. The 50th centile is her **mid-parental centile (MPC)**, If the curve continuously follows a centile somewhere between the 91st-9th centiles (**MPH** ± 8.5cm) it will still be within her **target centile range (TCR)** and her growth will be considered normal. NB This calculation is not appropriate if either parent is not of normal stature.

Now use the box on the back page to calculate this girl's adult height potential.

Calculate (and complete on back page) as follows:-

(a) = father's height
(b) = mother's height
(c) = sum of (a) and (b)
(d) = (c) ÷ 2
(e) = (d) - 7cm (**MPH**)
(f) = **MPC** - nearest centile to (e)
(g) = **TCR** (mid-parental height ± 8.5cm)

Arrow (h) the mid-parental height/centile and draw a vertical line above and below it to represent the target centile range.

(a)	_186_ cm
(b)	_156_ cm
(c)	_342_ cm
(d)	_171_ cm
(e)	_164_ cm	(f) _50th_ centile
(g)	_91st_ centile – _9th_ centile

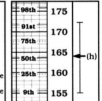

98th — 175
91st — 170
75th
50th — 165 ◄— (h)
25th — 160
9th — 155

references and acknowledgements

papers
1. Do growth chart centiles need a face lift? (TJ Cole) *BMJ* 1994; *308*: 641-2
2. Cross-sectional stature and weight reference curves for the UK, 1990 (JV Freeman, TJ Cole, S Chinn, PRM Jones, EM White, MA Preece) *ARCH DIS CHILD* 1995; 73: 17-24
3. Growth Charts for ethnic populations in the UK (S Chinn, TJ Cole, MA Preece, R Rona) *The Lancet* March 23rd 1996; 347: 839-840
Compilation: Institute of Child Health, London (Freeman JV et al). *Data sources:* British Size Surveys, Loughborough Consultants Ltd (Jones PRM, Norgan NG, Hunt MJ, Hooper RH); National Study of Health and Growth (Chinn S, Rona RJ); ONS National Heights and Weight Survey, 1980 & National Diet and Nutrition Survey, 1995; Tayside Growth Study (White EM et al); MRC Dunn Nutrition Group, Cambridge (Lucas A, Paul AA, Whitehead RG); MRC Human Genetics Unit, Edinburgh (Ratcliffe SG, Butler GE); UCH, London, 1000 births 1987/88 (Colley NV, Hanson GL), Rosie Hospital, Cambridge (Glazebrook C, Rennie JM) & Northern RHA birth data (Wariyar UK); Chard 1976-1988 Normal Puberty Longitudinal Study (Dunger DB, Cameron N, Baines-Preece J, Cox L, Preece MA)

0191 455 4286

Designed and Published by
© CHILD GROWTH FOUNDATION 1996/1
(Charity Reg. No 274325)
2 Mayfield Avenue,
London W4 1PW

Printed and Supplied by
HARLOW PRINTING LIMITED
Maxwell Street ◊ South Shields
Tyne & Wear ◊ NE33 4PU

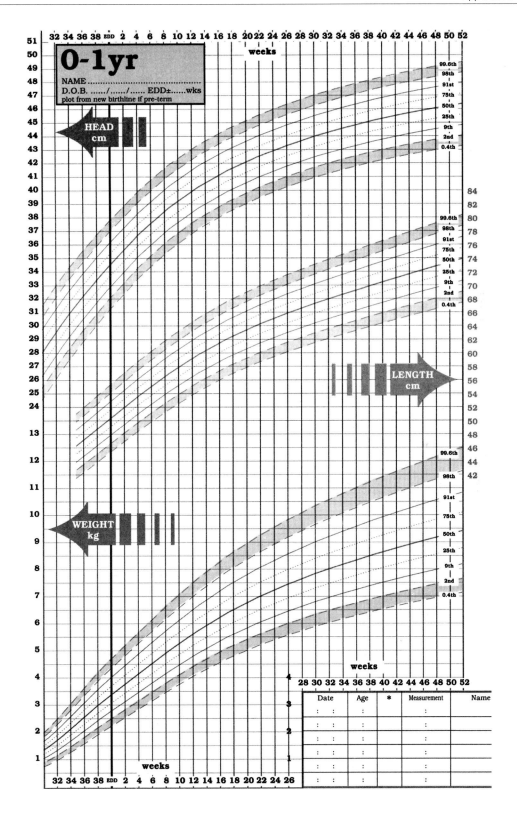

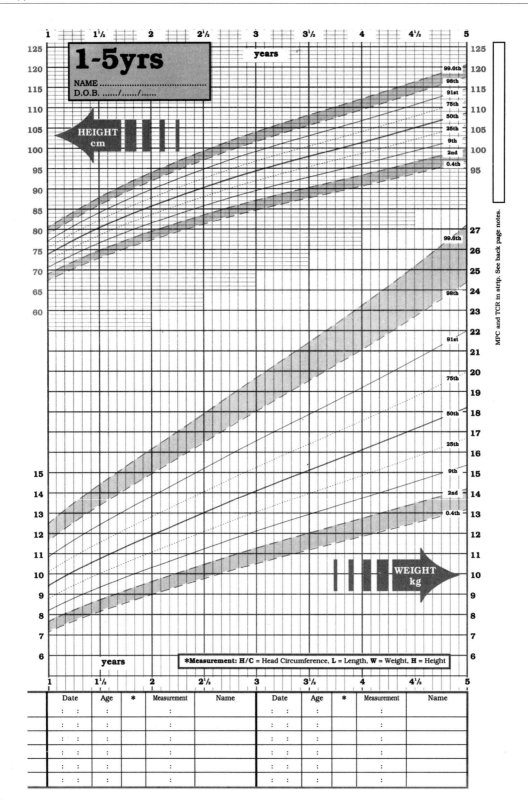

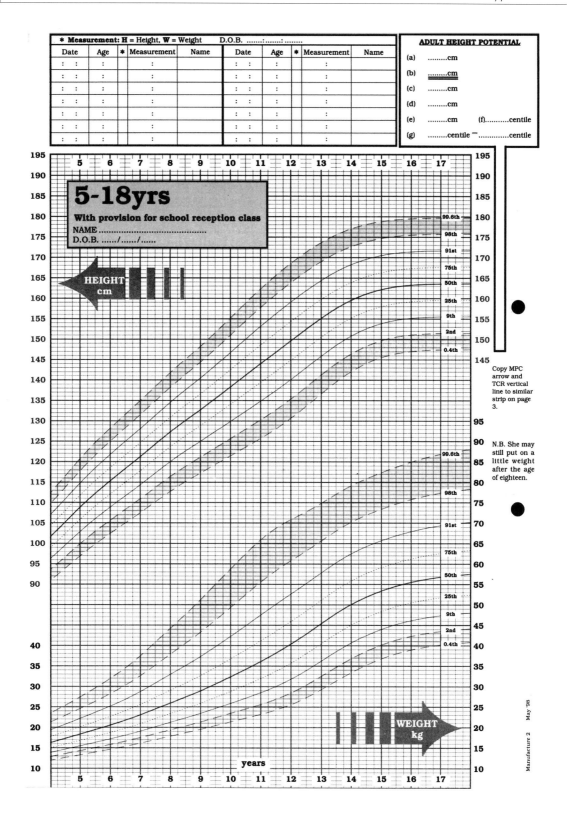

* Measurement: **H** = Height, **W** = Weight				D.O.B. ....:.......:........				
Date	Age	*	Measurement	Name	Date	Age	*	Measurement	Name
: :	:	:	:		: :	:	:	:	
: :	:	:	:		: :	:	:	:	
: :	:	:	:		: :	:	:	:	
: :	:	:	:		: :	:	:	:	
: :	:	:	:		: :	:	:	:	
: :	:	:	:		: :	:	:	:	
: :	:	:	:		: :	:	:	:	

ADULT HEIGHT POTENTIAL

(a) ....cm
(b) ....cm
(c) ....cm
(d) ....cm
(e) ....cm   (f)...........centile
(g) ....centile − ....centile

5-18yrs

With provision for school reception class

NAME..
D.O.B. ....../....../.....

HEIGHT cm

99.6th
98th
91st
75th
50th
25th
9th
2nd
0.4th

Copy MPC arrow and TCR vertical line to similar strip on page 3.

N.B. She may still put on a little weight after the age of eighteen.

99.6th
98th
91st
75th
50th
25th
9th
2nd
0.4th

WEIGHT kg

years

Manufacture 2   May '98

• Please place a sticker (if available) otherwise write in space provided.

Surname

First names

NHS no: Local no

G.P.   Code

H.V.   Code

BOYS
GROWTH CHART
(BIRTH - 18 YEARS)

United Kingdom cross-sectional reference data : 1996/1

D.O.B. ...... : ...... : ......   WEEKS GESTATION ....

HOSPITAL COMPUTER No. ....

pre-term

for a boy born before 37 completed weeks, draw a vertical "pre-term" line at the appropriate week and plot measurements from this line for at least twelve months. For all later deliveries plot from the EDD (Estimated Delivery Date) line.

measurements

weight: an infant or toddler should always be weighed naked on a self-calibrating or regularly calibrated scale. An older child should be weighed with the minimum of clothing.

head circumference: head circumference measurements should be taken from midway between the eyebrows and the hairline at the front of the head and the occipital prominence at the back. Appropriate thin plastic or metal tape should be used: sewing tape or paper tape is not recommended for this purpose.

supine length: an infant:- a child up to approximately 18 months - should be measured supinely (on his back) by two people with equipment featuring both a headboard and moveable footboard. Whilst one person holds the head against the headboard, with the head facing upwards in the Frankfurt plane*, a second person measures the length by bringing the footboard up to the heels. The downward pressure on the child's knees to ensure that the legs are flat will not endanger hip dislocation.

standing height: standing height should be measured against an appropriate vertical measure, door or wall free from radiators, pipes or large skirting board. The feet should be together with the heels, buttocks and shoulder blades touching the vertical and the head positioned in the Frankfurt plane*. To ensure that the maximum height is taken, upward pressure to the mastoid processes should be considered.

*The Frankfurt plane is an imaginary line from the centre of the ear hole to the lower border of the eye socket.

guidelines for recording, plotting and referral

Record the measurement using the boxes on this chart immediately you have taken it. Enter the date, specify the measurement in the box with the asterisk (i.e. **H/C** = head circumference, **H** = height, **L** = length, **W** = weight) and name your entry. You might find it helpful to enter his current age in the appropriate column. Plot each measurement on the grid with a well defined dot. Trace the growth curve with a line but leave the dots clearly visible. A normal growth curve is one that always runs roughly on/parallel to one of the printed centile lines. If it doesn't, consider these guidelines:-

Refer a boy whose height falls above the 99.6th or below the 0.4th centile line or outside his Target Centile Range (TCR). Refer him also if, pre-school, his growth curve veers upwards/downwards over the period 12-18 months by the width of one centile band or, post school entry, by $^2/_3$ of a band. If, prior to school entry, the curve veers by only $^2/_3$ of a band or, subsequently, by $^1/_2$ a band, flag the child for recall in 12 months and refer if the trend continues. Respond to parental concern about a child's growth, irrespective of the current centile, by monitoring height over a period of at least nine months and follow the criteria above. *(Source: BSPED September 1996)*

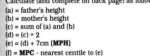

Date	Age	*	Measurement	Name
14 : 03 : 93	$^9/_{12}$	L	72 : 5 cm	John Smith
14 : 03 : 93	$^9/_{12}$	H/C	46 : cm	John Smith
14 : 03 : 93	$^9/_{12}$	W	9 : 3 kg	John Smith
: :		:	:	

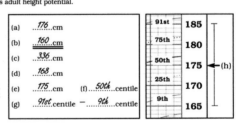

adult height potential

The table and illustrations below show how the adult height potential of a boy is calculated. They show that he is following his genetic pattern and that his growth curve should border the 50th centile to reach 175cm as an adult - **mid-parental height (MPH)**. The 50th centile is his **mid-parental centile (MPC)**. If the curve continuously follows a centile somewhere between the 91st-9th centiles (**MPH** ± 10cm) it will still be within his **target centile range (TCR)** and his growth will be considered normal. NB This calculation is not appropriate if either parent is not of normal stature.

Now use the box on the back page to calculate this boy's adult height potential.

Calculate (and complete on back page) as follows:-

(a) = father's height
(b) = mother's height
(c) = sum of (a) and (b)
(d) = (c) ÷ 2
(e) = (d) + 7cm (**MPH**)
(f) = **MPC** - nearest centile to (e)
(g) = **TCR** (mid-parental height ± 10cm)

Arrow (h) the mid-parental height/centile and draw a vertical line above and below it to represent the target centile range.

(a) ...*176*..cm
(b) ...*160*..cm
(c) ...*336*..cm
(d) ...*168*..cm
(e) ...*175*..cm   (f) .....*50th*....centile
(g) ...*91st*...centile – ....*9th*....centile

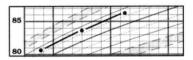

references and acknowledgements

papers
1. Do growth chart centiles need a face lift? (TJ Cole) *BMJ* 1994; 308: 641·2
2. Cross-sectional stature and weight reference curves for the UK, 1990 (JV Freeman, TJ Cole, S Chinn, PRM Jones, EM White, MA Preece) *ARCH DIS CHILD* 1995; 73: 17-24
3. Growth Charts for ethnic populations in the UK (S Chinn, TJ Cole, MA Preece, R Rona) *The Lancet* March 23rd 1996; 347: 839-840
Compilation: Institute of Child Health, London (Freeman JV et al). *Data sources:* British Size Surveys, Loughborough Consultants Ltd (Jones PRM, Norgan NG, Hunt MJ, Hooper RH); National Study of Health and Growth (Chinn S, Rona RJ); ONS National Heights and Weight Survey, 1980 & National Diet and Nutrition Survey, 1995; Tayside Growth Study (White EM et al); MRC Dunn Nutrition Group, Cambridge (Lucas A, Paul AA, Whitehead RG); MRC Human Genetics Unit, Edinburgh (Ratcliffe SG, Butler GE); UCH, London, 1000 births 1987/88 (Colley NV, Hanson GL), Rosie Hospital, Cambridge (Glazebrook C, Rennie JM) & Northern RHA birth data (Wariyar UK); Chard 1976-1988 Normal Puberty Longitudinal Study (Dunger DB, Cameron N, Baines-Preece J, Cox L, Preece MA)

Designed and Published by
© CHILD GROWTH FOUNDATION 1996/1
(Charity Reg. No 274325)
2 Mayfield Avenue,
London W4 1PW

Printed and Supplied by
HARLOW PRINTING LIMITED
Maxwell Street ◊ South Shields
Tyne & Wear ◊ NE33 4PU

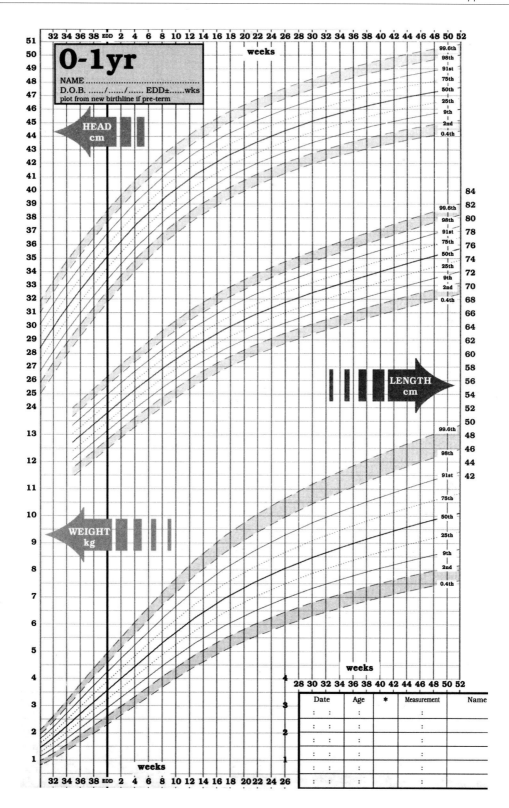

0-1yr

NAME ....
D.O.B. ..../......./........ EDD±......wks
plot from new birthline if pre-term

HEAD cm

LENGTH cm

WEIGHT kg

weeks

Date	Age	*	Measurement	Name
: :	:		:	
: :	:		:	
: :	:		:	
: :	:		:	
: :	:		:	
: :	:		:	

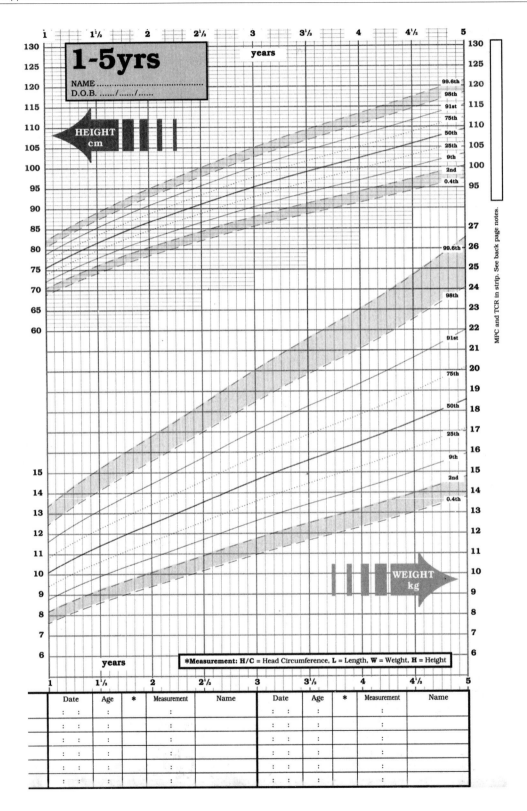

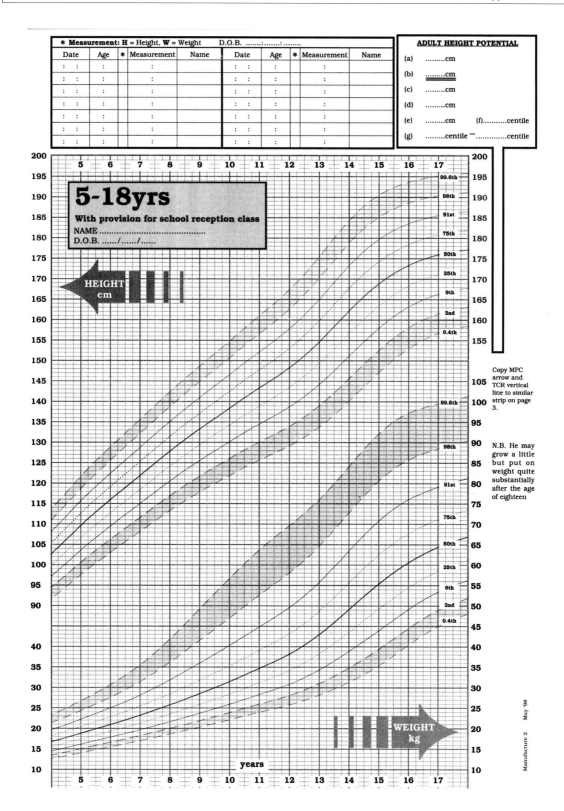

* **Measurement: H** = Height, **W** = Weight   D.O.B. ....:.......:........

Date	Age	*	Measurement	Name	Date	Age	*	Measurement	Name
: :	:		:		: :	:		:	
: :	:		:		: :	:		:	
: :	:		:		: :	:		:	
: :	:		:		: :	:		:	
: :	:		:		: :	:		:	
: :	:		:		: :	:		:	

ADULT HEIGHT POTENTIAL

(a) ....cm

(b) ....cm

(c) ....cm

(d) ....cm

(e) ....cm   (f)..........centile

(g) ....centile ⁻ ....centile

5-18yrs

With provision for school reception class

NAME ....

D.O.B. ..../......./......

HEIGHT cm

99.6th
98th
91st
75th
50th
25th
9th
2nd
0.4th

99.6th
98th
91st
75th
50th
25th
9th
2nd
0.4th

Copy MPC arrow and TCR vertical line to similar strip on page 3.

N.B. He may grow a little but put on weight quite substantially after the age of eighteen

years

WEIGHT kg

Manufacture 2   May '98

Referral guidelines

Consider referral for any girl whose BMI falls above the 99.6th centile/below the 0.4th centile as significantly over/underweight even on the basis of a single measurement. It is possible that a girl whose BMI falls in the tinted areas should also be referred. However, during infancy large but transient changes in centile may occur due to the shape of the charts, and these changes are normal. It should be remembered that the earlier the age of the second rise, the greater the risk of future obesity. Remember also that while BMI has a high correlation with relative fatness or leanness it is actually assessing the weight-to-height relationship: **this may give misleading results in girls who are very stocky and muscular who might appear obese on the BMI alone.**

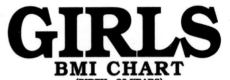

GIRLS
BMI CHART
(BIRTH - 20 YEARS)
United Kingdom cross-sectional reference data : 1995/1

Name...

NHS No. ☐☐☐ ☐☐☐ ☐☐☐☐

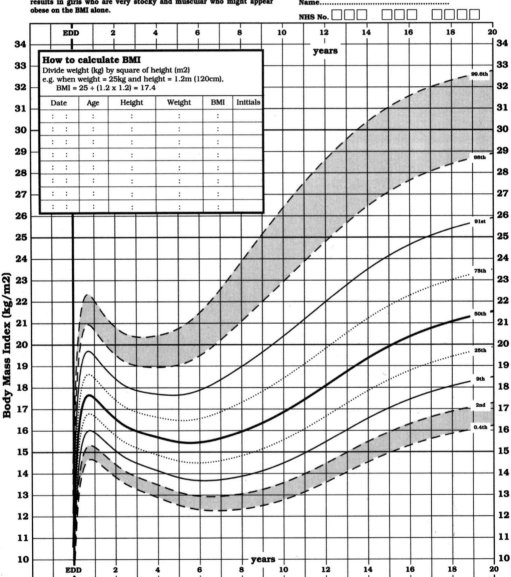

How to calculate BMI
Divide weight (kg) by square of height (m2)
e.g. when weight = 25kg and height = 1.2m (120cm),
    BMI = 25 ÷ (1.2 x 1.2) = 17.4

Date	Age	Height	Weight	BMI	Initials
: :	:	:	:	:	
: :	:	:	:	:	
: :	:	:	:	:	
: :	:	:	:	:	
: :	:	:	:	:	
: :	:	:	:	:	

Reference
Body Mass Index reference curves for the UK, 1990 (TJ Cole, JV Freeman, MA Preece) *Arch Dis Child* 1995; **73**: 25-29

Designed and Published by
© CHILD GROWTH FOUNDATION 1995/1
(Charity Reg. No 274325)
2 Mayfield Avenue,
London W4 1PW

Printed by
HARLOW PRINTING LIMITED
Maxwell Street ◊ South Shields
Tyne & Wear ◊ NE33 4PU
Tel: 0191 455 4286 Fax: 0191 427 0195

Referral guidelines

Consider referral for any boy whose BMI falls above the 99.6th centile/below the 0.4th centile as significantly over/underweight even on the basis of a single measurement. It is possible that a boy whose BMI falls in the tinted areas should also be referred. However, during infancy large but transient changes in centile may occur due to the shape of the charts, and these changes are normal. It should be remembered that the earlier the age of the second rise, the greater the risk of future obesity. Remember also that while BMI has a high correlation with relative fatness or leanness it is actually assessing the weight-to-height relationship: **this may give misleading results in boys who are very stocky and muscular who might appear obese on the BMI alone.**

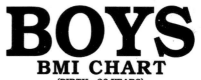

BOYS
BMI CHART
(BIRTH - 20 YEARS)
United Kingdom cross-sectional reference data : 1995/1

Name...

NHS No. ☐☐☐ ☐☐☐ ☐☐☐☐

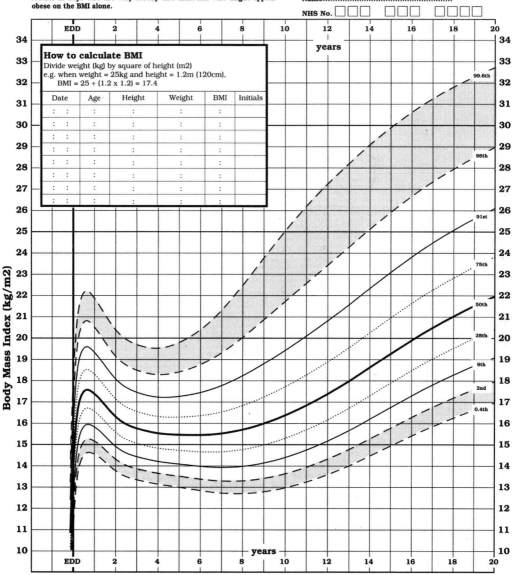

How to calculate BMI

Divide weight (kg) by square of height (m2)
e.g. when weight = 25kg and height = 1.2m (120cm),
$\quad$ BMI = 25 ÷ (1.2 x 1.2) = 17.4

Date	Age	Height	Weight	BMI	Initials
: :	:	:	:	:	
: :	:	:	:	:	
: :	:	:	:	:	
: :	:	:	:	:	
: :	:	:	:	:	
: :	:	:	:	:	
: :	:	:	:	:	

Reference

Body Mass Index reference curves for the UK, 1990 (TJ Cole, JV Freeman, MA Preece) *Arch Dis Child* 1995; **73**: 25-29

Designed and Published by
© CHILD GROWTH FOUNDATION 1995/1
(Charity Reg. No 274325)
2 Mayfield Avenue,
London W4 1PW

Printed by
HARLOW PRINTING LIMITED
Maxwell Street ◊ South Shields
Tyne & Wear ◊ NE33 4PU
Tel: 0191 455 4286 Fax: 0191 427 0195

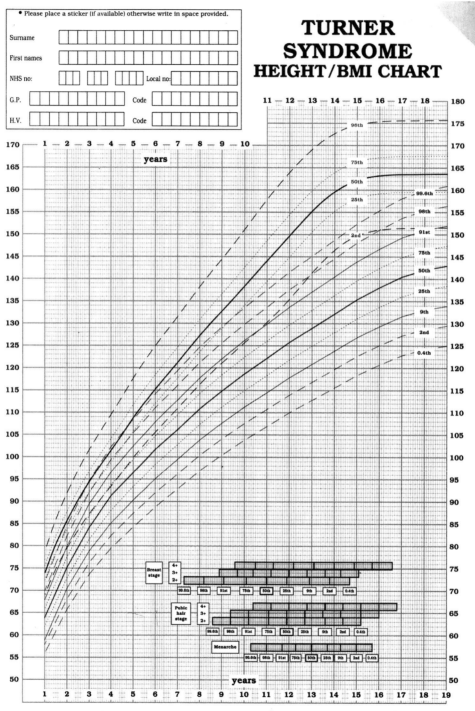

• Please place a sticker (if available) otherwise write in space provided.

Surname

First names

NHS no: Local no:

G.P.   Code

H.V.   Code

TURNER SYNDROME HEIGHT/BMI CHART

Designed and Published by
© CHILD GROWTH FOUNDATION 1997/1
(Charity Reg. No. 274325)
2 Mayfield Avenue,
London W4 1PW

Printed by and Supplied by
HARLOW PRINTING LIMITED
Maxwell Street ◊ South Shields
Tyne & Wear ◊ NE33 4PU

DATA BOXES FOR INSERTION OF WEIGHT, HEAD CIRCUMFERENCE, LENGTH, HEIGHT AND BMI

Date	Age	Measurement	BMI	Name/Initials
: :	: :	:	:	:
: :	: :	:	:	:
: :	: :	:	:	:
: :	: :	:	:	:
: :	: :	:	:	:
: :	: :	:	:	:
: :	: :	:	:	:
: :	: :	:	:	:
: :	: :	:	:	:
: :	: :	:	:	:
: :	: :	:	:	:
: :	: :	:	:	:
: :	: :	:	:	:
: :	: :	:	:	:
: :	: :	:	:	:
: :	: :	:	:	:

Date	Age	Measurement	BMI	Name/Initials
: :	: :	:	:	:
: :	: :	:	:	:
: :	: :	:	:	:
: :	: :	:	:	:
: :	: :	:	:	:
: :	: :	:	:	:
: :	: :	:	:	:

How to calculate BMI

Divide weight (kg) by the square of length/height (m²)

example
weight = 25kg
length/height = 1.2m

equation
25 ÷ (1.2 x 1.2)
= 17.4

Data: 1990

Manufacture 1 Apr '99

REFERENCES

Growth Curve for girls with Turner Syndrome (AJ Lyon, MA Preece, DB Grant) *ARCH DIS CHILD* 1985; 60: 932-935
Body Mass Index reference curves for the UK, 1990 (TJ Cole, JV Freeman, MA Preece) *Arch Dis Child* 1995; **73**: 25-29

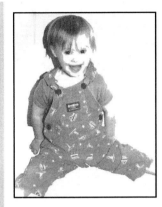

GIRLS

DOWN'S SYNDROME GROWTH CHART

UK/Republic of Ireland cross-sectional reference: 2000

STICKER

These charts are based on data from around 6000 measurements of 1100 children living throughout the UK and Republic of Ireland (Styles et al - in preparation). Growth can be charted from term to 18 years. Children with significant cardiac disease or other major pathology were excluded from the study population. In addition, data for those born before 37 completed weeks were excluded up to age two. The charts are therefore representative of healthy children with Down's syndrome growing in the U.K. and Republic of Ireland.

The charts were commissioned by the UK Down's Syndrome Medical Interest Group (DSMIG) and the data collected by Dr Mary Styles on DSMIG's behalf. The centiles were compiled under the guidance of Professor Michael Preece with statistical analysis provided by Professor Tim Cole, both of the Institute of Child Health, London. Data were analysed by Cole's LMS method. Dr Styles' data collection was funded by the Child Growth Foundation and remains the copyright of DSMIG.

PCHR - The charts are also available in A5 format for inclusion with the special PCHR Down's syndrome insert.

Preterm babies - We do not as yet have sufficient information to compile centiles for preterm babies with Down's syndrome. Measurements for those born before 37 completed weeks should not be plotted on the charts until the expected date of delivery (EDD) is reached. Thereafter they should be charted relative to EDD for at least a year. Those born at 38 weeks or later should be charted in the normal way from the EDD line.

More information about growth monitoring for children with Down's syndrome is included in the Medical Surveillance Guidelines for people with Down's Syndrome produced by the Down's Syndrome Medical Interest Group.

Overweight and underweight - Action guidelines:
Many older children with Down's syndrome are overweight and this is clearly reflected in this study population. Hence this reference data should not be used as a standard that children should aim to achieve, As with all children weight must be related to stature. Any child aged 5-18 years whose weight falls within the shaded area above the 75th centile should be charted on the BMI chart (see right). Those above the 98th centile on the BMI charts are significantly overweight and referral for further assessment and guidance should be considered.

Of those falling below the 2nd centile on the height and weight charts some will have major pathology, but some may be failing to thrive for other reasons - eg because of feeding difficulties. Again such children may need further assessment and guidance.

How to calculate BMI (Body Mass Index)

Divide weight (kg) by square of length/height (m²)
e.g. when weight = 25kg and length/height = 1.2m (120cm),
   BMI = 25 ÷ (1.2 x 1.2) = 17.4

Date	Age	Height	Ht²	Weight	BMI (Wt÷Ht²)	Initials
: :	: :	:	:	:	:	:
: :	: :	:	:	:	:	:
: :	: :	:	:	:	:	:
: :	: :	:	:	:	:	:
: :	: :	:	:	:	:	:
: :	: :	:	:	:	:	:
: :	: :	:	:	:	:	:

BMI CHART

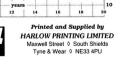

Printed and Supplied by
HARLOW PRINTING LIMITED
Maxwell Street ◊ South Shields
Tyne & Wear ◊ NE33 4PU

Girls' Down's Syndrome charts
Reprinted with permission from Jennifer Dennis and the Down's Syndrome Medical Interest Group.

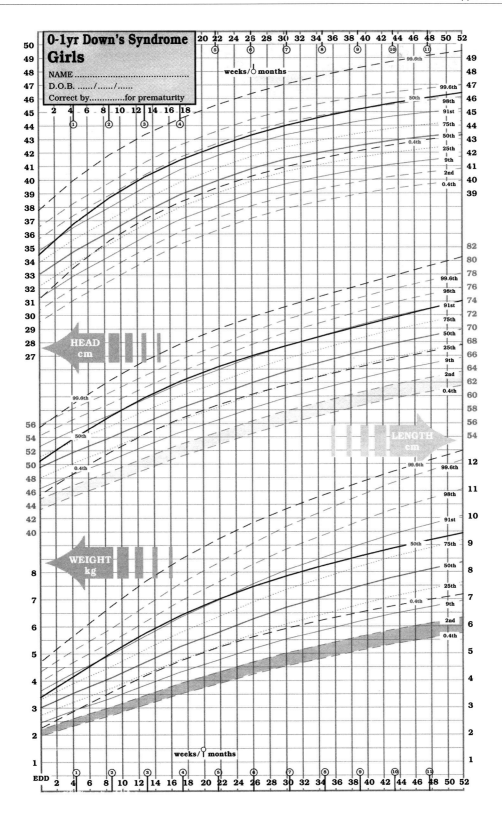

0-1yr Down's Syndrome Girls

NAME ....

D.O.B. ....../....../......

Correct by..............for prematurity

weeks/○ months

HEAD cm

LENGTH cm

WEIGHT kg

weeks/♀ months

EDD

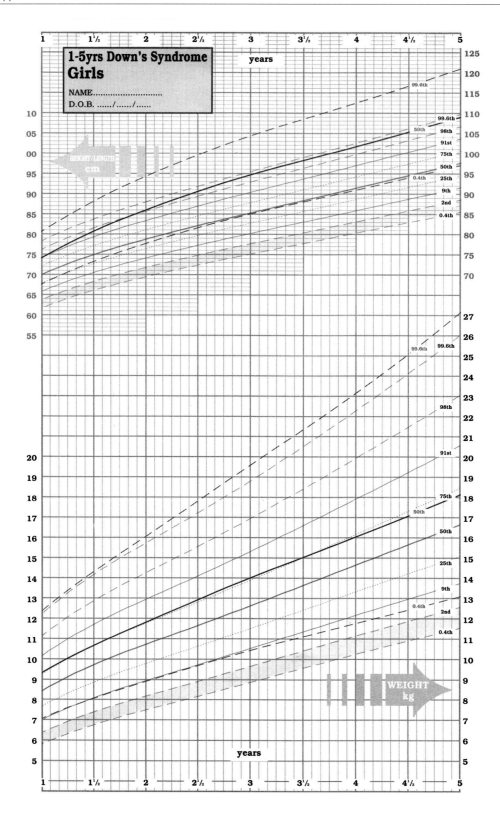

1-5yrs Down's Syndrome
Girls

NAME............................
D.O.B. ..../......./......

years

HEIGHT/LENGTH cm

WEIGHT kg

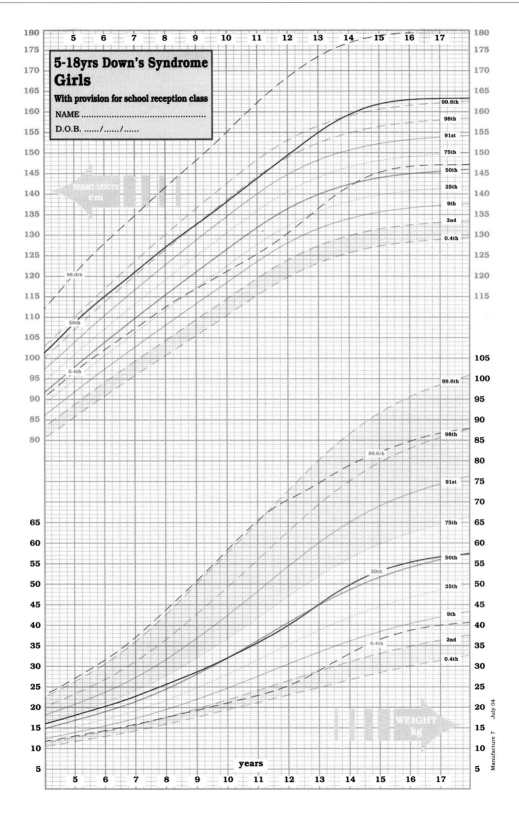

5-18yrs Down's Syndrome
Girls

With provision for school reception class

NAME ....

D.O.B. ....../....../......

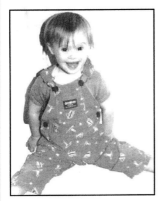

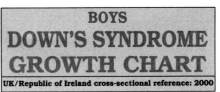

BOYS
DOWN'S SYNDROME
GROWTH CHART

UK/Republic of Ireland cross-sectional reference: 2000

STICKER

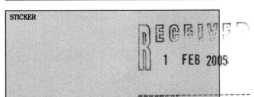

RECEIVED
1 FEB 2005

These charts are based on data from around 6000 measurements of 1100 children living throughout the UK and Republic of Ireland (Styles et al - in preparation). Growth can be charted from term to 18 years. Children with significant cardiac disease or other major pathology are excluded from the study population. In addition, data for those born before 37 completed weeks were excluded up to age two. The charts are therefore representative of healthy children with Down's syndrome growing in the U.K. and Republic of Ireland.

The charts were commissioned by the UK Down's Syndrome Medical Interest Group (DSMIG) and the data collected by Dr Mary Styles on DSMIG's behalf. The centiles were compiled under the guidance of Professor Michael Preece with statistical analysis provided by Professor Tim Cole, both of the Institute of Child Health, London. Data were analysed by Cole's LMS method. Dr Styles' data collection was funded by the Child Growth Foundation and remains the copyright of DSMIG.

PCHR - The charts are also available in A5 format for inclusion with the special PCHR Down's Syndrome insert.

Preterm babies - We do not as yet have sufficient information to compile centiles for preterm babies with Down's syndrome. Measurements for those born before 37 completed weeks should not be plotted on the charts until the expected date of delivery (EDD) is reached. Thereafter they should be charted relative to EDD for at least a year. Those born at 38 weeks or later should be charted in the normal way from the EDD line.

More information about growth monitoring for children with Down's syndrome is included in the Medical Surveillance Guidelines for people with Down's Syndrome produced by the Down's Syndrome Medical Interest Group. These are available from the address given below.

Overweight and underweight - Action guidelines:
Many older children with Down's syndrome are overweight and this is clearly reflected in this study population. Hence this reference data should not be used as a standard that children should aim to achieve, As with all children weight must be related to stature. Any child aged 5-18 years whose weight falls within the shaded area above the 75th centile on the BMI chart (see right). Those above the 98th centile on the BMI charts are significantly overweight and referral for further assessment and guidance should be considered.

Of those falling below the 2nd centile some will have major pathology, but some may be failing to thrive for other reasons - eg because of feeding difficulties. Again such children may need further assessment and guidance.

How to calculate BMI (Body Mass Index)
Divide weight (kg) by square of length/height (m²)
e.g. when weight = 25kg and length/height = 1.2m (120cm),
    BMI = 25 ÷ (1.2 x 1.2) = 17.4

Date	Age	Height	Ht²	Weight	BMI (Wt÷Ht²)	Initials
: :	:	:	:	:	:	
: :	:	:	:	:	:	
: :	:	:	:	:	:	
: :	:	:	:	:	:	
: :	:	:	:	:	:	
: :	:	:	:	:	:	
: :	:	:	:	:	:	

BMI CHART

(BMI chart: years 6 to 20 on x-axis, Body Mass Index (kg/m²) 10 to 34 on y-axis, centile curves labelled 99.6th, 98th, 91st, 75th, 50th, 25th, 9th, 2nd, 0.4th; Data: 1990)

© Down's Syndrome Medical Interest Group (DSMIG) 2000
Children's Centre City Hospital Campus
Nottingham
NG5 1PB

Printed and Supplied by
HARLOW PRINTING LIMITED
Maxwell Street ◊ South Shields
Tyne & Wear ◊ NE33 4PU

Boys' Down's Syndrome charts
Reprinted with permission from Jennifer Dennis and the Down's Syndrome Medical Interest Group.

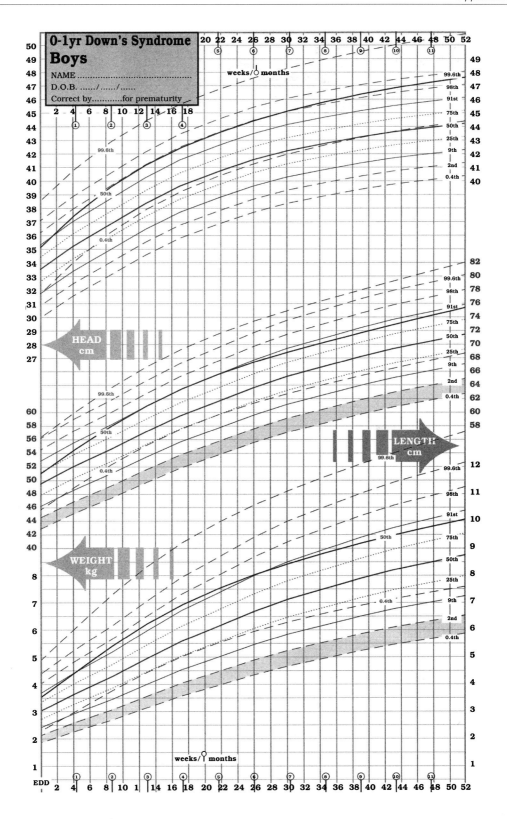

0-1yr Down's Syndrome
Boys

NAME ....
D.O.B. ....../....../......
Correct by............for prematurity

weeks/○ months

HEAD cm

LENGTH cm

WEIGHT kg

weeks/○ months

EDD

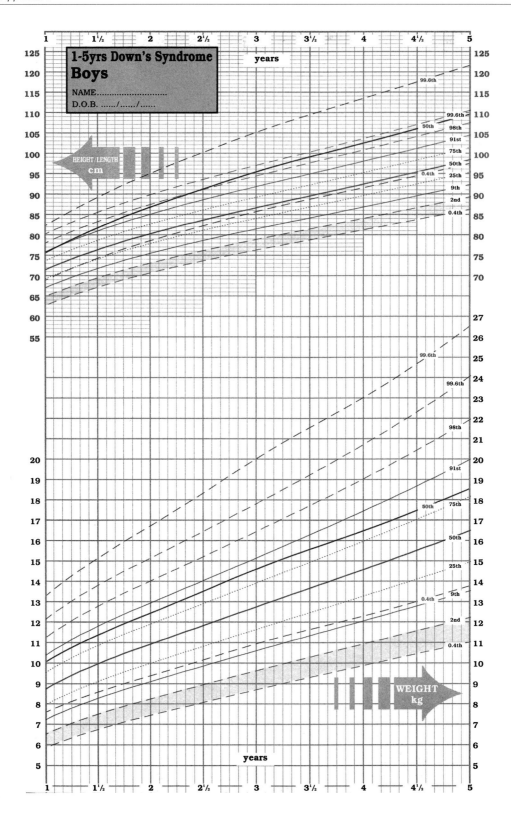

1-5yrs Down's Syndrome
Boys

NAME..............................
D.O.B. ..../......./......

years

HEIGHT/LENGTH
cm

WEIGHT
kg

years

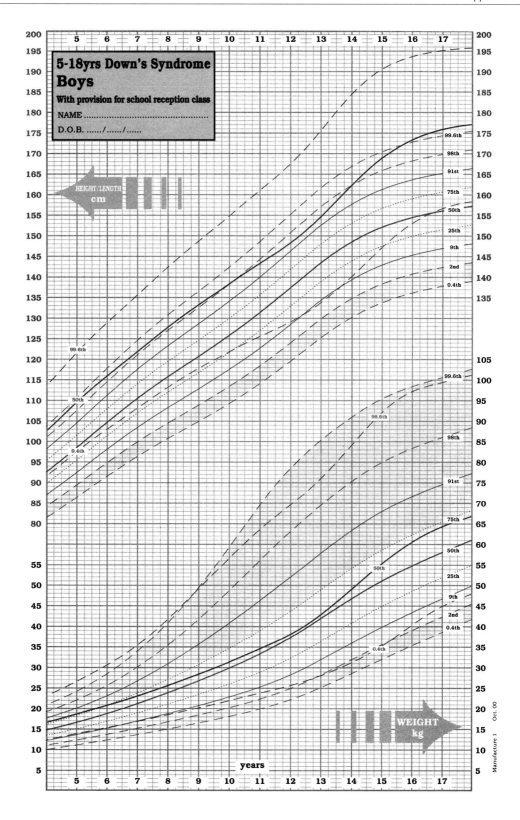

5-18yrs Down's Syndrome Boys
With provision for school reception class

NAME ....
D.O.B. ....../....../......

HEIGHT/LENGTH cm

WEIGHT kg

years

Manufacture 1

Oct. 00

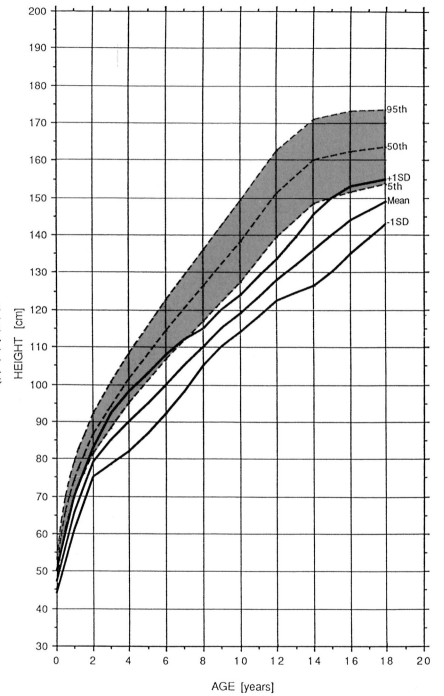

Growth curve for height in females with Noonan syndrome compared to normal values (dashed lines). Data obtained in 48 Noonan syndrome females from a collaborative retrospective review. Witt DR et al; Clin Genet 30:150, 1986.

Girls' Noonan Syndrome charts

Reprinted from Witt D.R. *et al. Clinical Genetics* (1986) **30**, 150, with permission from Blackwell Publishing Ltd.

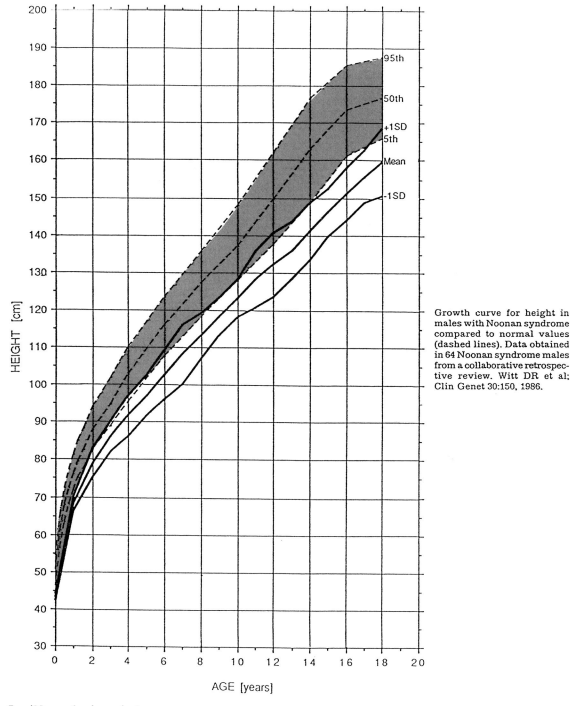

Growth curve for height in males with Noonan syndrome compared to normal values (dashed lines). Data obtained in 64 Noonan syndrome males from a collaborative retrospective review. Witt DR et al; Clin Genet 30:150, 1986.

Boys' Noonan Syndrome charts

Reprinted from Witt D.R. *et al*. *Clinical Genetics* (1986) **30**, 150, with permission from Blackwell Publishing Ltd.

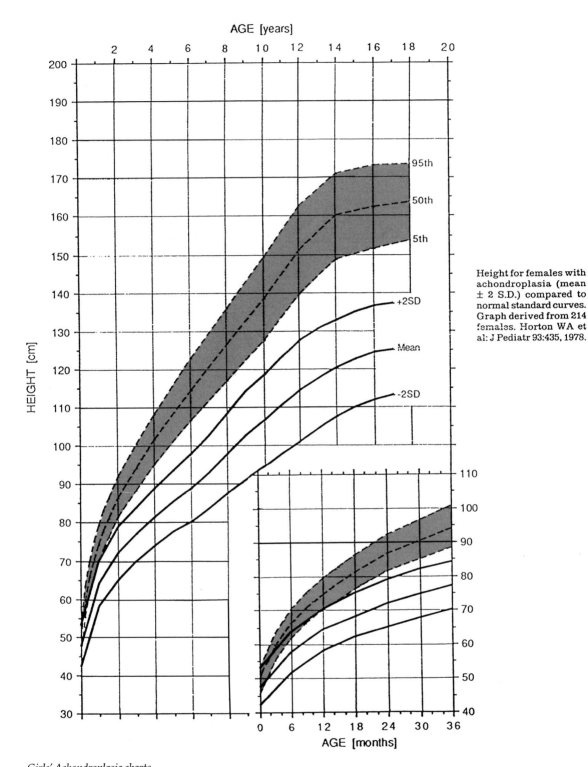

Girls' Achondroplasia charts
Reprinted from Horton W.A. *et al.*, Growth in achondroplasia, *Journal of Pediatrics* (1978) **93**, 435, with permission from Elsevier.

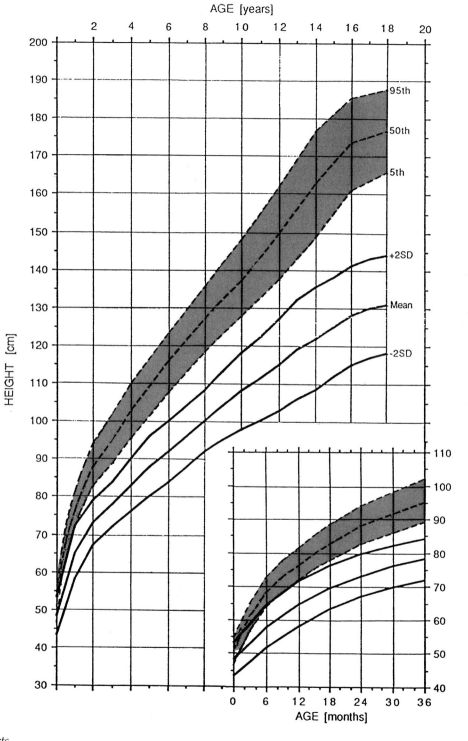

Boys' Achondroplasia charts
Reprinted from Horton W.A. *et al.*, Growth in achondroplasia, *Journal of Pediatrics* (1978) **93**, 435, with permission from Elsevier.

CAH therapy card

NHS
Greater Glasgow

CAH THERAPY CARD

The owner of this card has the condition **Congenital adrenal hyperplasia** also known as **CAH** or **Adrenogenital syndrome.**

Name ....

Address ....

....

DoB .... Hospital number ....

Hospital consultant: ....

Useful telephone numbers:

Hospital switchboard: ....
Ward ....
Dr A ....
Dr B ....
Endocrine Nurse ....
Endocrine Ward ....

GP's name / address / tel no ....

....

....

JCH/Med III 20556 / 41959 / 44656

Instructions for Hospital Doctor

Dear Doctor,

If this child is brought to hospital by the parents as an emergency the following management is advised:

- Insert an I.V. cannula
- Take blood for U's and E's, glucose, and perform any other appropriate tests (e.g. urine culture)
- Check glucostix or dextrostix
- Give _____ mg hydrocortisone intravenously as bolus (unnecessary if parent has already given I.M. hydrocortisone)
- Commence I.V. infusion of 0.45% saline and 5% dextrose at maintenance rate (extra if child is dehydrated). Add potassium depending on electrolyte results.
- Commence hydrocortisone infusion (50mg hydrocortisone in 50ml normal saline via syringe pump) at _____ ml/hour
- **Important!** If blood glucose/glucostix is < 2.5mmol, give bolus of 2ml/kg of 10% dextrose
- If child is drowsy, hypotensive and peripherally shut down with poor capillary return give 20 ml/kg of normal saline stat.

Please contact named consultant at Yorkhill and inform of admission.   *Thank you*

What to do if your child is unwell

1. In the event of *mild to moderate illness*, e.g. cold, cough, sore throat, flu, tummy upset, double the total daily dose of hydrocortisone and give this doubled dose in 3 equal portions (morning, afternoon and evening) for the duration of the illness.

   The fludrocortisone dose should stay the same.

   i.e Hydrocortisone dose _____ x 3 per day

2. If your child
   • *does not get better* after you have increased the tablets, or
   • *feels drowsy*, or
   • *is unable to take the tablets orally* (e.g. due to continued vomiting),

   the hydrocortisone must be given by injection (intra-muscular).

   Please check that this is not past the expiry date

   The dose of hydrocortisone injection is _____

3. If your child continues to be ill and does not seem to be getting better, telephone the hospital and say that you are bringing him/her up for admission.

   Please bring this card with you and show it to the doctor.

Dose to be taken in

Morning	Afternoon	Evening

Current treatment

Fill in details of the drugs your child is taking, with the dates of any dose changes.

Date	Drug	Tablet size

Index

Notes: Please note that entries in *italics* refer to figures and those in **bold** refer to tables.